CANNABIS: COLLECTED CLINICAL PAPERS
VOLUME 1
MARIJUANA: MEDICAL PAPERS 1839–1972

As a full-time research consultant at the N.I.M.H. Center of Narcotics and Drug Abuse Studies, Dr. Tod Mikuriya discovered just how much the English and American medical profession has known about cannabis for the past 130 years. Having access to priceless original documents, he has compiled this authoritative and fascinating collection of medical papers on marijuana. From 1839, when the herb was first introduced into the Western pharmacopoeia, to present research with THC, the anthology offers rich insights into the whole social history of medicine.

The studies published herein convey a wide variety of critical information, ranging from laboratory tests performed on animals and human subjects, to anthropological descriptions of marijuana use by African women during labor. A number of unusual and seldom-seen illustrations—from pharmaceutical catalogues in the days when Parke Davis and others marketed legal marijuana as a cure for coughs and corns—are both instructive and entertaining. In the section of clinical and pharmacological studies, a deep look is taken at the range of therapeutic effects attributed to a plant which has had prescribed medical uses for more than 2700 years, and is currently used by an estimated 250 million people.

If not always conclusive, these studies nonetheless dramatically show that marijuana has potentially great medical value. The impressive accumulation of information regarding it has been unfortunately relegated to the dust bin for decades by puritanical legislators and medical practitioners ignorant or unheeding of existing scholarship in the field. The final chapter analyzes the reasons behind the 1937 Tax Act which outlawed the use of marijuana, driving it underground, and offers some disturbing conclusions based on hitherto unpublished official hearings and interviews with former government officials.

Amidst the marijuana referendums, judicial challenges, and states vs. federal legislation, Marijuana: Medical Papers provides essential information—most of it never before available except in scarce, out-of-print medical journals—on a topic of tremendous current interest.

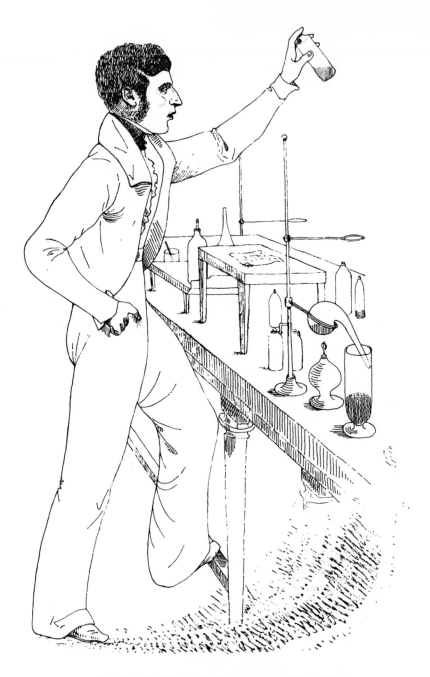

W.B. O'SHAUGHNESSY M.D.

Professor of Chemistry and Natural Philosophy.

Medical College Calcutta

T. Black Asiatic Lith Prof.

CANNABIS: COLLECTED CLINICAL PAPERS

VOLUME ONE

MARIJUANA: MEDICAL PAPERS 1839–1972

EDITED BY
TOD H. MIKURIYA, M.D.

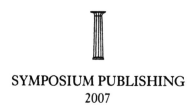

SYMPOSIUM PUBLISHING
2007

Cannabis: Collected Clinical Papers
Volume 1: Marijuana: Medical Papers 1839–1972
Volume 2: Cannabis: Clinical Papers
Volume 3: Cannabis: Collected Works of Tod H. Mikuriya, M.D.

Published by Symposium Publishing
an imprint of Blue Dolphin Publishing
P.O. Box 8, Nevada City, CA 95959
Orders 1-800-643-0765
Web: www.bluedolphinpublishing.com

ISBN: 1-57733-167-2 / 978-1-57733-167-4 hardcover
ISBN: 1-57733-219-9 / 978-1-57733-219-0 softcover

This edition was originally published privately in 1973 by Medi-
Comp Press under the title *Marijuana: Medical Papers 1839–1972*

Library of Congress Catalog Card Number 72-87736

First Symposium printing, November, 2007

Printed in the United States of America

To my parents:
Tadafumi and Anna Schwenk Mikuriya

Acknowledgments

My thanks and appreciation to:

Kathy Goss, compiler, scholar, typist, etc.

Bob Barker, of the Fitz Hugh Ludlow Memorial Library, for dedicated efforts coordinating production.

Nancy, my wife, critic, financial backer, supporter, etc.

Alex Shulgin, chemical wizard of psychoactive drugs, forensic toxicology, etc., for proof-reading and clarifying Section V with all those cryptic chemical structures.

The librarians at the National Library of Medicine for finding O'Shaughnessy's picture, which I'd sought for five years.

The librarians of the University of California, San Francisco, School of Medicine Library Historical Collection for helping me find the obscure.

Al Berger of *Medical World News* for documenting and defining the Defense Department's secret cannabinoid research during 1954–59 with his usual probing competence.

Larry Noggle for the layout of the chapters containing chemical formulae.

Dana Reemes for layout and indexing.

Michael Horowitz for kindly proof-reading the galleys.

Michael Aldrich for illustrations and comments.

Bill Rock for last-minute assistance.

Hendra & Howard for photocomposing.

Amorphia for help with production.

E. A. Gladman Memorial Foundation for diverse assistance.

Reprint Acknowledgments

The editor wishes to thank the following publishers and authors for their kind permission to quote from their works: Parke, Davis and Company and L. M. Wheeler, Ph.D., for his letter; The American Pharmaceutical Association for "The Physiological Activity of Cannabis Sativa"; J. B. Lippincott Company and R. P. Walton, M.D., for "Description of the Hashish Experience" and for "Marihuana: Therapeutic Application"; *Lancet* for "The Use of Indian Hemp in the Treatment of Chronic Chloral and Chronic Opium Poisoning" and for "Therapeutical Uses and Toxic Effects of Cannabis Indica"; The Federation of American Societies for Experimental Biology and Jean P. Davis, M.D., for "Antiepileptic Action of Marihuana Active Substances"; The Ronald Press and S. Allentuck, M.D., for "Medical Aspects: Symptoms and Behavior"; *The British Journal of Psychiatry* and Frances Ames, M.D., for "A Clinical and Metabolic Study of Acute Intoxication with Cannabis Sativa and Its Role in the Model Psychosis"; *Science* and A. T. Weil, M.D., for "Clinical and Psychological Effects of Marijuana in Man"; *Science* for "Clinical and Physiological Notes on the Action of Cannabis Indica"; J. B. Lippincott Company for "Dispensatory of the United States of America, 20th Ed."; *Bulletin of the New York Academy of Medicine* for "Marihuana"; Springer-Verlag, Berlin, Heidelberg & New York, for "The Active Principles of Cannabis and the Pharmacology of the Cannabinols"; *Journal of Psychedelic Drugs*, Haight-Ashbury Medical Clinic of San Francisco, and Alexander T. Shulgin, Ph.D., for "Recent Developments in Cannabis Chemistry"; David Musto, M.D., for "The 1937 Marihuana Tax Act."

Table of Contents

Preface   xi

Introduction   xiii

I   FROM EAST TO WEST   1

On the Preparation of the Indian Hemp or Gunja   3
    W. B. O'Shaughnessy, M.D. (1839)

II   PERSONAL EXPERIENCES AND SPECULATIONS   31

On the Haschisch or Cannabis Indica   33
    J. Bell, M.D. (1857)

Cannabis Indica Poisoning   51
    J. C. O'Day, M.D. (1899)

Two Cases of Poisoning by Cannabis Indica   55
    J. Foulis, M.D., F.R.C.P.Ed. (1900)

Letter from L. M. Wheeler, Ph.D.   67

The Physiological Activity of Cannabis Sativa   69
    H. C. Hamilton, M.S., et al. (1913)

Description of the Hashish Experience   83
    R. P. Walton, M.D. (1938)

III   THERAPEUTIC EXCURSIONS   115

Report of the Ohio State Medical Committee
on Cannabis Indica (1860)   117

The Use of Indian Hemp in the Treatment of
Chronic Chloral and Chronic Opium Poisoning   141
    E. A. Birch, M.D. (1889)

Therapeutical Uses and Toxic Effects of
Cannabis Indica   145
    J. R. Reynolds, M.D. (1890)

Cannabis Indica as an Anodyne and Hypnotic   151
    J. B. Mattison, M.D. (1891)

Marihuana: Therapeutic Application   159
    R. P. Walton, M.D. (1938)

Antiepileptic Action of Marihuana Active
Substances   167
    J. P. Davis, M.D., and H. H. Ramsey, M.D.
    (1949)

Cannabis Substitution as an Adjunctive Thera-
peutic Tactic in the Treatment of Alcoholism   169
    T. H. Mikuriya, M.D. (1969)

IV   RECENT ACUTE CLINICAL STUDIES   177

"La Guardia Report": Medical Aspects   179
   S. Allentuck, M.D. (1944)

A Clinical and Metabolic Study of Acute
Intoxication with Cannabis Sativa and Its Role
in the Model Psychosis   213
   F. Ames, M.D. (1958)

Clinical and Psychological Effects of Marijuana
in Man   255
   A. T. Weil, M.D., et al. (1968)

Comparison of the Effects of Marijuana and
Alcohol on Simulated Driving Performance   281
   A. Crancer, Ph.D., et al. (1969)

V   CHEMICAL AND PHARMACOLOGICAL STUDIES   291

Clinical and Physiological Notes on the Action
of Cannabis Indica   293
   H. A. Hare, M.D. (1887)

A Contribution to the Pharmacology of
Cannabis Indica   301
   C. R. Marshall, M.D. (1898)

Dispensatory of the United States of America,
20th Ed.: Cannabis Indica   333
   J. P. Remington, Ph.M., F.C.S., et al. (1918)

Marihuana   345
   R. Adams, Ph.D. (1942)

The Active Principles of Cannabis and the
Pharmacology of the Cannabinols   375
   S. Loewe, Ph.D. (1940)

Recent Developments in Cannabis Chemistry   397
   A. T. Shulgin, Ph.D. (1972)

VI   SOCIAL ORIGINS OF THE MARIJUANA LAWS   417

The 1937 Marihuana Tax Act   419
   D. Musto, M.D. (1971)

Glossary   442

Conversion Tables   444

Biographical Notes   446

Author Index   450

Subject Index   454

Preface

The orientation of this book is primarily medical. The described uses of marijuana were for healing or scientific purposes. Save for historical aspects of the prohibitory Marihuana Tax Act of 1937, social use is described in a minority of the papers and only in passing.

This diverse collection of papers represents some of the better professional journal articles concerning the medicinal applications and scientific properties of marijuana products.

The scope of topics included in this collection of papers culled from medical and scientific sources is necessarily wide. The study of a drug with complex pharmacological effects in concert with the diversity of human circumstance produces a wide spectrum of data.

Some of the papers suffer from lack of documentation and difficult, archaic, or colloquial language. In order to understand some of the chemical and pharmacological papers, understanding of biochemistry is needed.

As a psychiatrist, I was tempted to include material from influential and colorful literary origins. Descriptive experiential use started with Dr. Francois Rabelais's "The Herb Pantagruelion" in about 1530; it was re-introduced into European literature through the studies of J. J. Moreau de Tours in the early 1840s; it was popularized by Bayard Taylor, Theophile Gautier, Charles Baudelaire, and Fitz Hugh Ludlow in the 1850s and '60s. Dr. Victor Robinson carried this romantic intellectual tradition into the mid-1940s.

To attempt to include the lesser known but important literary works not published elsewhere would swell this anthology to an unwieldy size and detract from its usefulness as a medical reference.

The introspective accounts of practitioners' and scientists' personal use were influenced by contemporary literary figures who appear in a large proportion, especially in the earlier papers. Personal experimentation and description were once held to be an integral part of drug research.

The accounts of the adventures of the researcher, colleague, and patient serve to remind the reader of the constancy of the human psyche over the years. In the research lab, at the bedside, or at the controls of a locomotive, thoughtful scientists and clinicians describe their experiences and observations.

Despite the advent of technology, these intelligent observations articulately described in the past must not be forgotten. Failure to heed previous insights results in superfluous repetition, stupidity through ignorance and resultant failure.

Browsing through the book one cannot help but be struck by the fact that, although scientific tools have become more sophisticated, human nature has not. Ingenuity and clarity of thinking shine beyond the years, making us more humble in the realization that what is contemporary is not necessarily the best or uniquely innovative.

THM
Berkeley, California
1973

Introduction

Medicine in the Western World has forgotten almost all it once knew about therapeutic properties of marijuana, or cannabis.

Analgesia, anticonvulsant action, appetite stimulation, ataraxia, antibiotic properties and low toxicity were described throughout medical literature, beginning in 1839, when O'Shaughnessy introduced cannabis into the Western pharmacopoeia.

As these findings were reported throughout Western medicine, cannabis attained wide use. Cannabis therapy was described in most pharmacopoeial texts as a treatment for a variety of disease conditions.

During the second half of the 1800s and in the present century, medical researchers in some measure corroborated the early reports of the therapeutic potential of cannabis. In addition, much laboratory research has been concerned with bioassay, determination of the mode of action, and attempts to solve the problems of insolubility in water and variability of strength among different cannabis specimens.

"Recreational" smoking of cannabis in the twentieth century and the resultant restrictive federal legislation have functionally ended all medical uses of marijuana.

In light of such assets as minimal toxicity, no buildup of tolerance, no physical dependence, and minimal autonomic disturbance, immediate major clinical reinvestigation of cannabis preparations is indicated in the management of pain, chronic neurologic diseases, convulsive disorders, migraine headache, anorexia, mental illness, and bacterial infections.

Recently declassified secret U.S. Defense Department studies reconfirm marijuana's congeners to have therapeutic utility.

Cannabis indica, Cannabis sativa, Cannabis americana, Indian hemp and marijuana (or marihuana) all refer to the same plant. Cannabis is used throughout the world for diverse purposes and has a long history characterized by usefulness, euphoria or evil—depending on one's point of view. To the agriculturist cannabis is a fiber crop; to the physician of a century ago it was a valuable medicine; to the physician of today it is an enigma; to the user, a euphoriant; to the police, a menace; to the traffickers, a source of profitable danger; to the convict or parolee and his family, a source of sorrow.

This book is concerned primarily with the medicinal aspects of cannabis.

The Chinese emperor Shen-nung is reported to have taught his people to grow hemp for fiber in the twenty-eighth century B.C. A text from the period 1500–1200 B.C. documents a knowledge of the plant in China—but not for use as fiber. In 200 A.D., the use of cannabis as an analgesic was described by the physician Hoa-tho.[44]

In India the use of hemp preparations as a remedy was described before 1000 B.C. In Persia, cannabis was known several centuries before Christ. In Assyria, about 650 B.C., its intoxicating properties were noted.[44]

Except for Herodotus' report that the Scythians used the smoke from burning hemp seeds for intoxication, the ancient Greeks seemed to be unaware of the psychoactive properties of cannabis. Dioscorides in the first century A.D. rendered an accurate morphologic description of the plant, but made no note of intoxicating properties.[10]

In the thirteenth and fourteenth centuries, Arabic writers described the social use of cannabis and resultant cruel but unsuccessful attempts to suppress its non-medical use.[44]

Although Galen described the use of the seeds for creating warmth, he did not describe the intoxicating qualities of hemp. Of interest is the paucity of references to hemp's intoxicating properties in the lay and medical literature of Europe before the 1800s.[44]

The therapeutic use of cannabis was introduced into Western medicine in 1839, in a forty-page article by W. B. O'Shaughnessy, a thirty-year-old physician serving with the British in India.[27] His discussion of the history of the use of cannabis products in the East reveals an awareness that these drugs had not only been used in medicine for therapeutic purposes, but had also been used for recreational and religious purposes.

O'Shaughnessy is not primarily known for his discovery of hemp drugs, but rather for his basic studies on intravenous electrolyte therapy in 1831, and his introduction of the telegraph into India in the 1850s.[26]

After studying the literature on cannabis and conferring with contemporary Hindu and Mohammedan scholars O'Shaughnessy tested the effects of various hemp preparations on animals, before attempting to use them to treat humans. Satisfied that the drug was reasonably safe, he administered preparations of cannabis extract to patients, and discovered that it had analgesic and sedative properties. O'Shaughnessy successfully relieved the pain of rheumatism and stilled the convulsions of an infant with this strange new drug. His most spectacular success came, however, when he quelled the wrenching muscle spasms of tetanus and rabies with the fragrant resin. Psychic effects resembling a curious delirium, when an overdose was given, were treated with strong purgatives, emetics with a blister to the nape of the neck, and leeches on the temples.[27]

The use of cannabis derivatives for medicinal purposes spread rapidly throughout Western medicine, as is evidenced in the report of the Committee on Cannabis Indica of the Ohio State Medical Society, published in 1860. In that report physicians told of success in treating stomach pain, childbirth psychosis, chronic cough, and gonorrhea with hemp products.[25] A Dr. Fronmueller, of Fuerth, Ohio, summarized his experiences with the drug as follows:

> I have used hemp many hundred times to relieve local pains of an inflammatory as well as neuralgic nature, and judging from these experiments, I have to assign to the Indian hemp a place among the so-called hypnotic medicines next to opium; its effects are less intense, and the secretions are not so much suppressed by it. Digestion is not disturbed; the appetite rather increased; sickness of the stomach seldom induced; congestion never. Hemp may

consequently be employed in inflammatory conditions. It disturbs the expectoration far less than opium; the nervous system is also not so much affected. The whole effect of hemp being less violent, and producing a more natural sleep, without interfering with the actions of the internal organs, it is certainly often preferable to opium, although it is not equal to that drug in strength and reliability. An alternating course of opium and Indian hemp seems particularly adapted to those cases where opium alone fails in producing the desired effect.[25]

Because cannabis did not lead to physical dependence, it was found to be superior to the opiates for a number of therapeutic purposes. Birch, in 1889, reported success in treating opiate and chloral addiction with cannabis,[5] and Mattison in 1891 recommended its use to the young physician, comparing it favorably with the opiates. He quoted his colleague Suckling:

> With a wish for speedy effect, it is so easy to use that modern mischief-maker, hypodermic morphia, that they [young physicians] are prone to forget remote results of incautious opiate giving.
>
> Would that the wisdom which has come to their professional fathers through, it may be, a hapless experience, might serve them to steer clear of narcotic shoals on which many a patient has gone awreck.
>
> Indian hemp is not here lauded as a specific. It will, at times, fail. So do other drugs. But the many cases in which it acts well, entitle it to a large and lasting confidence.
>
> My experience warrants this statement: cannabis indica is, often, a safe and successful anodyne and hypnotic.[23]

In their study of the medical applications of cannabis, physicians of the nineteenth century repeatedly encountered a number of difficulties. Recognizing the therapeutic potential of the drug, many experimenters sought ways of overcoming these drawbacks to its use in medicine, in particular the following:

Cannabis products are insoluble in water.

The onset of the effects of medicinal preparations of cannabis takes an hour or so; its action is therefore slower than that of many other drugs.

Different batches of cannabis derivatives vary greatly in strength; moreover, the common procedure for standardization of cannabis samples, by administration to test animals, is subject to error owing to variability of reactions among the animals.

There is wide variation among humans in their individual responses to cannabis.

Despite these problems regarding the uncertainty of potency and dosage and the difficulties in mode of administration, cannabis has several important advantages over other substances used as analgesics, sedatives, and hypnotics:

The prolonged use of cannabis does not lead to the development of physical dependence.[11, 13, 14, 24, 39, 44]

There is minimal development of tolerance to cannabis products.*[11, 13, 14, 24, 44]

Cannabis products have exceedingly low toxicity.[9,21,22,24] (The oral dose required to kill a mouse has been found to be about 40,000 times the dose required to produce typical symptoms of intoxication in man.)[21]

Cannabis produces no disturbance of vegetative functioning, whereas the opiates inhibit the gastrointestinal tract, the flow of bile and the cough reflex.[1,2,24,44,46]

Besides investigating the physical effects of medicinal preparations of cannabis, nineteenth-century physicians observed the psychic effects of the drug in its therapeutic applications.[4,27,33] They found that cannabis first mildly stimulates, and then sedates the higher centers of the brain. Hare suggested in 1887 a possible mechanism of cannabis' analgesic properties:

> During the time that this remarkable drug is relieving pain a very curious psychical condition manifests itself; namely, that the diminution of the pain seems to be due to its fading away in the distance, so that the pain becomes less and less, just as the pain in a delicate ear would grow less and less as a beaten drum was carried farther and farther out of the range of hearing.
>
> This condition is probably associated with the other well-known symptom produced by the drug; namely, the prolongation of time.[16]

Reynolds, in 1890,[33] summed up thirty years of his clinical experience using cannabis, finding it useful as a nocturnal sedative in senile insomnia, and valuable in treating dysmenorrhea, neuralgias including tic douloureux and

---

* Loewe notes a slight "beginner's habituation" in dogs, during the first few trials with the drug, as the only noticeable tolerance effect.[20]

tabetic symptoms, migraine headache and certain epileptoid or choreoid muscle spasms. He felt it to be of uncertain benefit in asthma, alcoholic delirium and depressions. Reynolds thought cannabis to be of no value in joint pains that were aggravated by motion and in cases of true chronic epilepsy.

Reynolds stressed the necessity of titrating the dose of each patient, increasing gradually every third or fourth day, to avoid "toxic" effects:

> The dose should be given in minimum quantity, repeated in not less than four or six hours, and gradually increased by one drop every third or fourth day, until either relief is obtained, or the drug is proved, in such case, to be useless. With these precautions I have never met with any toxic effects, and have rarely failed to find, after a comparatively short time, either the value or the uselessness of the drug.[33]

Concerning migraine headache, Osler stated in his text: Cannabis indica is probably the most satisfactory remedy.[11,28]

In his definitive survey of the literature and report of his own studies, deceptively titled *Marihuana, America's New Drug Problem,* Walton notes that cannabis was widely used during the latter half of the nineteenth century, and particularly before new drugs were developed:

> This popularity of the hemp drugs can be attributed partly to the fact that they were introduced before the synthetic hypnotics and analgesics. Chloral hydrate was not introduced until 1869 and was followed in the next thirty years by paraldehyde, sulfonal and the barbitals. Antipyrine and acetanilide, the first of their particular group of analgesics, were introduced about 1884. For general sedative and analgesic purposes, the only drugs commonly used at this time were the morphine derivatives and their disadvantages were very well known. In fact, the most attractive feature of the hemp narcotics was probably the fact that they did not exhibit certain of the notorious disadvantages of the opiates. The hemp narcotics do not constipate at all, they more often increase than decrease appetite, they do not particularly depress the respiratory center even in large doses, they rarely or never cause pruritis or cutaneous eruptions and, most important, the liability of developing addiction is very much less than with opiates.[44]

The use of cannabis in American medicine was seriously affected by the increased use of opiates in the latter half of the nineteenth century. With the introduction of the hypodermic syringe into American medicine from England in 1856 by Barker and Ruppaner, the use of the faster acting, water-soluble opiate drugs rapidly increased. The Civil War helped to spread the use of opiates in this country; the injected drugs were administered widely—and often indiscriminately—to relieve the pain of maimed soldiers returning from combat. (Opiate addiction was once called the "army disease."[41]) As the use of injected opiates increased, cannabis declined in popularity.

Cannabis preparations were still widely available in legend and over-the-counter forms in the 1930s. Crump* in 1931 mentioned the proprietaries "Piso's Cure," "One Day Cough Cure" and "Neurosine" as containing cannabis.[44] In 1937 Sasman listed twenty-eight pharmaceuticals containing cannabis.[36] Cannabis was still recognized as a medicinal agent in that year, when the committee on legislative activities of the American Medical Association concluded as follows:

> ... there is positively no evidence to indicate the abuse of cannabis as a medicinal agent or to show that its medicinal use is leading to the development of cannabis addiction. Cannabis at the present time is slightly used for medicinal purposes, but it would seem worthwhile to maintain its status as a medicinal agent for such purposes as it now has. There is a possibility that a re-study of the drug by modern means may show other advantages to be derived from its medicinal use.[32]

Meanwhile, in Mexico, the poor were smoking marijuana to relax and to endure heat and fatigue. (Originally marijuana was the Mexican slang word for the smoking preparation of dried leaves and flowering tops of the Cannabis sativa plant—the indigenous variety of the hemp plant.)

The recreational smoking of marijuana may have started in this country in New Orleans in about 1910, and continued on a small scale there until 1926, when a newspaper ran a six-part series on the use of the drug.[44] The fad subsequently spread up the Mississippi and throughout the United States, faster than local and state laws could be passed to discourage it. The use of "tea" or "muggles" blossomed into a minor

---

* Chairman, Investigating Committee, American Medical Association.

"psychedelic revolution" of the 1920s Narcotics officers encouraged the enactment of local prohibitory laws and eventually succeeded in bringing about restrictive Federal legislation. In 1937 Congress passed the Marihuana Tax Act, the finale to a series of prohibitory acts in the individual states. Under the new laws, the already dwindling use of cannabis as a therapeutic substance in medicine was brought to a virtual halt. In 1941, cannabis was dropped from the *National Formulary and Pharmacopoeia.*

Around the time of the passage of the Marihuana Tax Act, Walton postulated sites of action for cannabis drugs. Cortical areas, he found, are affected at low dosage, while at high dosage there seems to be a depressant effect on the thalamocortical pathways. Hyperemia of the brain appears to be a local phenomenon, unless centers controlling vasodilation might be located in the thalamo-cortical region. Similar possible mechanisms are suggested for the phenomenon of mild hypoglycemia, usual hunger and thirst and occasional lacrimation and nausea.[44]

Despite restrictive legislation, a few medical researchers have had the opportunity to continue the investigation of the therapeutic applications of cannabis in recent years. In his study of the medical applications of cannabis for Mayor La Guardia's committee, Dr. Samuel Allentuck reported, among other findings, favorable results in treating withdrawal of opiate addicts with tetrahydrocannabinol (THC), a powerful purified product of the hemp plant.[1,24]

An article in 1949, buried in a journal of chemical abstracts, reported that a substance related to THC controlled epileptic seizures in a group of children more effectively than diphenylhydantoin (Dilantin®), a most commonly prescribed anticonvulsant.[9]

A number of experimenters, believing that cannabis products might be of value in psychiatry, have investigated the applications of various forms of them in the treatment of mental disorders. Cannabis had been used in the nineteenth century to treat mental illness.[19,25,45,46] However, aside from some rather equivocal clinical studies, primarily in the treatment of depression,[29,30,35,39] and another report of success in treating withdrawal from alcohol and opiate addiction,[42] no significant contemporary psychiatric studies involving cannabis therapy have been reported to date.

Many current "authoritative" publications unequivocally state that there is no legitimate medical use for marijuana. As compared with the 1800s, this century has seen very little medical research on the array of some twenty chemicals that are found in the hemp plant.[37]

Today's readers may tend to be skeptical about a report of a cure for gonorrhea published over a century ago.[19,25] Such findings may bear reinvestigation, however, in the light of a report from Czechoslovakia in 1960 that cannabidiolic acid, a product of the unripe hemp plant, has bacteriocidal properties.[7] Some of the therapeutic applications reported in the early medical papers have been corroborated by later investigators, but for the most part the therapeutic aspects of cannabis remain to be re-explored under modern clinical conditions.

In the past twenty years, clinical and basic research on cannabis have dwindled to practically nothing. The record of tax stamps issued by the Federal Bureau of Narcotics for cannabis research, as compared with those for research on narcotic drugs, tells the story of the twenty-year "drought" in the investigation of cannabis products:[43]

	Users for Purposes of Research, Instruction, or Analysis	
Year	Narcotic Drugs	Marijuana
1938	....	5
1941	94	..
1943	....	43
1946	323	..
1948	....	87
1951	1078	..
1953	....	18
1956	284	..
1958	....	6
1961	344	..
1965	431	16

The rising non-medical use of marijuana both floated and was buoyed by the "psychedelic revolution" of the mid 1960s. The panicked reaction included a renewed scientific interest in the drug.

Eleven studies funded by the National Institute of Mental Health in 1967 concerning cannabis were either specialized animal experiments, part of an observational sociologic study of a number of drugs, or explorations of chemical detection methods. No human studies were included.

Of the fifty-six projects funded during the next fiscal years 1968–69 only two used humans.[52] The next year was somewhat less cautious with eight out of thirty-five projects devoted to clinical studies.[53]

Some of the preliminary results are in from these studies. Much is still unpublished.

According to Harris, the toxicity factor of marijuana derivatives is over two hundred and that chronic smoking of marijuana is less harmful to the lungs than tobacco cigarettes.[49]

Domino described the cross tolerance of THC and alcohol in pigeons[47] corroborating Jones' clinical observations.[50,51] These rediscoveries demand therapeutic trial.

In August 1971 certain secret Defense Department documents were declassified. While at NIMH as a consulting research psychiatrist in 1967 I had become aware of the existence of clandestine research at Edgewood Arsenal in Maryland.

From 1954–59 Dr. Van M. Sim was in charge of the project. He reported to *Medical World News*: "Marijuana . . . is probably the most potent anti-epileptic known to medicine today."[49]

Dr. Harold F. Hardman, then with the Defense contracting group at the University of Michigan's Department of Pharmacology reported effects of profound hypothermia and felt marijuana derivatives to be potentially quite useful in brain and traumatic surgery.[48]

The principal focus was, however, on the possible use of THC homologs as incapacitating agents. Besides the aforementioned government agency and university, the private sector was represented by the Arthur D. Little Company of Cambridge, Massachusetts.[55]

Recently in the course of a study of effects on driving, it was incidentally discovered that cannabis lowers intraocular pressure, thus being possibly useful in the treatment of glaucoma.[56]

Thus, a helix is made. Modern technologic methods confirm O'Shaughessy's observations 130 years ago. After swinging away from the knowledge of marijuana's properties through the worship of new synthetics, an unrelated rise of marijuana use socially, illegalization and removal from availability for clinical use, medicine rediscovers marijuana.

The flame of knowledge is at a low ebb, kept alive by isolated scientists and clinicians; it is now being rekindled by these recent circumscribed revelations.

Unless existing restrictive state and federal laws governing marijuana are changed, there will be no future for either modern scientific investigation or controlled clinical trial by present-day methods.

The tide is turning. The Federal Bureau of Narcotic and Dangerous Drugs, National Institute of Mental Health and The Food and Drug Administration Joint Committee recently authorized human therapeutic trial of cannabis products. We may now look forward to reinvestigation of the numerous possible medical uses of marijuana.[54]

A concerted effort is indicated for full-scale investigations where knowledge is lacking. Acute and chronic effects of cannabis should be restudied by modern methods. Metabolic pathways of action and detoxification need exploration by the pharmaceutical means of today. Chronic toxicity studies must be undertaken to examine possible long-term effects of cannabis use.*

Medical science must again confront the problems of cannabis' insolubility in water and its variable strength. Since human and animal responses vary a great deal, individual doses must be titrated. The popular "double blind" type of study methods will require revision. The reporting of personal drug experience was once acceptable to the scientific community.[15,22,25,29,34,39,44] Humans who are drug "sophisticates" will again become indispensable to psychoactive drug research, as wine tasters are to the wine industry, for only humans can verbally report the subtle and complex effects of these substances.

---

* Cunningham in 1893 found no gross central nervous system changes with chronic administration of hemp drugs to primates over several months.[8]

Government agencies having stimulated little significant clinical research in this field, the pharmaceutical industry should take the initiative in starting basic research and clinical studies into the purified congeners of cannabis for their chemical properties, pharmacologic qualities and therapeutic applications.

Possible Therapeutic Applications of
Tetrahydrocannabinols and Like Products

Analgesic-hypnotic [16,18,19,23,25,27,33,45]

Appetite stimulant [18,25,27]

Antiepileptic-antispasmodic [9,18,27,33,40,45,49]

Prophylactic and treatment of the neuralgias, including migraine and tic douloureux [3,16,17,18,19,23,25,28,31,33,38,40,45]

Antidepressant-tranquilizer [6,16,18,19,23,25,31,33,40,45]

Antiasthmatic [18,25,45]

Oxytocic [25,45]

Antitussive [3,16,25,38,45]

Topical anesthetic [8]

Withdrawal agent for opiate and alcohol addiction [5,23,24,38,42,45,47,50,51]

Childbirth analgesic [12]

Antibiotic [7]

Intraocular hypotensive [56]

Hypothermogenic [48]

Medicine, being an empiric art, has not hesitated in the past to utilize a substance first used for recreational purposes,* in the pursuit of the more noble purposes of healing, relieving pain and teaching us more of the workings of the human mind and body. The active constituents of cannabis appear to have remarkably low acute and chronic toxicity factors and might be quite useful in the management of many chronic disease conditions. More reasonable laws and regulations controlling psychoactive drug research are required to permit significant medical inquiry to begin so that we can fill the large gaps in our knowledge of cannabis.

---

* Morton "discovered" ether for anesthetic purposes after observing medical students at "ether frolics" in 1846. (Howard W. Haggard: *Devils, Drugs and Doctors,* Harper and Row, New York, 1929, p. 99.)

REFERENCES

1. Adams, Roger: Marihuana, Bulletin of the New York Academy of Medicine, 18:705–29, Nov. 1942.

2. Ames, Frances: A clinical and metabolic study of acute intoxication with cannabis sativa and its role in the model psychoses, J. of Mental Science, 104:972–99, Oct. 1958.

3. Anderson, G. S. D.: Remarks on the remedial virtues of cannabis indica, or Indian hemp, Boston Med. and Surg. J., 67:427–30, 1863.

4. Bell, John: On the haschisch or cannabis indica, Boston Med. and Surg. J., 56:209–16, 229–36, 1857.

5. Birch, Edward A.: The use of Indian hemp in the treatment of chronic chloral and chronic opium poisoning, Lancet, 1:625, 30 Mar. 1889.

6. Boyd, E. S., and Merritt, D. A.: Effects of a tetrahydrocannabinol derivative on some motor systems in the cat, Arch. Internat. de Pharmacodynamie et de Therapie, 153:1–12, 1965.

7. CIBA Foundation Study Group, Hashish—Its Chemistry and Pharmacology, 1964, pp. 45, 49.

8. Cunningham, D. D.: Report by Brigade-Surgeon—Lieut. Col. D. D. Cunningham, F.R.S., C.I.E., on the nature of the effects accompanying the continued treatment of animals with hemp drugs and with dhatura; *from* Report of the Indian Hemp Drugs Commission, 1893–4, Government Central Printing Office, Simla, India, 1894, Vol. 3, pp. 192–96.

9. Davis, J. P., and Ramsey, H. H.: Antiepileptic action of marihuana-active substances, Federat. Proc., 8:284–85, Mar. 1949.

10. Dioscorides, Pedanius: The Greek Herbal of Dioscorides, Edited by Robert T. Gunther, Hafner Publishing Co., New York, 1959, pp. 390–91.

11. Eddy, N. B., Halbach, H., Isbell, H., and Seevers, M. H.: Drug dependence: its significance and characteristics. Psychopharmacology Bull., 3:1–12, July 1966.

12. Effects of alcohol and cannabis during labor, JAMA, 94:1165, 1930.

13. Goodman, L. S., and Gilman, A.: The Pharmacological Basic of Therapeutics, 2nd Edition, Macmillan, New York, 1955.

14. Goodman, L. S., and Gilman, A.: The Pharmacological Basis of Therapeutics, 3rd Edition, Macmillan, New York, 1965.

15. Hamilton, H. C., Lescohier, A. W., and Perkins, R. A.: The physiological activity of cannabis sativa. Comparison of extracts from Indian and American-grown drug upon human subjects, J. Amer. Pharm. Assoc., 2:22–30, 1913.

16. Hare, Hobart Amory: Clinical and physiological notes on the action of cannabis indica, Therap. Gaz., 11:225–28, 1887.

17. Hare, H. A., and Chrystie, W.: A System of Practical Therapeutics, Lee Brothers and Co., Philadelphia, 1892, Vol. 3.

18. Indian Materia Medica, edited by A. K. Nadkarni, Popular Book Depot, Bombay, 1954.

19. Lilly's Hand Book of Pharmacy and Therapeutics, Eli Lilly and Co., Indianapolis, 1898, p. 32.

20. Loewe, S.: The active principles of cannabis and the pharmacology of the cannabinols, Archiv fur Experim. Pathologie und Pharmakologie, 211:175–93, 1950.

21. Loewe, S.: Studies on the pharmacology and acute toxicity of compounds with marihuana activity, J. Pharmacol. and Experim. Therap., 88:154–61, Oct. 1946.

22. Marshall, C. R.: A contribution to the pharmacology of cannabis indica, JAMA, 31:882–91, 15 Oct. 1898.

23. Mattison, J. B.: Cannabis indica as an anodyne and hypnotic, St. Louis Med. and Surg. J., 61:265–71, Nov. 1891.

24. Mayor's Committee on Marihuana, The Marihuana Problem in the City of New York, Jaques Cattell, Lancaster, Pa., 1944.

25. McMeens, R. R.: Report of the committee on cannabis indica; from Transactions of the Fifteenth Annual Meeting of the Ohio State Medical Society, Follett, Foster and Co., Columbus, Ohio, 1860, pp. 75–100.

26. Moon, J. B.: Sir William Brooke O'Shaughnessy—the foundations of fluid therapy and the Indian telegraph service. New Eng. J. of Med., 276:283–84, 2 Feb. 1967.

27. O'Shaughnessy, W. B.: On the preparations of the Indian hemp, or gunjah, Trans. Med. and Phy. Soc., Bengal, 71-102, 1838–40; 421–61, 1842.

28. Osler, W., and McCrae, T.: Principles and Practice of Medicine, 8th Edition, D. Appleton and Co., New York, 1916, p. 1089.

29. Parker, C. S., and Wrigley, F.: Synthetic cannabis preparations in psychiatry: (1) synhexyl, J. of Mental Science, 96:176–79, 1950.

30. Pond, D. A.: Psychological effects in depressive patients of the marihuana homologue synhexyl, J. Neurol. Neurosurg, Psychiat., 11:271–79, 1948.

31. Ratnam, E. V.: Cannabis indica, J. of the Ceylon Branch of the Brit. Med. Assoc., 13:30–34, 1916.

32. Report of the Committee on Legislative Activities, JAMA, 108:2214–15, 1937.

33. Reynolds, J. Russell: Therapeutical uses and toxic effects of cannabis indica, Lancet, 1:637–38, 22 Mar. 1890.

34. Robinson, Victor: An Essay on Hasheesh—Historical and Experimental, L. H. Ringer, New York, 1912.

35. Rolls, E. J., and Stafford-Clark, D.: Depersonalization treated by cannabis indica and psychotherapy, Guy's Hospital Report, 103:330–36, 1954.

36. Sasman, Marty: Cannabis indica in pharmaceuticals, J. of the N.J. Med Soc., 35:51–52, Jan. 1938.

37. Shulgin, Alexander T.: personal communication, 1968.

38. Stevens, A. A.: Modern Materia Medica and Therapeutics, W. B. Saunders and Co., Philadelphia, 1903, pp. 77-78.

39. Stockings, G. Taylor: A new euphoriant for depressive mental states, Brit. Med J., 1:918-22, 28 June 1947.

40. Suckling, C. W.: On the therapeutic value of Indian Hemp, Brit. Med. J., 2:12, 1881.

41. Terry, C. E., and Pellens, M.: The Opium Problem, Bureau of Social Hygiene, Inc., New York, 1928, pp. 53-93.

42. Thompson, L. J. and Proctor, R. C.: The use of pyrahexyl in the treatment of alcoholic and drug withdrawal conditions, N. Carolina Med. J., 14:520-23, Oct. 1953.

43. U.S. Treasury Dept., Bureau of Narcotics, Traffic in Opium and Other Dangerous Drugs for the Year Ended Dec. 31, 1965, U.S. Printing Office, Washington, 1966, pp. 55-56.

44. Walton, Robert P.: Marihuana: America's New Drug Problem, J. B. Lippincott, Philadelphia, 1938, pp. 1-18, 86-157.

45. Waring, Edward John: Practical Therapeutics, Lindsay and Blakiston, Philadelphia, 1874, pp. 157-61.

46. Wood, G. B., and Bache, F.: The Dispensatory of the United States of America, 12th Edition, J. B. Lippincott, Philadelphia, 1866, pp. 379-82.

47. Domino, Edward F., Neuropharmacological Studies of Marijuana—Some Synthetic and Natural THC Derivatives in Animals and Man, 1971. Unpublished. 54 pp.

48. Hardman, Harold F., Domino, Edward F. and Seevers, Maurice T. General Pharmacological Actions of Synthetic Tetrahydrocannabinol Derivatives, 1971. Unpublished.

49. Berger, Alfred D., Marijuana. Med. World News, July 16, 1971, pp. 37-43.

50. Jones, Reese T., Psychological Studies of Marijuana and Alcohol in Man. Psychopharmacologia 18,108-117, 1970.

51. Jones, Reese T., Tetrahydrocannabinol and the Marijuana Induced Social "High" or the Effects of the Mind on Marijuana. Ann. N.Y. Acad. Sci., 1972. In press.

52. Grants Active During Fiscal Years 1968 and 1969 Center for Studies in Narcotics and Drug Abuse. National Institute of Mental Health, 1969. Unpublished.

53. Ibid., 1970.

54. Bozetti, Louis: personal communication, January, 1972.

55. Arthur D. Little Company, New Incapacitating Agents—Quarterly Report 15/16 Supplement. Preclinical Pharmacology and Toxicology of Candidate Agent 226, 169. Papers on Tetrahydrocannabinols —Cleared for public release. The National Technical Information Service, Department of Commerce, 1971.

56. Hepler, R. S. and Frank, I. R. Marihuana Smoking and Intraocular Pressure. JAMA, Sept. 6, 1971. Vol. 217, no. 10.

ON THE PREPARATIONS

OF THE

INDIAN HEMP, OR GUNJAH

(CANNABIS INDICA);

THEIR EFFECTS ON THE ANIMAL SYSTEM IN HEALTH, AND THEIR UTILITY IN
THE TREATMENT OF TETANUS AND OTHER CONVULSIVE DISEASES

By W. B. O'SHAUGHNESSY, M.D.,

Assistant-Surgeon, and Professor of Chemistry, &c.

In the Medical College of Calcutta.

Presented October, 1839.

The narcotic effects of Hemp are popularly known in the south of Africa, South America, Turkey, Egypt, Asia Minor, India, and the adjacent territories of the Malays, Burmese, and Siamese. In all these countries Hemp is used in various forms, by the dissipated and depraved, as the ready agent of a pleasing intoxication, In the popular medicine of these nations, we find it extensively employed for a multitude of affections. But in Western Europe, its use either as a stimulant or as a remedy, is equally unknown. With the exception of the trial, as a frolic, of the Egyptian ' Hasheesh,' by a few youths in Marseilles, and of the clinical use of the wine of Hemp by Mahneman, as shewn in a subsequent extract, I have been unable to trace any notice of the employment of this drug in Europe.

Much difference of opinion exists on the question, whether the Hemp so abundant in Europe, even in

I

FROM EAST TO WEST

Although there was widespread trafficking in opium by the Western powers in Asia in the eighteenth and nineteenth centuries, trafficking in marijuana products was apparently not considered worthwhile from an exploitative point of view. The widespread growth and cultivation of cannabis for its mental effects went virtually unnoticed.

In 1839, W. B. O'Shaughnessy, M.D., a thirty-year-old graduate of the medical school in Edinburgh, under service to the British East India Company, published the following monograph. Marking the introduction of marijuana into western medicine as a therapeutic tool, O'Shaughnessy's monograph provides a summary of all the knowledge available to him and reviews his experiments with animals before he performed human experiments with diseases, including rheumatism, cholera, rabies, and tetanus.

Some seven years before, at the end of his medical training in Scotland, O'Shaughnessy invented intravenous fluid and electrolyte replacement therapy during a cholera epidemic. In the years following the publication of this article, he went on to publish a pharmacopoeia of Indian medicines. He then changed careers, becoming an engineer, and brought the telegraph to India, a service which led to his being knighted. He then returned to England, changed his name, and was married thrice before dying at the age of eighty-one.

On the Preparations of the Indian Hemp, or Gunjah

By W.B. O'SHAUGHNESSY

The narcotic effects of Hemp are popularly known in the south of Africa, South America, Turkey, Egypt, Asia Minor, India, and the adjacent territories of the Malays, Burmese, and Siamese. In all these countries Hemp is used in various forms, by the dissipated and depraved, as the ready agent of pleasing intoxication. In the popular medicine of these nations, we find it extensively employed for a multitude of affections. But in Western Europe, its use either as a stimulant or as a remedy, is equally unknown. With the exception of the trial, as a frolic, of the Egyptian 'Hasheesh,' by a few youths in Marseilles, and of the clinical use of the wine of Hemp by Mahneman, as shewn in a subsequent extract, I have been unable to trace any notice of the employment of this drug in Europe.

Much difference of opinion exists on the question, whether the Hemp so abundant in Europe, even in high northern latitudes, is identical in specific characters with the Hemp of Asia Minor and Hindostan. The extraordinary symptoms produced by the latter depend a resinous secretion with which it abounds and which seems totally absent in the European kind. As the closest physical resemblance or even identity exists between both plants, difference of climate seems to me more than sufficient to account for the absence of the resinous secretion, and consequent want of narcotic power in that indigenous in colder countries.

In the subsequent article I first endeavour to present an

Reprinted from *Transactions of the Medical and Physical Society of Bengal,* 1838–40, pp. 421–461.

adequate view of what has been recorded of the early history, the popular uses and employment in medicine of this powerful and valuable substance. I then proceed to notice several experiments which I have instituted on animals, with the view to ascertain its effects on the healthy system; and, lastly, I submit an abstract of the clinical details of the treatment of several patients afflicted with hydrophobia, tetanus, and other convulsive disorders, in which a preparation of Hemp was employed with results which seem to me to warrant our anticipating from its more extensive and impartial use no inconsiderable addition to the resources of the physician.

In the historical and statistical department of the subject, I owe my cordial thanks for most valuable assistance to the distinguished traveller, the Syed Keramut Ali, Mootawulee of the Hooghly Imambarrah, and also the the Hakim Mirza Abdul Rhazes of Teheran, who have furnished me with interesting details regarding the consumption of Hemp in Caudahar, Cabul, and the countries between the Indus and Herat. The Pundit Modoosudun Goopto has favoured me with notices of the remarks on these drugs in the early Sanscrit authors on Materia Medica;—to the celebrated Kamalakantha Vidyadanka, the Pundit of the Asiatic Society, I have also to record my acknowledgments;—Mr. DaCosta has obligingly supplied me with copious notes from the 'Mukzun-ul-Udwieh,' and other Persian and Hindee systems of Materia Medica. For information relative to the varieties of the drug, and its consumption in Bengal, Mr. McCann, the Deputy Superintendent of Police, deserves my thanks;—and lastly, to Dr. Goodeve, to Mr. Richard O'Shaughnessy, to the late Dr. Bain, to Mr. O'Brien of the Native Hospital, and Nobinchunder Mitter, one of my clinical clerks, I am indebted for the clinical details with which they have enriched the subject.

Botanical characters, chemical properties, production. *Botanical Description*—Assuming with Lindley and other eminent writers that the *Cannabis sativa* and *Indica* are identical, we find that the plant is dioecious, annual, about three feet high, covered over with a fine pubescence; the stem is erect, branched, bright green, angular; leaves alternate or opposite, on long weak petioles; digitate, scabrous, with linear, lanceolate, sharply serrated leaflets, tapering into a long, smooth, entire point; stipules subulate; clusters of

flowers axillary, with subulate bractes; males lax and drooping, branched and leafless at base; females erect, simple and
leafy at the base. ♂ Calyx downy, five parted, imbricated.
Stamens five; anthers large and pendulous. ♀ Calyx covered
with brown glands. Ovary roundish, with pendulous ovule,
and two long filiform glandular stigmas; achenium ovate, one
seeded.—*v. Lindley's Flora Medica, p. 299.*

The fibres of the stems are long and extremely tenacious,
so as to afford the best tissue for cordage, thus constituting
the material for one of the most important branches of
European manufactures.

The seed is simply albuminous and oily, and is devoid of
all narcotic properties.

Chemical Properties—In certain seasons, and in warm countries, a resinous juice exudes, and concretes on the leaves,
slender stem, and flowers; the mode of removing this juice
will be subsequently detailed. Separated and in masses it
constitutes the *Churrus** of Nipal and Hindostan, and to this
the type, or basis of all the Hemp preparations, are the
powers of these drugs attributable.

The resin of the Hemp is very soluble in alcohol and ether;
partially soluble in alkaline; insoluble in acid solutions; when
pure, of a blackish grey colour; hard at 90°; softens at higher
temperatures, and fuses readily;—soluble in the fixed and in
several volatile oils. Its odour is fragrant and narcotic; taste
slightly warm, bitterish, and acrid.

The dried Hemp plant which has flowered, and *from which
the resin has not been removed*, is called *Gunjah*. It sells from
twelve annas to one rupee seer, in the Calcutta bazars, and
yields to alcohol twenty per 100 of resinous extract, composed of the resin (*churrus*) and green colouring matter
(*Chloro-phille*). Distilled with a large quantity of water,
traces of essential oil pass over, and the distilled liquor has
the powerful narcotic odour of the plant. The *gunjah* is sold
for smoking chiefly. The bundles of *gunjah* are about two
feet long, and three inches in diameter, and contain 24 to 36
plants. The colour is dusky green—the odour agreeably
narcotic—the whole plant resinous and adhesive to the touch.
The larger leaves and capsules without the stalks, are called

* For very fine specimens of *churrus*, I have to express my thanks to
Dr. Campbell, late assistant Resident at Nipal.

'Bangh Subjee or Sidhee.' They are used for making an
intoxicating drink, for smoking, and in the conserve or
confection termed *Majoon*. *Bang* is cheaper than *gunjah*, and
though less powerful, is sold at such a low price, that for one
pice enough can be purchased to intoxicate an experienced
person.

According to Mr. McCann's notes, the *gunjah* consumed in
Bengal is chiefly brought from Mirzapúr and Ghazeepore,
being extensively cultivated near Gwalior and in Tirboot. The
natives cut the plant when in flower, allow it to dry for three
days, and then lay it in bundles, averaging one seer weight
each, which are distributed to the licensed dealers. The best
kind are brought from Gwalior and Bhurtpore, and it is also
cultivated of good quality in a few gardens around Calcutta.
In Jessore, I am informed, the drug is produced of excellent
quality, and to a very considerable extent of cultivation.

In Central India and the Saugor territory, and in Nipal,
churrus is collected during the hot season, in the following
singular manner:—Men clad in leathern dresses run through
the Hemp-fields, brushing through the plant with all possible
violence; the soft resin adheres to the leather, is subsequently
scraped off, and kneaded into balls, which sell from five to
six rupees the seer. A still finer kind, the *momeea* or waxen
churrus, is collected by the hand in Nipal and sells for nearly
double the price of the ordinary kind. In Nipal, Dr.
McKinnon informs me, the leathern attire is dispensed with,
and the resin is gathered on the skins of naked coolies. In
Persia, it is stated by Mirza Abdool Rhazes that the *churrus* is
prepared by pressing the resinous plants on coarse cloths, and
then scraping it from these, and melting it in a pot with a
little warm water. He considers the *churrus* of Herat as the
best and most powerful of all the varieties of the drug.

Popular uses.   The preparations of Hemp are used for the purpose of
intoxication as follow:

Sidhee, subjee, and *bang* (synonymous) are used with
water as a drink, which is thus prepared. About three tola
weight, 540 troy grains, are well washed with cold water,
then rubbed to powder, mixed with black pepper, cucumber
and melon seeds, sugar, half a pint of milk, and an equal
quantity of water. This is considered sufficient to intoxicate

an habituated person. Half the quantity is enough for a novice. This composition is chiefly used by the Mahomedans of the better classes.

Another recipe is as follows:

The same quantity of *sidhee* is washed and ground, mixed with black pepper, and a quart of cold water added. This is drank at one sitting. This is the favorite beverage of the Hindus who practice this vice, especially the Birjobassies, and many of the rajpootana soldiery.

From either of these beverages intoxication will ensue in half an hour. Almost invariably the inebriation is of the most cheerful kind, causing the person to sing and dance, to eat food with great relish, and to see aphrodisiac enjoyments. In persons of quarrelsome disposition it occasions, as might be expected, an exasperation of their natural tendency. The intoxication lasts about three hours, when sleep supervenes. No nausea or sickness of stomach succeeds, nor are the bowels at all affected; next day there is slight giddiness and vascularity of the eyes, but no other symptom worth recording. *Gunjah* is used for smoking alone—one rupee weight, 180 grains, and a little dried tobacco are rubbed together in the palm of the hand with a few drops of water. This suffices for three persons. A little tobacco is placed in the pipe first, then a layer of the prepared *gunjah*, then more tobacco, and the fire above all.

Four or five persons usually join in this debauch. The hookah is passed round, and each person takes a single draught. Intoxication ensues almost instantly, and from one draught to the unaccustomed—within half an hour, and after four or five inspirations to those more practised in the vice. The effects differ from those occasioned by the *sidhee*. Heaviness, laziness, and agreeable reveries ensue, but the person can be readily roused, and is able to discharge routine occupations, such as pulling the punkab, waiting at table, &c.

The *Majoon*, or Hemp confection, is a compound of sugar, butter, flour, milk and *sidhee* or *bang*. The process has been repeatedly performed before me by Ameer, the proprietor of a celebrated place of resort for Hemp devotees in Calcutta, and who is considered the best artist in his profession. Four ounces of *sidhee*, and an equal quantity of *ghee* are placed in an earthen or well-tinned vessel, a pint of water added, and the whole warmed over a charcoal fire. The mixture is constantly stirred until the water all boils away, which is known by the crackling noise of the melted butter on the sides of the vessel. The mixture is then removed from the fire, squeezed through cloth while hot—by which an oleaginous solution of the active principles and colouring matter of the Hemp is obtained—and the leaves, fibres, &c. remaining on the cloth are thrown away.

The green oily solution soon concretes into a buttery mass, and is then well washed by the hand with soft water, so long as the water becomes coloured. The colouring matter and an extractive substance are thus removed, and a very pale green mass, of the consistence of simple ointment, remains. The washings are thrown away: Ameer says that these are intoxicating, and produce constriction of the throat, great pain, and very disagreeable and dangerous symptoms.

The operator then takes 2 lbs. of sugar, and adding a little water, places it in a pipkin over the fire. When the sugar dissolves and froths, two ounces of milk are added; a thick scum rises and is removed; more milk and a little water are added from time to time, and the boiling continued about an hour, the solution being carefully stirred until it becomes an adhesive clear syrup, ready to solidify on a cold surface; four ounces of tyre (new milk dried before the sun) in fine powder, are now stirred in, and lastly the prepared butter of Hemp is introduced, brisk stirring being continued for a few minutes. A few drops of attur of roses are then quickly sprinkled in, and the mixture poured from the pipkin on a flat cold dish or slab. The mass concretes immediately into a thin cake, which is divided into small lozenge-shaped pieces. A seer thus prepared sells for four rupees: one drachm by weight will intoxicate a beginner; three drachms one experienced in its use: the taste is sweet, and the odour very agreeable.

Ameer states that there are seven or eight *majoon* makers in Calcutta—that sometimes, by special order of customers, he introduces stramonium seeds, but never nux-vomica; that all classes of persons, including the lower Portuguese, or 'Kala Feringhees,' and especially their females, consume the drug; that it is most fascinating in its effects, producing extatic happiness, a persuasion of high rank, a sensation of flying— voracious appetite, and intense aphrodisiac desire. He denies that its continued use leads to madness, impotence, or to the

numerous evil consequences described by the Arabic and
Persian physicians. Although I disbelieve Ameer's statements
on this point, his description of the immediate effect of
majoon is strictly and accurately correct.

Most carnivorous animals eat it greedily, and very soon
experience its narcotic effects, becoming ludicrously drunk,
but seldom suffering any worse consequences.

The preceding notice suffices to explain the subsequent
historical and medicinal details. I premise the historical, in
order to shew the exact state of our knowledge of the
subject, when I attempted an investigation.

Although the most eminent of the Arabic and Persian
authors concur in referring the origin of the practice of Hemp
intoxications to the natives of Hindoostan, it is remarkable
that few traces can be detected of the prevalence of the vice
at any early period in India.

The Pundit Modoosudun Gooptu finds that 'Tajni guntu,'
a standard treatise on Materia Medica, which he estimates
vaguely at 600 years' date, gives a clear account of this agent.
Its synonyms are *'Bijoya,' 'Ujoya,'* and *'Joya,'* names which
mean promoters of success; *'Brijputta,'* or the strengthener,
or the strong-leaved; *'Chapola,'* the causer of a reeling gait;
'Ununda,' or laughter moving; *'Hursini,'* the exciter of sexual
desire. Its effects on man are described as excitant, heating
astringent. It is added that it 'destroys phlegm, expels
flatulence, induces costiveness, sharpens the memory, increases eloquence, excites the appetite, and acts as a general
tonic.'

The 'Rajbulubha,' a Sanscrit treatise of rather later date,
alludes to the use of Hemp in gonorrhoea, and repeats the
statements of the 'Rajniguntu.' In the Hindu Tantra, or a
religious treatise, teaching peculiar and mystical formulae and
rites for the worship of the deities, it is said moreover, that
sidhee is more intoxicating than wine.

In the celebrated 'Susruta,' which is perhaps the most
ancient of all Hindu medical works, it is written that persons
labouring under catarrh should, with other remedies, use
internally the *bijoya* or *sidhee.* The effects however are not
described.

The learned Kamalakantha Vidyalanka has traced notice of
Hemp in the 5th chapter of *Menu,* where Brahmins are

Historical details—
Notice of Hemp,
and its popular
uses by the
Sanscrit, Arabic,
and Persian
writers.

prohibited to use the following substances, *plandoo* or onions; *gunjara* or *gunjah*; and such condiments as have strong and pungent scents.

The Persian and Arabic writers are however far more voluminous and precise in their accounts of these fascinating preparations. In the 1st vol. of De Sacy's 'Crestomathie Arabe,' we find an extremely interesting summary of the writings of Takim Eddin Makrizi on this subject. Lane has noticed it too with his usual ability in his admirable work 'The Modern Egyptians.' From these two sources, the MS. notes of the Syed Keramut Ali and Mr. DaCosta, and a curious paper communicated by our friend Mirza Abdool Rhazes, a most intelligent Persian Physician, the following epitome is compiled.

Makrizi treats of the Hemp in his glowing description of the celebrated Canton de la Timbaliere, or ancient pleasure grounds, in the vicinity of Cairo. This quarter, after many vicissitudes, is now a heap of ruins. In it was situated a cultivated valley named Djoneina, which we are informed was the theatre of all conceivable abominations. It was famous above all for the sale of the *Hasheeha*, a drug still greedily consumed by the dregs of the populace, and from the consumption of which sprung the excesses which led to the name of 'Assassin,' being given to the Saracens in the Holy Wars. The history of the drug the author treats of thus: The oldest work in which Hemp is noticed is a treatise by Hasan, who states that in the year 658 (Mahometan era), the Sheikh Djafar Shirazi, a monk of the order of Haider, learnt from his master the history of the discovery of Hemp. Haider, the chief of ascetics and self-chasteners, lived in rigid privation on a mountain between Nishabor and Romah, where he established a monastery of Fakirs. Ten years he had spent in this retreat, without leaving it for a moment, till one burning summer's day, when he departed alone to the fields. On his return an air of joy and gaiety was imprinted on his countenance; he received the visits of his brethren, and encouraged their conversation. On being questioned, he stated that struck by the aspect of a plant which danced in the heat as if with joy, while all the rest of the vegetable creation was torpid, he had gathered and eaten of its leaves. He led his companions to the spot, all ate, and all were similarly excited. A tincture of the Hemp leaf in wine or spirit seems to have been the favorite formula in which the Sheikh Haider indulged himself. An Arab poet sings of Haider's *emerald* cup; an evident allusion to the rich green colour of the tincture of the drug. The Sheikh survived the discovery ten years, subsisting chiefly on this herb, and on his death his disciples by his desire planted it in an arbour about his tomb.

From this saintly sepulcher the knowledge of the effects of Hemp is stated to have spread into Khorasan. In Chaldea it was unknown until 728, during the reign of the Khalif Mostansir Billah: the kings of Drmus and Bahrein then introduced it into Chaldea, Syria, Egypt, and Turkey.

In Khorasan, however, it seems that the date of the use of Hemp is considered to be far prior to Haider's era. Biraslan, an Indian pilgrim, the contemporary of Cosröes,* is believed to have introduced and diffused the custom through Khorasan and Yemen. In proof of the great antiquity of the practice, certain passages in the works of Hippocrates may be cited, in which some of its properties are clearly described; but the difficulty of deciding whether the passages be spurious or genuine renders the fact of little value. Dioscorides (lib. ij. cap. 169) describes Hemp, but merely notices the emollient properties of its seeds—its intoxicating effects must consequently be regarded as unknown to the Greeks prior to his era, which is generally agreed to be about the second century of the Christian epoch, and somewhat subsequent to the life time of Pliny.

In the narrative of Makrizi we also learn that oxymel and acids are the most powerful antidotes to the effect of this narcotic; next to these, emetics, cold bathing, and sleep; and we are further told that it possesses diuretic, astringent, and specially aphrodisiac properties. Ibn Beitar was the first to record its tendency to produce mental derangement, and he even states that it occasionally proves fatal.

In 780 M. E. very severe ordinances were passed in Egypt against the practice: the Djoneina garden was rooted up, and all those convicted of the use of the drug were subjected to

* By this term is probably meant the first of the Sassanian dynasty, to whom the epithet of 'Khusrow' or Cosroes, equivalent to Kaiser, Caesar, or Czar, has been applied in many generations. This dynasty endured from A.D. 202 to A.D. 635—*vide note* 50 to *Lane's translation of the Arabian Nights, vol. ii, p. 226.*

the extraction of their teeth; but in 799 the custom re-established itself with more than original vigour. Makrizi draws an expressive picture of the evils this vice then inflicted on its votaries—'As its consequence, general corruption of sentiments and manners ensued, modesty disappeared, every base and evil passion was openly indulged in, and nobility of external form alone remained to these infatuated beings.'

Medicinal properties assigned to Hemp by the ancient Arabian and Persian writers, and by modern European authors. In the preceding notice of Makrizi's writings on this subject, we have confined ourselves chiefly to historical details, excluding descriptions of supposed medicinal effects. The Mukzunul-Udwieh and the Persian MS. in our possession, inform us as to the properties which the ancient physicians attributed to this powerful narcotic.

In Mr. DaCosta's MS. version of the chapter on Hemp in the Mukzun-ul-Udwieh, *churrus*, we are informed, if smoked through a pipe, causes torpor and intoxication, and often proves fatal to the smoker; three kinds are noticed, the *garden*, *wild* and *mountain*, of which the last is deemed the strongest—the seeds are called *sheaduna* or *shaldaneh* in Persia. These are said to be 'a compound of opposite qualities, cold and dry in the third degree; that is to say, stimulant and sedative, imparting at first a gentle reviving heat, and then a considerable refrigerant effect.'

The contrary qualities of the plant, its stimulant and sedative effects, are prominently dwelt on. 'They at first exhilirate the spirits, cause cheerfulness, give colour to the complexion, bring on intoxication, excite the imagination into the most rapturous ideas, produce thirst, increase appetite, excite concupiscence. Afterwards the sedative effects begin to preside, the spirits sink, the vision darkens and weakens; and madness, melancholy fearfulness, dropsy, and such like distempers, are the sequel—and the seminal secretions dry up. These effects are increased by sweets, and combatted by acids.'

The author of the *Mukzun-ul-Udwieh*, further informs us—

'The leaves make a good snuff for deterging the brain; the juice of the leaves applied to the head as a wash, removes dandrin and vermin; drops of the juice thrown into the ear allay pain, and destroy worms or insects. It checks diarrhoea; is useful in gonorrhoea; restrains seminal secretions, and is diuretic. The bark has a similar effect.'

'The powder is recommended as an external application to fresh wounds and sores, and for causing granulations; a poultice of the boiled root and leaves for discussing inflammations, and cure of erysipelas, and for allaying neuralgic pains. The dried leaves bruised and spread on a castor oil leaf cure hydrocele and swelled testes. The *dose*, internally, is one *direm* or 48 grains. The antidotes are emetics, cow's milk, hot water, and sorrel wine.'

Alluding to its popular uses, the author dwells on the eventual evil consequences of the indulgence;—weakness of the digestive organs first ensues, followed by flatulency, indigestion, swelling of the limbs and face, change of complexion, diminution of sexual vigour, loss of teeth, heaviness, cowardice, depraved and wicked ideas, scepticism in religious tenet; licentiousness and ungodliness are also enumerated in the catalogue of deplorable results.

The medicinal properties of Hemp, in various forms are the subject of some interesting notes by Mirza Abdool Rhazes. 'It produces a ravenous appetite and constipation, arrests the secretions, except that of the liver, excites wild imagining, especially a sensation of ascending, forgetfulness of all that happened during its use, and such mental exaltation, that *the beholders attribute it to supernatural inspiration.*'

Mirza Abdool considers Hemp to be a powerful exciter of the flow of bile, and relates cases of its efficacy in restoring appetite—of its utility as an external application as a poultice with milk, in relieving haemorrhoids—and internally in gonorrhoea to the extent of a quarter drachm of *bangh*. He states also that the habitual smokers of Gunjah generally die of diseases of the lungs, dropsy, and anasarca—'so do the eaters of *majoon* and smokers of *sidhee*, but at a later period. The inexperienced on first taking it are often senseless for a day, some go mad, others are known to die.'

In the 35th chapter of the 5th vol. of Rumphius Herbarium Amboinense, p. 208, Ed. Amsterd. A.D. 1695, we find a long and very good account of this drug, illustrated by two excellent plates. The sub-joined is an epitome of Rumphius' article.

Rumphius first describes botanically the male and female Hemp plants, of which he gives two admirable drawings. He assigns the upper provinces of India as its *habitat*, and states it to be cultivated in Java and Amboyna. He then notices very briefly the exciting effects ascribed to the leaf, and to mixtures thereof with spices, camphor, and opium. He alludes doubtingly to its alleged aphrodisiac powers, and states that the kind of mental excitement it produces depends on the temperament of the consumer. He quotes a passage from Galen lib. i. (de aliment. occult.) in which it is asserted that in that great writer's time it was customary to give Hemp seed to the guests at banquets as promoters of hilarity and enjoyment. Rumphius adds, that the Mahomedans in his neighbourhood frequently sought for the male plant from his garden to be given to persons afflicted with virulent gonorrhoea, and with asthma, or the infection, what is popularly called, 'stitches in the side.'

He tells us, moreover, that the powdered leaves check diarrhoea, are stomachic, cure the malady named *Pitao*, and moderate excessive secretion of bile. He mentions the use of Hemp smoke as an enema in strangulated hernia, and of the leaves as an antidote to poisoning by orpiment. Lastly, he notices in the two subsequent chapters varieties of Hemp which he terms the *gunja sativa* and *gunja agrestis*. In the *Hortus Malabaricus* Rheede's article on the Hemp is a mere outline of Rumphius's statements.

Among modern European writers, the only information we could trace on the medicinal use of Hemp *in Europe,* is the recent work of Ness v. Esenbeck, from which the following is an extract kindly supplied by Dr. Wallich:—
"The fresh herb of the Hemp has a very powerful and unpleasant narcotic smell, and is used in the East in combination with opium, in the preparation of intoxicating potions, &c. It is probable that the *nepenthe* of the ancients was prepared from the leaves of this plant. Many physicians, Hahnemann among them, prescribe the vinous extract in various nervous disorders, where opium and hyoscyamus used to be employed, being less heating and devoid of bitterness.'*

No information as to the medicinal effect of Hemp exists in the standard work on Materia Medica, to which I have access. Soubeiran, Feé, Merat and de Lens in their admirable

* *Handbuch der Medicin. und Pharmac. Botanik,* von. F. Nees von. Estabeck et Dr. Carl Ebermaier, vol. 1, p. 338.

dictionary; Chevalier and Richard, Roques (Phytographie Medicale); Ratier and Henry (Pharmacopée Francaise); and the Dictionnaire des Sciences Medicales—are all equally silent on the subject.

In *Ainslie's Materia Indica*, 2d vol., we find three notices of the plant and its preparations.

At page 39 'Banghie,' (*Tamul*) with the Persian and Hindee synonymes of 'Beng' and 'Subjee,' is described as an intoxicating liquor prepared with the leaves of the *Gunjah* or Hemp plant.

Under the head *Gunjah*, Ainslie gives numerous synonymes, and tells that the leaves are sometimes prescribed in cases of diarrhoea; and in conjunction with turmeric, onions, and warm gingilie oil are made into an unction for painful protruded piles. Dr. Ainslie also gives a brief view of the popular uses, and botanical peculiarities of the plant.

Majoon lastly is described by Dr. Ainslie, page 176, as a preparation of sugar, milk, ghee, poppy seeds, flowers of the datura, powder of nux-vomica, and sugar. The true *majoon* however, as prepared in Bengal, contains neither datura, or nux-vomica. I have already described the process by which it has been manufactured before me.

In the *Journal de Pharmacie*, the most complete magazine in existence on all pharmaceutical subjects, we find Hemp noticed in several volumes. In the Bulletin de Pharmacie t. v. a. 1810, p. 400, we find it briefly described by M. Rouyer, apothecary to Napoleon, and member of the Egyptian scientific commission, in a paper on the popular remedies of Egypt. With the leaves and tops, he tells us, collected before ripening, the Egyptians prepare a conserve, which serves as the base of the *berch*, the *diasmouk*, and the *bernaouy*. Hemp leaves reduced to powder, and incorporated with honey, or stirred with water, constitute the *berch* of the poor classes.

The same work also, (Bulletin vol. 1. p. 523, x. 1809,) contains a very brief notice on the intoxicating preparations of Hemp, read by M. De Sacy before the Institute of France in July, 1809. M. De Sacy's subsequent analysis of Makrizi, of which I have given an outline, is however much more rich in details than the article in the Bulletin.

Such was the amount of preliminary information before me, by which I was guided in my subsequent attempts to gain more accurate knowledge of the action, powers, and possible medical applications of this extraordinary agent.

There was sufficient to show that Hemp possessed in small doses an extraordinary power of stimulating the digestive organs, exciting the cerebral system, of acting also on the generative apparatus. Larger doses, again, were shewn by the historical statements to induce insensibility, or to act as a powerful sedative. The influence of the drug in allaying pain was equally manifest in all the memoirs referred to. As to the evil sequelae so unanimously dwelt on by all writers; these did not appear to me so numerous, so immediate, or so formidable, as many which may be clearly traced to over-indulgence in other powerful stimulants, or narcotics, viz. alcohol, opium, or tobacco.

The dose in which the Hemp preparations might be administered, constituted of course one of the first objects of inquiry. Ibn Beitar had mentioned a *direm*, or 48 grains of *churrus*; but this dose seemed to me so enormous, that I deemed it expedient to proceed with much smaller quantities. How fortunate was this caution, the sequel will sufficiently denote.

Experiments of the author— Inferences as to the action of the drug on animals and man.

An extensive series of experiments on animals, was in the first place undertaken, among which the following may be cited:

Expt. 1.—Ten grains of Nipalese *churrus*, dissolved in spirit, were given to a middling-sized dog. In half an hour he became stupid and sleepy, dozing at intervals, starting up, wagging his tail, as if extremely contented; he ate some food greedily; on being called to, he staggered to and fro, and his face assumed a look of utter and helpless drunkenness. These symptoms lasted about two hours, and then gradually passed away; in six hours he was perfectly well and lively.

Expt. 2.—One drachm of *majoon* was given to a small-sized dog; he ate it with great delight, and in twenty minutes was ridiculously drunk; in four hours his symptoms passed away, also without harm.

Expt. 3, 4, & 5—Three kids had ten grains each of the alcoholic extract of *gunjah*. In one no effect was produced; in the second there was much heaviness and some inability to move; in the third a marked alteration of countenance was conspicuous, but no further effect.

Expt. 6.—Twenty grains were given, dissolved in a little spirit, to a dog of very small size. In a quarter of an hour he was intoxicated; in half an hour he had great difficulty of movement; in an hour he had lost all power over the hinder extremities, which were rather stiff but flexible; sensibility did not seem to be impaired, and the circulation was natural. He readily acknowledged calls by an attempt to rise up. In four hours he was quite well.

In none of these, or several other experiments, was there the least indication of pain, or any degree of convulsive movement observed.

It seems needless to dwell on the details of each experiment; suffice it to say that they led to one remarkable result.—That while carnivorous animals, and fish, dogs, cats, swine, vultures, crows, and adjutants, invariably and speedily exhibited the intoxicating influence of the drug, the graminivorous, such as the horse, deer, monkey, goat, sheep, and cow, experienced but trivial effects from any dose we administered.

Encouraged by these results, no hesitation could be felt as to the perfect safety of giving the resin of Hemp an extensive trial in the cases in which its apparent powers promised the greatest degree of utility.

The first cases selected were two of acute rheumatism, and one of that disease in the chronic form. In the two former but little relief had been derived from a fair trial of antiphlogistic measures, and Dover's powder with antimonials—In the last case sarsaparilla at first, and subsequently the Hemides-mus Indicus, with warm baths, had been tried without advantage. *Cases of Rheumatisi treated by*

On the 6th of November, 1838, one grain of the resin of Hemp was administered in solution at 2 P.M. to each of these three patients.

At 4 P.M. it was reported that one was becoming very talkative, was singing songs, calling loudly for an extra supply of food, and declaring himself in perfect health. The other two patients remained unaffected.

At 6 P.M. I received a report to the same effect, but stating that the first patient was now falling asleep.

At 8 P.M. I was alarmed by an emergent note from Nobinchunder Mitter, the clinical clerk on duty, desiring my immediate attendance at the Hospital, as the patient's symptoms were very peculiar and formidable. I went to the Hospital without delay, and found him lying on his cot quite insensible, but breathing with perfect regularity, his pulse and skin natural, and the pupils freely contractile on the approach of light.

Alarmed and pained beyond description at such a state of things, I hurried to the other patients, found one asleep, the third awake, intelligent, and free from any symptoms of intoxication or alarm.

Returning then to the first, an emetic was directed to be prepared, and while waiting for it, I chanced to lift up the patient's arm. The professional reader will judge of my astonishment, when I found that it remained in the posture in which I placed it. It required but a very brief examination of the limbs to find that the patient had, by the influence of this narcotic, been thrown into that strange and most extraordinary of all nervous conditions, into that state what so few have seen, and the existence of which so many still discredit—the genuine *catalepsy* of the nosologist.

It had been my good fortune years before to have witnessed two unequivocal cases of this disorder. One occurred in the female clinical ward in Edinburgh, under Dr. Duncan's treatment, and was reported by myself for the *Lancet* in 1828. The second took place in 1831, in a family with whom I resided in London. The case was witnessed by Dr. Silver, Mr. George Mills, and several other professional friends. In both these cases the cataleptic state was established in full perfection, and in both the paroxysm ran on each occasion a regular course, and terminated suddenly without any evil consequence.

To return to our patient. We raised him to a sitting posture, and placed his arms and limbs in every imaginable attitude. A waxen figure could not be more pliant, or more stationery in each position, no matter how contrary to the natural influence of gravity on the part.

To all impressions he was meanwhile almost insensible; he made no sign of understanding questions; could not be aroused. A sinapism to the epigastrium caused no sign of pain. The pharynx and its coadjutor muscles acted freely in the deglutition of the stimulant remedies which I thought it advisable to administer, although the manifest cataleptic state had freed me altogether of the anxiety under which I before laboured.

The second patient had meanwhile been roused by the noise in the ward, and seemed vastly amused at the strange aspect of the statue-like attitudes in which the first patient had been placed, when on a sudden he uttered a loud peal of laughter, and exclaimed that four spirits were springing with his bed into the air. In vain we attempted to pacify him, his laughter became momentarily more and more incontrollable. We now observed that the limbs were rather rigid, and in a few minutes more his arms or legs could be bent, and would remain in any desired position. A strong stimulant drink was immediately given, and a sinapism applied. Of the latter he made no complaint, but his intoxication led him to such noisy exclamations, that we had to remove him to a separate room; here he soon became tranquil, his limbs in less than an hour gained their natural condition, and in two hours he experienced himself perfectly well, and excessively hungry.

The first patient continued cataleptic till 1 P.M., when consciousness and voluntary motion quickly returned, and by 2 A.M. he was exactly in the same state as the second patient.

The third man experienced no effect whatever, and on further inquiry, it was found that he was habituated to the use of *gunjah* in the pipe.

On the following day it gave me much pleasure to find that both individuals, above mentioned, were not only uninjured by the narcotic, but much relieved of their rheumatism; they were discharged quite cured in three days after.

The fourth case of trial was an old muscular cooly, a rheumatic malingerer, and to him half a grain of Hemp resin was given in a little spirit. The first day's report will suffice for all.—In two hours the old gentleman became talkative and musical, told several stories, and sang songs to a circle of highly delighted auditors; ate the dinners of two persons subscribed for him in the ward, sought also for other luxuries we can scarcely venture to allude to, and finally fell soundly asleep, and so continued till the following morning. On the noonday visit, he expressed himself free from headache, or any other unpleasant sequel, and begged hard for a repetition of the medicine, in which he was indulged for a few days and then discharged.

In several cases of acute and chronic rheumatism admitted about this time, half-grain doses of the resin were given, with closely analogous effects;—alleviation of pain in most— remarkable increase of appetite in all—unequivocal aphro- disia, and great mental cheerfulness. In no one case did these effects proceed to delirium, or was there any tendency to quarrelling. The disposition developed was uniform in all, and in one was the headache or sickness of stomach a sequela of the excitement.

Case of Hydrophobia. A case now occurred in which the influence of a narcotic, capable either of cheering or of inducing harmless insensi- bility, would be fraught with blessings to the wretched patient.

On the 22nd November, at 9 A.M., a note in English was handed to me by my servant, entreating my assistance for the Hakim Abdullah, then at my gate, who had been bitten by a rabid dog, three weeks before, and who feared that the miserable consequences of the bite already had commenced. I found the poor man in a carriage, he was perfectly composed, though quite convinced of the desperate nature of his case. He told me that the evening before, on passing near a tank, he started in alarm, and since then was unable to swallow liquid. His eye was restless, suspicious, and wild; his features anxious, his pulse 125, his skin bedewed with cold moisture; he stated nevertheless that he wished for food and felt well; a small red and painful cicatrix existed on the left fore-arm.

He was immediately removed to the Hospital, where I accompanied him. By his own desire water was brought in a metallic vessel, which he grasped and brought near his lips;—never can I forget the indescribable horrors of the paroxysm which ensued. It abated in about three minutes, and morbid thirst still goading the unhappy man, he besought his servant to apply a moistened cloth to his lips. Intelligent and brave, he determinately awaited the contact of the cloth, and for a few seconds, though in appalling agony, permitted some drops to trickle on his tongue,—but then ensued a second struggle, which, with a due share of the callousness of my profession, I could not stand by to contemplate.

Two grains of Hemp resin in a soft pillular mass were

ordered every hour; after the third dose he stated that he felt commencing intoxication—he now chatted cheerfully on his case, and displayed great intelligence and experience in the treatment of the very disease with which he was visited. He talked calmly of drinking, but said it was in vain to try—but he could suck an orange; this was brought to him, and he succeeded in swallowing the juice without any difficulty.

The Hemp was continued till the sixth dose, when he fell asleep and had some hours' rest. Early the ensuing morning, however, Mr. Siddons, my assistant, was called up to him, and found him in a state of tumultuous agony and excitement: tortured by thirst he attempted to drink,—but I will spare the reader the details of the horrors which ensued.

The Hemp was again repeated, and again by the third dose the cheering alleviation of the previous day was witnessed. He ate a piece of sugar-cane, and again swallowed the juice—he partook freely of some moistened rice, and permitted a purgative enema to be administered. His pulse was nearly natural, the skin natural in every respect. His countenance was happy. On *one* subject only was he incoherent, and even here was manifested the powerful and peculiar influence of the narcotic. He spoke in raptures of the inmates of his *zenana* and his anxiety to be with them. We ascertained however that he had no such establishment.

Four days thus passed away, the doses of Hemp being continued. When he fell asleep, on waking the paroxysms returned, but were again almost immediately assuaged as at first. Meanwhile purgative enemata were employed, and he partook freely of solid food, and once drank water without the least suffering. But about 3 P.M. of the fifth day he sunk into profound stupor, the breathing slightly stertorous; in this state he continued, and without further struggle, death terminated his sufferings at 4 A.M. of the 27th November.

Reviewing the preceding summary of this interesting case, it seems evident that at least one advantage was gained from the use of the remedy;—the awful malady was stripped of its horrors; if not less fatal than before, it was reduced to less than the scale of suffering which precedes death from most ordinary diseases. It must be remembered too that in the first case ever so treated, I possessed no data to guide me as to the dose or manner of administration of the drug. The remarkable cases of tetanus detailed in the sequel, throw light on these important points, and will lead in future cases to the unhesitating administration of much larger quantities than at first I ventured to employ. I am not however rash enough to indulge the hope which involuntarily forces itself upon me, that we will ever from this narcotic derive an effectual remedy, for even a solitary case of this disease—but next to cure, the physician will perhaps esteem the means which enable him 'to strew the path to the tomb with flower,' and to divest of its *specific* terrors the most dreadful malady to which mankind is exposed.

While the preceding case was under treatment, and exciting the utmost interest in the school, several pupils commenced experiments on themselves, to ascertain the effects of the drug. In all, the state of the pulse was noted before taking a dose, and subsequently the effects were observed by two pupils of much intelligence. The result of several trials was, that in as small doses as the quarter of a grain, after an average interval of one hour, the pulse was increased in fulness and frequency; the surface of the body glowed; the appetite became extraordinary; vivid ideas crowded the mind; unusual loquacity occurred; and with scarcely any exception, great aphrodisia was experienced.

In one pupil, Dinonath Dhur, a retiring lad of very quiet habits, ten drops of the tincture, equal to a grain of the resin, induced in twenty minutes the most amusing effects I ever witnessed. A shout of laughter ushered in the symptoms, and a transitory state of cataleptic rigidity occurred for two or three minutes. Summoned to witness the effects, we found him enacting the part of a Raja giving orders to his couriers; he could recognize none of his fellow-students or acquaintances; all to his mind seemed as his own condition; he spoke of many years having passed since his student's days; described his teachers and friends with a piquancy which a dramatist would envy; detailed the adventures of an imaginary series of years, his travels, his attainment of wealth and power. He entered on discussions on religious, scientific, and political topics, with astonishing eloquence, and disclosed an extent of knowledge, reasoning, and a ready apposite wit, which those who knew him best were altogether unprepared for. For three hours and upwards he maintained the character he at first assumed, and with a degree of ease and dignity perfectly becoming his high situation. A scene more interesting it would be difficult to imagine. It terminated nearly as rapidly as it commenced, and no headache, sickness, or other unpleasant symptom followed the innocent excess.

In the symptoms above described we are unavoidably led to trace a close resemblance to the effects produced by the reputed inspiration of the Delphic Oracles—perhaps it would not be very erroneous to conclude, that it was referable to the same kind of excitement.

An epidemic cholera prevailing at this period, two of the students administered the tincture of Hemp in several cases of that disease, and cures were daily reported by its alleged efficacy. Dr. Goodeve was thus led to try it in several cases, and his report was in the highest degree favourable. The diarrhoea was in every instance checked, and the stimulating effect of the drug clearly manifested. The Durwan of the College, an athletic Rajpoot, was attacked, and came under my treatment after he had been ill seven hours; he was pulseless, cold, and in a state of imminent danger; the characteristic evacuations streaming from him without effort—half a grain of the Hemp resin was given, and in twenty minutes the pulse returned, the skin became warm, the purging ceased, and he fell asleep. In an hour he was cataleptic, and continued so for several hours. In the morning he was perfectly well, and at his duty as usual.

It is but fair to state, however, that the character of the epidemic was not at the time malignant. I admit the cases to be inconclusive, but I conceive them to be promising, and that they deserve the close attention of the practitioner.

I now proceed to notice a class of most important uses, in which the results obtained are of the character which warrants me in regarding the powers of the remedy as satisfactorily and incontrovertibly established. I allude to its use in the treatment of traumatic *tetanus*, or lock-jaw, next to hydrophobia, perhaps the most intractable and agonizing of the whole catalogue of human maladies.

The first case of this disease treated by Hemp was that of Ramjan Khan, aet. 30, admitted to the College Hospital on the 13th of December, 1838, for a sloughing ulcer on the back of the left hand. Five days previously a native empiric had applied a red hot *gool* (the mixture of charcoal and

Use in Cholera.

Use in Tetanus.

tobacco used in the hookah) to the back of the left wrist, as a remedy for chronic dysentery and spleen. The patient's brother was similarly cauterized on the same day. In both sloughing took place down to the tendons. Symptoms of tetanus occurred on the 24th of December. The brother who had refused to avail himself of European aid had been seized with tetanus at his own home four days previously, and died after three days' illness. On the 26th December, spasms set in and recurred at intervals of a few minutes; the muscles of the abdomen, neck, and jaw, became firmly, and permanently contracted. Large doses of opium with calomel having been administered for some hours, without the least alleviation of symptoms, and his case having on consultation been pronounced completely hopeless, I obtained Dr. Egerton's permission to subject the poor man to the trial of the Hemp resin. Two grains were first given at 2½ P.M., dissolved in a little spirit. In half an hour the patient felt giddy; at 5 P.M. his eyes were closed, he felt sleepy, and expressed himself much intoxicated.

He slept at intervals during the night, but on waking had convulsive attacks.

On the 27th, two grains were given every third hour—(a purgative enema was also administered, which operated three times); the stiffness of the muscles became much less towards evening, but the spasms returned at intervals as before. Pulse and skin natural.

28th.—Improved; is lethargic but intelligent. Spasms occasionally recur, but at much longer intervals, and in less severity.

29th.—Dose of Hemp increased to three grains every second hour. Symptoms moderating.

30.—Much intoxicated; continues to improve.

1st January 1839. A Hemp cataplasm applied to the ulcer, and internal use of remedy continued; towards evening was much improved; no permanent rigidity; had passed two *dysenteric stools.*

2nd Morning report. Has passed a good night, and seems much better. Hemp continued. *Evening report.* Doing remarkably well.

3rd, 4th, and 5th.—Continues to improve. Hemp resin in two grain doses every 5th hour.

6th, 5 A.M. Feverish; skin hot; pulse quick; all tetanic

symptoms gone; passing mucous and bloody stools; leeches to abdomen; starch and opium enema, with three grains acetate of lead, every second hour; tepid sponging to the body; Hemp omitted.

7th, 6 A.M. Still feverish; stools frequent, mucous; abdomen tender on pressure. No appetite. The ulcer sloughy, ragged, and offensive. Opium and acetate of lead continued. Abdomen leeched. Sore dressed with water. At noon there was slight rigidity of abdominal muscles; Hemp resumed. At 3 P.M. became intoxicated and hungry, ulcer extremely dry, foul, and abominably foetid; towards evening rigidity ceased. Hemp discontinued.

From this day the tetanus may be considered to have ceased altogether, but the dysenteric symptoms continued, despite of the use of opium and acetate of lead; the ulcer too proved utterly intractable. Some improvement in the dysenteric symptoms occurred from the 10th to the 15th, when natural stools were passed; he seemed gaining strength, but the wound was in no wise improved, the slough on the contrary threatened to spread, and two metacarpal bones lay loose in the centre of the sore; on consultation it was agreed to amputate the arm, but to this the patient peremptorily objected. The mortification now spread rapidly, and to our infinite regret, he died of exhaustion on the night of the 23rd January.

An unprejudiced review of the preceding details exhibits the sedative powers of the remedy in the most favourable light; and although the patient died, it must be remembered that is was of a different disease, over which it is not presumed that the Hemp possesses the least power.

The second case was that of Chunoo Syce, (treated by Mr. O'Brien at the Native Hospital) in whom tetanus supervened on the 11th December, after an injury from the kick of a horse. After an ineffectual trial of turpentine and castor oil in large doses, two grain doses of Hemp resin were given on the 26th November. He consumed in all 134 grains of the resin, and left the Hospital cured on the 28th December.

Third case. *Huroo*, a female aged 25, admitted to the Native Hospital on 16th December; had tetanus for the three previous days, the sequel of a cut on the left elbow received a fortnight before. Symptoms violent on admission. Turpentine and castor oil given repeatedly without effect; on the 16th and 17th, three grains of Hemp resin were given at bed-time. On the morning of the 18th she was found in a state of complete catalepsy, and remained so until evening, when she became sensible, and a tetanic paroxysm recurred. Hemp resumed, and continued in two grain doses every fourth hour. From this time till the third hour tetanic symptoms returned. She subsequently took a grain twice daily till the 8th of February, when she left the Hospital quite well.

Mr. O'Brien has since used the Hemp resin in five cases, of which four were admitted in a perfectly hopeless state. He employed the remedy in *ten grain doses* dissolved in spirit. The effect he describes as almost immediate relaxation of the muscles and interruption of the convulsive tendency. Of Mr. O'Brien's eight cases, four have recovered.

In the Police Hospital of Calcutta, the late Dr. Bain has used the remedy in three cases of traumatic tetanus, of these one has died and two recovered.

A very remarkable case has recently occurred in the practice of my cousin, Mr. Richard O'Shaughnessy. The patient was a Jew, aged 30, attacked with tetanus during the progress of a sloughing sore of the scrotum, the sequel of a neglected hydrocele. Three grain doses were used every second hour, with the effect of inducing intoxication, and suspending the symptoms. The patient has recovered perfectly, and now enjoys excellent health. The details of this case are given as a companion article to this paper.

Besides the preceding cases I have heard of two of puerperal trismus thus treated in native females. Both terminated fatally, an event which cannot discredit the remedy, when it is remembered that the Hindoo native females of all ranks are placed during, and subsequent to their confinement, in a cell within which large logs of wood are kept constantly ignited. The temperature of these dens I have found to exceed 130 of Fahrenheit's scale.

The preceding facts are offered to the professional reader with unfeigned diffidence, and to the inferences I feel disposed to derive from the consideration. To me they seem unequivocally to shew, that when given *boldly*, and in large doses, the resin of Hemp is capable of arresting effectually the progress of this formidable disease, and in a large proportion of cases of effecting a perfect cure.

The facts are such at least as justify the hope that the

virtues of the drug may be widely and severely tested in the multitudes of these appalling cases which present themselves in all Indian Hospitals.

A very interesting case of this disease has recently occurred in my private practice; the particulars of which I have the permission of the family to insert in this paper. Case of Infantile Convulsions.

A female infant, 40 days old, the child of Mr. and Mrs. J. L. of Calcutta, on the 10th September, had a slight attack of convulsions, which recurred chiefly at night for about a fortnight, and for which the usual purgative, warm baths, and a few doses of calomel and chalk were given without effect. On the 23rd the convulsive paroxysms became very severe and the bowels being but little deranged, two leeches were applied to the head. Leeches, purgatives, and opiates were alternately resorted to, and without the slightest benefit up to the 30th of September.

On that day the attacks were almost unceasing and amounted to regular tetanic paroxysms. The child had more-over completely lost appetite, and was emaciating rapidly.*

I had by this exhausted all the usual methods of treatment, and the child was apparently in a sinking state.

Under these circumstances I stated to the parents the results of the experiments I had made with the Hemp, and my conviction that it would relieve their infant, if relief could possibly be obtained.

They gladly consented to the trial, and a single drop of the spiritous tincture, equal to the one-twentieth part of a grain in weight, was placed on the child's tongue at 10 P.M. No immediate effect was perceptible, and in an hour and a half two drops more were given. The infant fell asleep in a few minutes, and slept soundly till 4 P.M. when she awoke, screamed for food, *took the breast freely*, and fell asleep again. At 9 A.M., 1st October, I found the child fast asleep, but easily roused; the pulse, countenance and skin perfectly natural. In this drowsy state she continued for four days totally free from convulsive symptoms in any form. (During this time the bowels were frequently spontaneously relieved, and the appetite returned to the natural degree.)

October 4th. At 1 A.M. convulsions returned, and con-

* The nurse, I should have mentioned, was changed early in the illness, and change of air resorted to on the river, but in vain.

tinued at intervals during the day; five drop doses of the tincture were given hourly. Up to midnight there were thirty fits, and forty-four drops of the tincture of Hemp were ineffectually given.

October 5th. Paroxysms continued during the night; at 11 A.M. it was found that the tincture in use during the preceding days had been kept by the servants in a small bottle with a paper stopper; that the spirit had evaporated, and the whole of the resin settled on the sides of the phial. The infant had in fact been taking drops of 'water' during the preceding day.

A new preparation was given in three drop doses during the 5th and 6th, and increased to eight drops; with the effect of diminishing the violence though not of preventing the return of the paroxysm.

On the 7th, I met Dr. Nicolson in consultation, and despairing of a cure from the Hemp, it was agreed to intermit its use, to apply a mustard poultice to the epigastrium, and to give a dose of castor oil and turpentine. The child, however, rapidly became worse, and at 2 P.M. a tetanic spasm set in, which lasted without intermission till 6½ P.M. A cold bath was given without solution of the spasm—the Hemp was therefore again resorted to, and the dose of 30 drops, equal to 1½ grains of the resin, given at once.

Immediately after this dose was given the limbs relaxed, the little patient fell fast asleep, and so continued for thirteen hours. While asleep, she was evidently under the narcotic influence of the drug.

On the 8th October, at 4 A.M., there was a severe fit, and from this hour to ten at night 25 fits occurred and 130 drops of the tincture were given in 80 drop doses, equal to 15 grains of the resin. It was now manifestly a struggle between the disease and the remedy, but at 10 P.M. she was again narcoticized, and from that hour no fit returned.

On the three following days there was considerable griping, and on administering large doses of almond oil, several small dark green lumps of the Hemp resin were voided, which gave effectual relief. The child is now (23rd November) in the enjoyment of robust health, and has regained her natural plump and happy appearance.

In reviewing this case several very remarkable circumstances present themselves. At first we find three drops, or one twentieth of a grain, causing profound narcoticism; subsequently we find 130 drops daily required to produce the same effect. The severity of the symptoms doubtless must be taken chiefly into account, in endeavouring to explain this circumstance. It was too soon for habit to gain ascendancy over the narcotic powers of the drug. Should the disease ever recur, it will be a matter of much interest to notice the quantity of the tincture requisite to afford relief. The reader will remember that this infant was but sixty days old when 130 drops were given in one day, of the same preparation of which ten drops had intoxicated the student Dinonath Dhur, who took the drug for experiment. 130 drops are equal again to 15 grains of the resin, one grain of which occasioned profound trance (or catalepsy) in two men labouring under rheumatism.

Before quitting this subject, it is desirable to notice the singular form of delirium which the incautious use of the Hemp preparations often occasions, especially among young men first commencing the practice. Several such cases have presented themselves to my notice. They are as peculiar as the 'delirium tremens,' which succeeds the prolonged abuse of spiritous liquors, but are quite distinct from any other species of delirium with which I am acquainted. *Delirium occasioned by continued Hemp inebriation.*

This state is at once recognized by the strange balancing gait of the patient's; a constant rubbing of the hands; perpetual giggling; and a propensity to caress and chafe the feet of all bystanders of whatever rank. The eye wears an expression of cunning and merriment which can scarcely be mistaken. In a few cases, the patients are violent; in many highly aphrodisiac; in all that I have seen, voraciously hungry. There is no increased heat or frequency of circulation, or any appearance of inflammation or congestion, and the skin and general functions are in a perfectly natural state.

A blister to the nape of the neck, leeches to the temples, and nauseating doses of tartar emetic with saline purgatives have rapidly dispelled the symptoms in all the cases I have met with, and have restored the patient to perfect health.

The preceding cases constitute an abstract of my experience on this subject, and which has led me to the belief that in Hemp the profession has gained an anti-convulsive remedy of the greatest value. Entertaining this conviction, be it true or false, I deem it my duty to publish it without any avoidable delay in order that the most extensive and the speediest trial may be given to the proposed remedy. I repeat what I have already stated in a previous paper—that were individual reputation my object, I would let years pass by, and hundreds of cases accumulate before publication, and in publishing I would enter into every kind of elaborate detail. But the object I have proposed to myself in the inquiries is of a very different kind. To gather together a few strong facts, to ascertain the limits which cannot be passed without danger, and then pointing out these to the profession, to leave their body to prosecute and decide on the subject of discussion, such seems to me the fittest mode of attempting to explore the medical resources which an untried Materia Medica may contain.

It may be useful to add a formula for making the preparation which I have employed.

The *resinous extract* is prepared by boiling the rich, adhesive tops of the dried *gunjah* in spirit (Sp. gr. 835,) until all the resin is dissolved. The tincture thus obtained is evaporated to dryness in a vessel placed over a pot of boiling water. The extract softens at a gentle heat, and can be made into pills without any addition.

The *tincture* is prepared by dissolving 3 grains of the extract in one drachm of proof spirit.

Doses, &c.—In *Tetanus* a drachm of the tincture every half hour until the paroxysms cease, or catalepsy is induced. In *Hydrophobia* I would recommend the resin in soft pills, to the extent of ten to twenty grains to be chewed by the patient, and repeated according to the effect. In *Cholera* ten drops of the tincture every half hour will be often found to check the vomiting and purging, and bring back the warmth of the surface;—my experience would lead me to prefer *small* doses of the remedy in order to excite rather than narcotise the patient.

II

PERSONAL EXPERIENCES AND SPECULATIONS

Unlike the often florid, voluptuary Romantic English and French chroniclers of hashish eating who enthralled the literary world, physicians took much more prosaic attitudes toward marijuana.

Bell concerns himself with personal reactions to the drug and reactions of different forms of mental illness to its therapeutic use. With a professional skepticism he tries to relate the effects to possible mechanisms of mental illness.

O'Day describes a personal incident; intoxicated by an overdose of a cough cure containing cannabis—at the controls of a locomotive.

Foulis recounts a "trip" of an art student and a medical student who had come under the spell of the then "high priest of drugs," De Quincey.

Today, if Doctors Hamilton, Lescohier, and Perkins had been able to find a publisher for the description of their antics in the lab at Parke, Davis & Company, they would quickly have been taken in custody by the narcotics police and remanded to durance vile. The "dope farm" located at Rochester, Michigan, would be burned, the implements seized as evidence, and the company bankrupted by Internal Revenue Service tax liens.

As it turned out, Dr. Lescohier went on to become the

president of the company. His colleagues went on to other successful careers.

Professor Walton wrote me some four years ago that he wasn't a bit surprised at his book being forgotten by the modern authors. He considers it a fact of scientific life that new work done on an old drug or principle is likely to overlook much of the past.

It is sad that this most comprehensive recent book, from which the excerpt beginning on page 83 is taken, is absent from most modern scientific reference lists.

On the Haschisch
or Cannabis Indica

BY JOHN BELL, M.D.

The various periodicals of this country have abounded, during the last few years, with accounts of the Haschisch; every experimenter giving the history of the effects it has had upon himself. In most cases this has been mingled with much fanciful and irrelevant matter. These notices have been confined almost exclusively to the various popular literary journals, but it has not received the attention it merits in those exclusively devoted to medicine. Under these circumstances, the following *résumé* of what has been written on the subject, seen through the medium of personal experience, may not be destitute of interest.

Among the nations professing Mahometanism, there are not a few substances used as substitutes for the alcoholic liquors interdicted by the author of that religion. They are everywhere the most inveterate users of tobacco, opium, coffee, and a variety of other narcotics less generally known. Among these latter, no one has recently attracted so much attention as the *Haschisch,* Cannabis Indica, or Indian Hemp. It is only within a few years, comparatively, that a knowledge of it has come to us, but it has been in general use for many centuries at the East, and reference is even thought to have been made to it by the ancient classic authors. The novelty of its effects and its apparent harmlessness have induced travellers in Egypt and Asia to experiment upon themselves, and a knowledge of it has thus found its way to the nations of the West. The defective pharmaceutic process employed by the inhabitants of its native countries, render its preparations of very different strength, and admixtures of various foreign

Reprinted from *The Boston Medical and Surgical Journal,* vol. lvi, no. 11, April 16, 1857, pp. 209–216; vol. lvi, no. 12, April 23, 1857, pp. 229–236.

substances make its effects uncertain. A specimen obtained from Damascus contained about twenty-five percent of opium, a considerable quantity of camphor and spices, and nearly half was a mixture of rancid butter and extract of hemp. The substance widely known in this country under the Arabic name of *Haschisch,* is obtained by boiling the leaves and flowers of the plant with butter, and, when pure and carefully prepared, is a very active preparation. The extracts prepared in this country from the Indian plant, contain all the properties of the *Haschisch,* and are every way preferable to it. The common hemp, though believed by botanists to be a variety of the same species as its Indian congener, is entirely destitute of the property which distinguishes the latter. This difference alone, if found to be permanent, would be sufficient to cause them to be regarded as distinct species.

The action of the drug is not confined to any single part of the system. It is an efficient but slow cathartic, an active diuretic and sudorific, and a most irresistible hypnotic in the latter stages of its action. But it is better known for its effect upon the nervous system; it is for this object that it is extensively employed in the East, and it is in this connection that it possesses its greatest interest. Abundant personal experience of it leads me to think that its peculiar effects upon the nervous system are only a secondary result of its action upon the mucous membrane throughout the whole track of the alimentary canal. The slowness of its action, not commencing in less than two hours after the dose is taken; the sensation of dryness, and afterward the abundant secretion in the throat and mouth; the heat throughout the abdomen; and the soreness which persists for several days; and, finally, the absence of any symptoms of nervous debility, when the immediate effects are gone; all point to this as its *modus operandi.* It would seem as though it were absorbed, and that in this process of being thrown off, it occasioned those phantasies which have caused it to be used as an intoxicating agent. In the dose usually recommended, of from one to three grains, it is absolutely inert: five grains is the smallest quantity from which any perceptible effects are to be expected, and generally more will be required. Few persons, perhaps, who have read the brilliant "Confessions of an English Opium Eater," have been without a fancy to experience the wonderful effects there described: all who have yielded to the desire, have been disappointed. If any one supposes the intoxication of *Haschisch* to be of the same nature, a few grains of the drug will most efficiently purge him of the idea. On the first trial, one is generally frightened at the intensity and violence of its action, and few will be disposed to carry the dose beyond ten grains. Indeed, most will be amply satisfied with having once experienced it. The following were the results of a moderately large dose of Tilden & Co.'s extract.

It was taken with coffee, which increases the effects of the hemp, and at the same time diminishes its duration, perhaps merely by promoting a more rapid absorption. For two hours no results at all were experienced. At this time a dryness seemed to commence at a particular spot in the throat, and a feeling of warmth throughout the abdomen. These were not the results of disordered sensation, for a clammy mucus soon began to be secreted, though the huskiness of the throat still remained. Up to this time, there was not the slightest excitement or confusion of thought. Suddenly, however, an idea having no connection with the train of thought passing in the mind at the time, appeared, as though suggested by another person, and then was gone again as suddenly as it came, leaving upon the mind much the same feeling as when one escapes from a dream or a deep reverie. The same thing was repeated two or three times, at intervals rapidly diminishing in length. Even now I can hardly believe but it was the result of strained attention to my physical sensations, for the gentle warmth of the abdomen was rapidly becoming a burning heat—still, however, not by any means unpleasant—and the dryness of the throat had extended to the tongue.

I had taken the drug with great scepticism as to its reputed action, or at any rate with the opinion that it was grossly exaggerated, and I accordingly made up my mind not to be "caught napping" in this way again, and to keep a careful watch over my thoughts. But while enforcing this resolution, as I supposed, I found myself, to my own astonishment, waking from a reverie longer and more profound than any previous. From scepticism, to the fullest belief of all I had read on the subject, was but a step. Its effects so far surpassed anything which words can convey, that I began to think I was on the verge of narcotic poisoning; yet, strange to say, there was not the slightest feeling of inquietude on that account. I resolved to walk into the street. While rising from the chair, another lucid interval showed that another dream had come and gone. While passing through the door, I was aware of having wandered again, but how or when I had permitted myself to fall into the reverie I was perfectly unconscious, and knew only that it seemed to have lasted an interminable length of time.

These singular attacks of mental disturbance recurred oftener, and lasted longer, till the lucid interval between was reduced to a mere instant's conscious duration of thought. This condition came on so rapidly, that in less than fifteen minutes from the time of my being aware of the first mental disturbance, the power of controlling the thoughts was almost completely lost. All ideas of time and space were especially bewildered, and I realized completely for the first time the ideas of some metaphysicians, that time, properly speaking, has no existence except in connection with a succession of mental operations or sensations. The most trivial circumstance, the slighest noise, gave rise to trains of thought, which went bounding from subject to subject, completely emancipated from the rules which ordinarily govern the mental operations, till suddenly some other circumstance would give an entirely new direction to them, and the last series of imaginations would seem to have lasted from eternity, even while the eye was fixed upon the clock, the hand of which had not perceptibly moved.

Now, a phenomenon still more singular began to exhibit itself. I felt that, in spite of all exertions, I was beginning to receive the suggestions of disordered fancy for real objective facts. Intellectually, I knew that the spinal column could not be a barometer, in which mercury had usurped the place of the spinal cord. Yet in another sense, over which the operations of the intellect were completely powerless, I felt that it was a barometer. An unpleasant sensation in the lumbar region suggested the idea of a heavy column of mercury pressing upon it, and at the time, and under the circumstances, the transition to the idea of the barometer was easy and natural. There was no balancing of arguments in the arrival at this conclusion; there was no half-way period of doubt and uncertainty, to emerge into full credence. At the instant the idea occurred at all, it commanded the assent, with the same fulness as when in perfect mental health does the idea of our own existence. The thought certainly occurred that it was a delusion, but it made no more impression than the suggestion would, that the sense of sight was a figment of the brain, and objects seen had no existence except in the imagination. This belief was not a transient one; it was the first hallucination to appear, and continued with varying degrees of intensity, as the thoughts were more or less occupied with other subjects, till all others had disappeared. The belief in the reality of the delusion was never for an instant absent; it pervaded the whole being, and was often the point on which the thoughts turned seemingly for a long time. The painful attempt to regulate these disturbed states of consciousness, was soon given up, and, half voluntarily, half by a species of moral compulsion, the whole psychical nature surrendered itself, without further struggle, to the fullest and most complete belief in the actual existence of a thousand hallucinations. During this time the thoughts were becoming more and more disordered; ideas, between which, apparently, there was not the slightest connection, thrust themselves in, till finally their rapid recurrence, and the loss of that sense of governing the mind which we ordinarily possess, induced the belief that I was the victim of diabolical agency—that some terrible demon had taken possession of my whole intellectual being, and identified himself with every thought, in the same way that a man might direct the physical movements of a child. The feeling of utter powerlessness to check the wild current of thought was complete, and there was a sensation as though, if there had been the ability, the will could not be exercised.

The firmest intentions were forgotten in an instant. There seemed to be no difference between the idea and the expression of it in words. A moment was long enough to forget whether it had been expressed or not. The sound of persons whispering in the room, brought with it the belief that they were laying some plot. It was not a vague suspicion that they were intending some injury, such as whispers and glances might excite in any one; but everything they had said—the particulars of the whole plot—were present, with the same vividness and overpowering conviction as they always are in true hallucinations.

The *fantasia* had now arrived at its height. It was an hour and a half since the first sensations of excitement and wandering commenced. About the same time passed before it had completely subsided. The mental phenomena in this stage were as remarkable as while the effects were coming on. One after another the delusions disappeared as rapidly as they came; not by any exercise of the gradually returning regularity of thought, but suddenly—with a bound—so that it was surprising to have believed, a moment before, what now appeared so absurd.

The whole time during which there is any perceptible difference from the normal state, is from three to five hours, according to the dose taken. The hemp resembles in its action some other medicines which are erroneously called cumulative. That is, a dose may be taken without producing any perceptible action; and on another occasion, a dose only a grain larger will act violently. Indeed, the effects of this agent seem to be of such a nature, that there is no resting place between its full action and none at all. A delusion, of the truth of which we are only half convinced, would be no delusion at all. Unlike opium, alcohol, and other narcotics of the order Solanaceae, it leaves behind it no mental confusion, headache, or other signs of a direct and powerful action upon the nervous system. The secretions of the alimentary canal, however, remain in an unnatural state for several days, and there is a slight oppression felt in the abdomen, if the dose has been at all large. During all the time of its action, there is a tendency to laugh, in spite of the delusions, which are almost uniformly of an unpleasant character. The feeling of buoyancy of spirits is somewhat the same as is caused by a slight dose of alcoholic stimulant.

Amid all the strange vagaries of the *Haschisch*, the mind preserves the power of taking cognizance of its condition, and to a certain extent of analyzing its operations. The memory of everything said and done is nearly perfect; but of the multitude of thoughts, only those making a more than commonly distinct impression are preserved.

Can this singular substance be put to any useful purpose, to illustrate any of the varied mental phenomena of health and disease? Is it worthy a place in the medical *armamentum*, from its action alone upon the mind?

The great advances made in the philosophy of medicine during the last half century, have been due almost entirely to the devotion with which pathology has been pursued. Instead of the ill-arranged and ill-understood assemblage of symptoms observed with scrupulous care, which went to make up the idea of a disease, we now direct our aim to strip it of everything fortuitous and to fix in the mind the type of the malady—those essential features which are uniformly the same under every variety of circumstances, and about which the more obvious symptoms cluster, like the drapery about a statue. In diseases of the mind, this has not been done: their seat and nature are too deep to be reached by the knife of the morbid anatomist. Esquirol, after a whole life devoted to the study of this subject, and after the most ample opportunities that have ever fallen to the lot of any individual, says, that "Pathological anatomy is yet silent as to the seat of madness; it has not yet demonstrated what is the precise alteration in the encephalon which gives rise to this disease." Nor has greater success obtained in the attempt to explain the relations and analogies of the various forms of insanity. The cause of the latter failure is sufficiently obvious. Theory has taken the place of fact. No competent individual who has experienced insanity in his own person, has written upon the disease. The insane themselves can rarely give a consistent account of their disease, even if they were qualified, by previous study and observation, to take the best advantage of their own mental state. Even our own observation of the disease is rarely complete: the minor degrees do not come under the care of the physician, and it is only when the more severe cases are evident to all, that friends will acknowledge its existence and submit the unfortunate patient to examination. How imperfect would be our ideas of grief, anger, or pain, if we could only observe their outward manifestations, or listen to a description of them by one who had suffered them! And yet this is all, and more than all that we can know of the intimate nature of insanity, of its connections and analogies, unless we have suffered it in our own persons. If we had never felt any of the passions, our diagnosis of them might perhaps be as perfect, and the empirical treatment as successful, as now; but a vagueness would necessarily pervade our mind as to their nature, and we should be liable to continual error in reasoning upon them. Southwood Smith well observes, that the symptom of fever termed *febrile restlessness* cannot be understood by any one who has not experienced it in person.

The most superficial observation of a case of mania, will

not fail to show many and strong points of resemblance to that of a person under the influence of a powerful dose of Cannabis Indica. In both there is the same excitement and abruptness of manner, the same rapidity and incoherence of thought, the same false convictions and lesions of the affective faculties. The following description, by Prichard, of an ordinary case of chronic mania, such as composes the greater number in the wards of every hospital, might apply, without the change of a word, to the condition of a person under the influence of the *Haschisch*. "It is, however, a state of great intellectual weakness, in which none of the operations of the mind are performed with energy or effect. The memory, the judgment, the powers of attention and combination, are so much impaired, that the individual is wholly inadequate to the duties of society, and incapable of any continued conversation; his actions and conduct are without steadiness and consistency, his thoughts are deficient in concentration and coherence."

There is no really important point in which these manifestations differ from the condition produced by the *Haschisch*. There is no error of judgment, no delusion or lesion of the will or moral faculties, which is seen in the former state, but what might take its rise in the latter. In this question, the difference of cause of the mental disturbance might at first sight appear an insuperable objection to reasoning from one condition to the other. But is insanity always produced by the same cause? On the contrary, there is no disease to which the human frame is subject, that acknowledges such a variety. There is hardly a physical or functional lesion of any tissue or organ, but may produce it by its reaction on the nervous system, and it is difficult to say whether the best or worst proclivities of our nature are oftenest regarded as the productive agents of the same mental disease. If opium and tobacco and alcohol may produce, by long use, without any apparent disease, a mental state which deserves the name of insanity, why may not the *fantasia* of hemp receive the same name? What reason, then, is there why we may not rely upon its revelations as so many views of the hidden workings of the spirit, in that gravest of all diseases? If this be allowed, the *Haschisch* may in a degree serve as a key to unlock some at least of the mysteries of mental pathology. Why may we not thus possess a means of studying the disease in question, better than we have of most others? We can apply to it the principles of experimental philosophy, and test it by the best of means upon the best of subjects. The idea of this application of the medicine originated with Dr. Moreau (de Tours), of Paris, a physician of large experience in his specialty, and whose work* on the subject possesses the highest interest, as presenting many views of insanity and kindred subjects, different from those commonly received.

In the study of insanity by this means, if there is any one fact impressed upon the mind more strongly than another, it is that of the essential unity of the whole psychical nature. It is impossible not to recognize the truth that the ordinary language of metaphysics is applicable to the explanation of morbid mental phenomena. The popular division into the intellect, the will, the instincts and the moral faculties, though having a show of precision, and absolutely necessary in common language, conveys too much. Such divisions are too distinct and disconnected to be true to nature. The minute organological divisions and hasty generalizations of the phrenologists are only the results of the same principle carried to a greater extent.

A few words upon each of the kinds of psychical disturbance caused by the *Haschisch* will conduce to the better understanding of its action, and of its relations with the analogous, or precisely similar phenomena of insanity.

Throughout the whole period of its effects, there is a sense of pleasurable excitement. By the French authors who have experimented and written on the subject,† this feeling is regarded as one of the most marked phenomena of the drug. Doubtless this was the case with them: with myself, it has never been so great as is generally represented.

It is true there is a strong tendency to laugh, but it is a laugh in which the feelings participate to a very slight degree. It is the same to whatever subject the thoughts are directed. In delusions of an agreeable or disagreeable character, there is the same smile. It is different entirely from that state of mental excitement, attended with pleasurable emotions, which is met with in the first stages of many cases of insanity. In such instances the sentiments of a pleasure are

---

* *Du Haschisch, et de l'aliénation mentale.*

caused by the most sanguine anticipations of success in every wild project. It is a feeling which would be very proper, did not its cause show too plainly the intellectual disturbance which pervades it. There is nothing like this in the effects of the *Haschisch*. The face does not as ordinarily prove a true index to the mind. While the thoughts do not pause long enough upon any subject for the feelings to be touched, the face is covered with smiles. Disagreeable anticipations and a joyful expression of countenance do not seem at all incongruous. It seems to be all on the surface, leaving the depths below unmoved. The condition is much the same as in dreams, when we are often surprised at our own callousness to all impressions of pleasure and pain: when good and bad fortune alike pass over us without exciting happiness or sorrow. Perhaps upon different temperaments, the action of the drug may be essentially different. My own experience of it has been sufficient to convince me that this sentiment of happiness may be completely lost in the crowd of other phenomena. It would have been hardly worth while to notice so slight a peculiarity, were it not that one of the most interesting of its proposed therapeutic uses is in connection with this property.

It has been proposed by M. Moreau to take advantage of this reputed action, to combat certain varieties of insanity connected with melancholy and depressing delusions. If a series of hallucinations of a pleasing character, or a state of pleasurable excitement, could be produced and kept up for a length of time, the change might become permanent. The morbid chain of thought might be broken, and the mind resume its healthy action upon the withdrawal of the medicine. Used in this way, the drug would seem to hold a middle place between medical agents as ordinarily used, and the moral discipline which is principally relied on at present. This proposed application is original with M. Moreau, but the idea of superseding melancholy by exciting pleasurable emotions, is certainly as old as the time of David, whose harp succeeded in driving the evil spirit out of Saul. Such means, in cases of true insanity, have in practice fallen into utter contempt. Music, *per se*, never has cured an insane patient in our times, or, as a late writer says, "music never cures insanity, except such cases as appear in the comic opera." Music may be, and unquestionably is, of value as one among the diversions and employments which take off the tedium of hospital life, and *pro tanto* occupy the space in the disordered mind, which would otherwise be absorbed in diseased acts and reflections. M. Moreau reports several instances of doubtful cures effected by the medicine, but confesses that his experience of its use is limited. The following cases from his work will illustrate its effects upon the variety of insanity in question. "Two patients suffering under melancholia, after five or six hours experienced a lively excitement, with all the characters of gaiety and sprightliness which we have observed. One especially, tormented by terrors of imagination and melancholy delusions, who had not spoken ten words a day for more than nine months, did not cease to chat and laugh and joke during the whole evening. I rarely found in his words any connection with the ideas which habitually occupied his attention. However, the excitment over, both fell again into their previous condition."

The use of the *Haschisch*, with this view, has not been extensive in this country—not so extensive as it deserves to be. It has been tried, however, in several of the insane hospitals, but the results have not been encouraging. Indeed, in most cases they have been completely null, so that the suspicion has been engendered that it does not possess the physiological action attributed to it. Nothing could be more unfounded; there is no article in the whole *materia medica* which, according to my observation, is more to be depended upon to induce its peculiar effects. But it must be given in doses much larger than those usually employed, that any effects may be experienced from it. We could hardly expect that cases having their origin in extensive physical disease, can be benefited in this manner, but in functional diseases of the brain, it certainly gives promise of possessing powers more directly useful than any other specific drug of the materia medica.

Every one is aware how much our ideas of time depend upon the rapidity of thought, and the degree of attention we give to passing events. While the mind is busily engaged in conversation or reading, we seem to lose all notion of the succession of events; we live in a world of ideas, retaining, however, an intimate sensation of the fact that we are only thinking. In this state we take no note of the passage of time; an hour is compressed into a minute. In dreaming, the mind is just as busily engaged, and yet we may magnify an instant into any conceivable limits. In the state of reverie, the same thing occurs, though to a less marked degree. The fact is familiar to every one that we may be awakened by some noise, and in the interval between sound sleep and complete wakefulness, we may pass through a long imaginary conversation, or an extended series of events, ending with some explosion or catastrophe, which on being completely awake, we are aware is only the noise which has awakened us. Our ideas of time, then, do not depend exclusively upon the succession of mental pictures. They are much more closely connected with the degree to which we identify ourselves with our thoughts. Just in proportion to their vividness and the extent to which they overcome our attention to the fact that we are thinking—not acting, just in such proportion does time correspond to what it would be, were the subject of our thoughts real objective facts. This sensation of the excessive duration of time, is perhaps the most remarkable and obvious of the effects of hemp, and the extent to which it is experienced may be regarded as the best means of regulating the dose. It is never absent, throughout the whole duration of the mental disturbance, and the deception is so complete and so disagreeable, that no one who has taken it need ever be in the slightest doubt as to whether he is experiencing its effects or not. In the higher degrees of its action all definite ideas of time are lost. Past, present and future exist no longer. The whole existence is concentrated in the train of thought we are engaged in. In dreaming, this change in the ideas of time is not unpleasant, for we cannot observe the discrepancy between our present and former sensations. The following case of insanity, where all proper notions of time were lost, is abridged from Moreau. "A young lady, during the first few days of an attack of maniacal excitement, believed that she had no longer any age. She imagined herself to have lived at every historic epoch to which memory carried her. Those about her were reproached with having stolen her measure of time. Her mother was acknowledged as such no longer, for the reason that she could not have a mother younger than herself." Another believed himself to be God, because he had existed from eternity. Under the influence of *Haschisch*, the ideas of time may be regulated by the intellect, and consequently one is never led astray, except when the attention is

directed to another subject; while this is the case, the sensation of immense duration of time is continually and
intimately present. Without having experienced it, no one can
form the slightest idea of its vividness and reality.

The errors in regard to space are dependent ·for their
existence upon those of time, and are of much the same
nature. During the existence of the *fantasia*, an object does
not appear more distant than under ordinary circumstances.
But while the hand is stretched forth to take it, and we are
conscious that the movement is executed with ordinary
rapidity, such a length of time has passed away, that only the
exercise of reflection and the direct evidence of the sense of
sight, can convince us that the hand has not moved through a
space corresponding to the time it seems to have been in
motion.

The deception is never so complete as that in regard to
time; a glance of the eye corrects it, but it rules again as soon
as the head is turned. It is in this circumstance that insanity
differs from the delirium of an ordinary dose of hemp. In the
former, and in cases of large doses of the latter, the sense of
sight does not correct the delusion. The sensations coming
from the eye are overruled by the reality of those having
their origin in the imagination. It is only during the occasional lucid moments of *Haschisch* that the judgment can be
exercised, or the eye directed to an object to appreciate its
circumstances. Not that the muscles are paralyzed, but the
will does not put them in motion. As in an ordinary reverie,
the vacant stare shows that the mind does not take cognizance of the objects towards which the eyes are directed.

The first effects of it upon the intellectual faculties, are a
gradual loss of power to direct the thoughts. The sense which
is ever present in mental health, that we are responsible for
what passes in our minds, is lost. This loss is never partial as
to any single thought. We do not perceive this power to be
gradually slipping away so that we can mark each step of its
departure, but suddenly, like lightning, it occurs to us that,
the moment before, some thought came into the mind by a
channel very different from ordinary. To use a well-under-
stood manner of speaking, we have nothing to do with its
presence—it came there of itself. In small doses, its effects are
limited to this degree of mental disturbance. If the quantity
taken has been larger, these attacks recur oftener and oftener,

the experimenter losing and regaining the consciousness of directing the course of thought many times in a minute. When under the highest degree of its action, the glimpses of the fact that our thoughts are not our own, are few in number and momentary in duration. In this state of veritable mania, ideas come and go with a rapidity completely inconceivable in ordinary mental conditions. Some glide through the mind without seeming to make any impression at all; others become realities as perfect as though admitted through the senses. Yet in all this overthrow of the governing power, there is a certain degree of connection in the succession of ideas. But the attention is so slightly concentrated upon even the most vivid of them, that the slightest occurrence, the movement of a hand or a word addressed to us, sweeps them away in an instant. We live in the thought that is uppermost at the time; those which are past are as nothing, and we take no thought of what the future are to be. Intentions formed the moment before, are lost. If we wish to say anything, the chances are equal that it will be forgotten—buried by the succeeding idea. Let one in this state attempt to write, and he will produce a composition similar to what is often seen by those practically acquainted with hospitals for the care of the insane. Broken phrases, words without the least connection, with occasionally a few sentences having some obviously connected ideas at bottom, make a compound highly characteristic.

The conversation is more connected than the writing, for it is better able to keep up with the thoughts. In both there is some connection in the mind of the individual; while one word or part of a sentence is being written, a multitude are gone, and when the pen comes to a stop, it goes on again with the train of thought which is present at the instant, without endeavoring to go back and take up the thread which is lost. In talking, one feels compelled to finish the sentence without an instant's hesitation; if the word which expresses the meaning does not occur, another is substituted for it without reference to its signification. If we hesitate, the train of thought is overwhelmed by the rushing tide of ideas, which never waits for utterance. The connection between successive conceptions, however, is not always perceptible to the individual, even in the slight degree referred to above. A large portion seem to be mere isolated pictures, drawn alike from memory, from imagination and from incidents which happen to be taking place at the time, but all strangely confused and equally transient in the impression they make. This mental state is so similar to many cases of insanity, that it would be difficult, if not impossible, to distinguish them without having recourse to their duration and the causes which produced them. The extreme rapidity and vividness of thought are absolutely identical with the most observable phenomena of that disease.

Mania is by far the most hopeful species of insanity, in respect to its prognosis, while dementia is the most hopeless. It has been thought that in cases of mental disease, tending to fall into the latter state, the powerful stimulation of the hemp might perhaps arrest the downward course, and place the patient in a state more amenable to treatment, and consequently more hopeful, as regards chances of ultimate cure. With these ideas in view, it has been administered in very heroic doses in all stages of hebetude. But the mind in this condition seems to have completely lost its wonted resiliency: it responds no longer to what were once powerful stimuli. In this state the hemp produces no perceptible effects, in the more advanced stages, and only the slightest change in any. All hopes of benefit resulting from its administration in these cases, have been abandoned by the author, himself, of the proposition—a sure proof of its utter want of any probability of value.

But the most interesting of the effects of the hemp are in connection with the subject of delusions. It is in reference to these that it can be put to the best use in assisting to understand the workings of disease. There are very few cases of insanity but exhibit delusions at some period of their course, and there are not a few persons, ordinarily reputed sane, who are subject to them. A clear understanding of them will conduce, more than anything else, to a full understanding of those mental states which are spoken of under the collective term insanity. Their importance will justify a closer examination than any of the other morbid mental manifestations, caused by the drug of which we are speaking.

Before the time of Esquirol, all the mistakes of madness were included under one term. He saw reason to divide them into two classes—illusions and hallucinations; the first taking their origin chiefly in a disordered condition of the senses,

the latter depending exclusively upon intellectual disturbance. These distinctions of the great master have been
adopted by most succeeding authors who have written upon
the subject. Whether these divisions are founded in nature,
and show evidence enough to demand adoption, we shall
presently examine. In the mean time, a few words on the
origin of hallucinations in addition to what has been said
before. They have the same relation to disorders of the
intellect that ordinary states of consciousness do to healthy
manifestations of that function. There is no word which gives
any better idea of the process by which these figments of the
brain come to be regarded as facts, than there is of the way in
which we come to believe so strongly in our own existence,
or the existence of the objects we feel or see. There is certainly not the slightest similarity between hallucinations and
ordinary mistakes in regard to the existence of facts. One
pre-supposes the exercise of the memory; the other acts without it and even defies it. The circumstances under which they
have their origin are as varied as the hallucinations themselves. Many seem to be purely intellectual, at least the chain
which connects them with the external world is too long and
complicated to be followed. Some idea, disconnected
perhaps, or having a very loose connection with those preceding it, assumes the attributes of reality, and for the future
it is an idea no longer, but becomes a fact, and is reasoned
and acted upon as such. The great majority of the hallucinations of the insane have this origin. Their fears and suspicions, their strange actions, their pride and humility, are
often founded upon some belief which they act upon but do
not disclose. Perhaps in many instances it is too vague to be
put into words. A thought suggested by another may be
adopted in the same way and become a thought and finally a
belief of our own. Some sensation of pain or uneasiness in a
particular part of the body turns the thoughts in that direction, and forthwith a delusion is established. This is pecu-
liarly apt to be the case in hypochondria, where the stomach
being in most cases the peccant organ, is believed to be the
abode of some reptile. Esquirol relates cases of a woman
suffering under chronic peritonitis, who believed the Pope
was holding a council in her belly; of a military officer who
had rheumatism in the knee, and believed there was a robber
confined in it. These last, however, he gives as instances of his

variety of illusions, though in this he is not followed by other writers, who confine themselves exclusively to the five senses.

The idea of illusions is perhaps too stongly fixed, by the ability and influence of writers who have acknowledged their existence, to be easily refuted. There are certainly no such phenomena among all the varieties of psychical disturbance caused by taking the hemp, though there are delusions which if observed in another and judged by the rules laid down by writers on mental pathology, would be considered as striking instances of them. There is never the slightest lesion of the sentient extremities of the nerves, so far as I have experienced. The senses are as perfect as ever, and the information given to the mind is as correct as though the latter were in its natural condition. It is in the disordered state of the psychical system that we must look for the origin of all insane delusions, whether having reference to objects of sense or not. There is no ground for the distinction that has been made between hallucinations and delusions. On this subject Ray* says, "that the functions of the senses are sometimes greater perverted, there can be no question; but it needs more evidence than we yet have to prove that such perversions have much if any part in producing these illusions." The principal arguments for the existence of sensory illusions are of this kind: a person may have continually before him some vision, as long as his eyes are open, but upon shutting them the delusion disappears. Or it may last during the day and disappear at night, or *vice versa*. It is inferred from such cases, which are sufficiently numerous, that the whole difficulty is in the sentient extremities of the sensory nerves, and that as soon as these cease to act, the object seen disappears. The true explanation of these and similar cases seems to be this. The mere contact of light with the retina gives rise to ideas, perhaps immediately, perhaps through a crowd of others preceding them, which are taken for verities. And all this, while the objects within view are seen as well as ever. But the sensations caused by sight are too feeble and receive too little attention to compete with the vividness of those supplied by the perverted intellect. The facility with which the evidence of the former is passed by, and credence given to the latter, is astonishing and inexplicable to one who has not experienced it in his own person. Esquirol mentions the

* *Medical Jurisprudence of Insanity.*

case of an individual who, under the influence of such a delusion, took a window for a door, walked through it and was precipitated from the third story to the ground. If there had been the slightest doubt in the mind of this person, the uncertainty would have saved him. He must have seen what was before him, but pre-occupied with the notion of the door, the evidence of the eyes made no impression. The hearing is passed by in the same way, but still oftener, for sounds are rarely so continuous as objects of sight. A person under the influence of hemp may carry on a tolerably well-connected conversation, till suddenly he makes some remark which shows that it is made in reference to his own thoughts, rather than to anything which has been said before. He confounds what is passing in his own imagination with the thoughts of others, and consequently attributes to them motives and intentions which they do not possess. His memories of the past and anticipations of the future are drawn from the same inexhaustible fountain. Add to these false premises, false reasoning, warped affections and a disordered will, and the picture of insanity is complete.

Any one who, under the influence of Cannabis Indica, has seen what the human mind is capable of becoming, cannot but feel a lively interest in those who are suffering under mental alientation; he cannot but look with hope to it, as a means of more fully comprehending what is the most distressing of finite calamities, and he cannot but think that a substance, the action of which is so powerful and unique, will be found, when fully understood, to possess valuable therapeutic virtues. But this point can only be set at rest by a series of experiments more careful and extended than has yet been made.

Cannabis Indica Poisoning

BY J.C. O'DAY, M.D.

Believing an experience I once had with cannabis indica to be of interest to some of the readers of the *Plexus*, will be my apology for contributing this article.

It has never been the inclination of the writer to indulge the feeling of egotism; and as the pronoun "I" may appear frequently, you will please bear in mind my desire of accurately and truthfully recounting the event as it actually occurred.

Some few years prior to my taking up the study of medicine, I was employed in northwestern Pennsylvania as locomotive engineer on the Bradford, Bordell & Kinzua Railway. My run was to double the road with the way freight.

One day I pulled into Bradford suffering with an attack of acute bronchitis, and, having a few minutes to spare, ran over to a corner drugstore to consult the clerk about my cough. He recommended Piso's Cure for Consumption, and I bought a bottle and returned to my engine.

Taking a mouthful of the cure I completed the shifting of the freight cars in the yard and made up my train for the trip out. This consumed about one-half hour. Before leaving the yard the conductor (George Caswell) came to the engine telling me we had two car loads of cinders in our train and instructed me to stop at "Hard Scrable" that the Italian section hands might unload the cinders.

My cough was very distressing, and so, as we sped along, I made frequent requisition on the bottle. The more I partook the more I had need to partake.

We had covered about seven miles of the road when I

Reprinted from *The Plexus*, 1899–1900, pp. 325–328.

suddenly became aware that I had been dreaming, and that I had forgotten that the responsibility for the safety of the engine and the train rested on my shoulders. The realization of this responsibility shocked me, but did not dispel an illusion that one of my legs was larger than the top of the smoke-stack, my arms like ponderous levers and my hands capable of encircling a flour barrel.

Just then my fireman yelled, "O'Day, what is the matter with you?" and the conductor came clambering over the tender, calling to me to know why I had not stopped at Hard Scrable to allow the unloading of the cinders. About this time I began to realize that I had been imbibing too freely of Piso's Cure, and made a desperate effort to concentrate my mind on my work. I reversed my engine and backed away toward the dumping spot. Looking back I was astonished to find that my train appeared to be more than a mile long, and that the Italian shovelers on the loads of cinders were expanding into enormous misty phantoms.

The sight unnerved me, and I again forgot to stop at Hard Scrable. So wrapped up in the novelty of my new surroundings was I that I forgot my place at the lever until the conductor came forward the second time and told the fireman I must be going crazy. This sobered me somewhat and the ashes were at last dumped at the desired place.

Before starting again I began to wander away into a land of giants and monsters, and fearing that some erratic impulse might seize me I told the fireman to watch me closely and to take charge of the engine if he saw anything wrong with me.

As I responded to the signal to go ahead, I noticed the great length of my engine. The telegraph poles shot upward until their cross arms pierced the blue vault above. Dogs as large as Durham bulls ran out and barked at us as we passed. Flocks of English sparrows with spread of wing greater than the condor rose from the road-bed and flew away. I had run over the road day and night for some years, until I knew every whistling post, but things did not have the old familiar look, and I could not tell whether I was running up grade or down, and was curious to see what the next curve would reveal. The cab grew to enormous proportions, and the fireman stood at his post more than one hundred feet away.

After what seemed to be days of running, and when we had covered what seemed hundreds of miles of track, I began to realize that we were nearing Kinzua Junction, and I slowed up.

The effects of the drug were wearing away and were soon gone, so that I knew how to handle my engine, and persons and objects shrank down to their old proportions.

The intoxication did not last more than three-quarters of an hour.

When a student of medicine in Baltimore, I ran across Prof. H. C. Wood's classic description of cannabis indica intoxication, as experienced by himself, and immediately attributed my peculiar sensations and illusions to hemp in the Cure for Consumption.

A medical journal published in India has recently made very free use of Dr. Wood's article in describing the effects of the drug on its habitués, who, it claims, are becoming very numerous in that country.

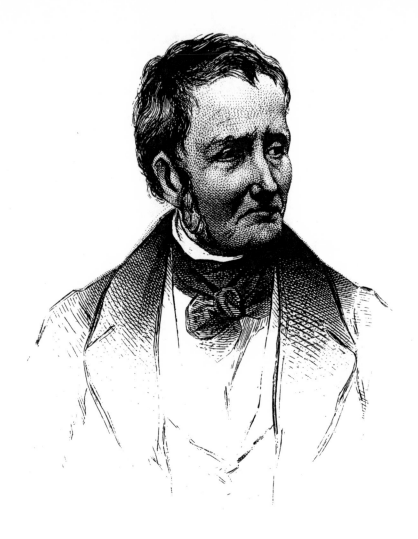

Very truly yours,

Thomas De Quincey

"My brother chose as a fitting subject to exite the dreamy, imaginative state of which we were in quest, De Quincey's famous 'Confessions,' from which he read aloud."

Two Cases of Poisoning by Cannabis Indica

BY JAMES FOULIS, M.D., F.R.C.P.Ed.

One night at the beginning of this year, about 11:30 P.M. a young gentleman rang me up, and asked me to go as quickly as possible to see his two brothers, who, he said, were both suffering from some poison. I at once asked, what kind of poison—was it opium? My young friend could only remember that his brothers had spoken of a drug which had a name like "Hash." I at once suspected "cannabis indica," or "Hashish," so I hurriedly looked at one or two medical books to refresh my memory as to symptoms and treatment in such a case of poisoning. On the way to the house I met a medical friend (Dr. C.), who had been sent for as the nearest medical man, and he was now on his way to bring me as quickly as possible to the patients. He had just left the patients, and he said to me he did not think there was any danger to life, though they were greatly excited, and were evidently suffering from the effects of a large dose of cannabis indica, or Indian hemp. These facts he had gathered from what he heard from one of the patients a few minutes before our meeting.

As I was well acquainted with both patients, I had great hopes I should soon find out all about the drug they had taken; and if the drug was Indian hemp, it would be comforting to tell them there was little or no danger from it. I requested Dr. C. to accompany me to the house of the patients, in case help would be needed.

The patients were brothers, A. and B. A. was twenty-two years of age, a medical student in his third year; B. was twenty years of age, an art student, quite a philosopher in his way, and of a highly strung and sensitive nature. Both were

Reprinted from *Edinburgh Medical Journal*, vol. 8, 1900, pp. 201–210.

tall, powerful fellows, nearly six feet in height. On entering
the dining-room, where our patients were, we saw an extraordinary sight. A. and B. were only partially dressed. A. was
hanging tightly on to B., who was rushing round the dining-
room table in a very excited state, wildly throwing about his
arms and singing in a most jovial manner. They were alone in
the room when we entered. A. was evidently doing his best to
control B., both were panting for breath, while B. was singing
out loudly in a most excited manner. A. looked pale and
depressed, as if overweighted by some sense of heavy responsibility. Both in mind and body B. was in a state of extraordinary excitement. He appeared as if he could not talk fast
enough, and as if his arms and legs were acting automatically,
while A. hung like a dead-weight on the back of his brother,
doing his best to control the awful restlessness. As Dr. C. and
I entered the dining-room, B. was rushing wildly round the
room, and A., in an almost exhausted condition, was hanging
as a dead-weight on the back of his brother with his arms
clasped tightly round his body. Dr. C. went quietly to an
arm-chair and sat down, while I went up towards the
brothers, who at once recognised me, and seemed to be wild
with joy at my appearance on the scene.

The younger brother, B., threw his arms round me in a
loving embrace, and spoke most kindly and even tenderly to
me; and then all of a sudden he began to quote poetry, and in
an excited manner asked me which poet I liked best, naming
several, one after another—the brother A. calmly looking on,
and regaining his breath after the recent struggles. A perfect
torrent of words and poetic sentences was showered on to
my face in this moment of excitement, and then B. rushed
off again round the table, with his brother after him,
endeavouring to control him, as before.

I also did my best to control A., making the mistake of
trying to argue with him as to such foolish conduct. This
seemed to excite B. very much, and he made a rush at Dr. C.
as if to strike him, and it required all my own power and that
of A. to calm B. I then went upon the opposite plan, and
agreed with A. in everything, and gradually B. became less
excited. I then gave Dr. C. the hint to slip quietly out of the
room, and told him to get the young brother to go off at
once for a cab, as I had made up my mind that both patients
would be better for a night in the Infirmary.

It is necessary here to state that the parents of our patients were at this time in the country, after an attack of influenza, for a change of air, and that the only relative in the house besides the youngest boy was a sister, who at this particular hour was fast asleep, and happily unconscious, in a room at the very top of the house.

As soon as Dr. C. left the house and the young boy had gone for a cab, I thought of an emetic for my patients. I could not find mustard; but I had in my pocket a bottle of ipecacuanha wine, a large dessert-spoonful of which I persuaded B. to swallow. As it was nearly two hours since the drug had been swallowed, I had little hopes that an emetic would do good, and it was not possible for me to give an antidote to cannabis indica. I therefore decided to stay with my patients until I could safely get them to bed, either in their own house or in the Infirmary. For a full quarter of an hour after this our time was spent in rushing round the room, accompanying B. as he dashed about his arms and legs, and as he talked and sang and quoted poetry incessantly. A. looked quite tired out. He was quite conscious, and able to talk sensibly regarding the situation; but it was impossible to get B. to do anything else than dance and sing and talk. I saw an open penknife on the dining-room table when I entered the room at first; this I took possession of. At last we heard the cab drive up to the front door. It was now snowing hard, and the air was very cold. A. put on his coat and cap, and after some trouble we managed to get B. to put on his coat and hat, and then with a rush we all bundled into the cab, and I told the cabman to drive rapidly to the Infirmary. A. and I got B. into a corner of the cab, where we partly held him down, for fits of excitement came upon him at simple suggestions, and it was most difficult to prevent him from becoming violent. Fortunately B. and I were great friends, and my plan of humouring and agreeing with him had a soothing effect upon him.

After what seemed a terribly long journey, we at last reached the Infirmary at about 1 A.M., in the midst of a heavy snow-storm, and we at once went into the medical waiting-room and rang up the resident medical officer.

During our journey to the Infirmary, A. was very depressed. His head hung down, and I saw him continually feeling his pulse; and he frequently asked me if he was going to die. On the other hand, B. was very lively during the journey—songs and poetic quotations would come out, in spite of a tendency to yawn occasionally. I rather thought the dessert-spoonful of ipecacuanha wine was now nauseating him slightly, but he did not vomit. The medical officer was greatly puzzled by B.'s symptoms, and began questioning him. This greatly excited B., who went at the doctor. The latter quickly retreated to a corner of the room, while A. and I took possession of B. once more.

The doctor told us there were no private wards to be had, and that the only beds vacant for such a case were in the D.T. Ward. This was rather trying to my patients, especially to A. but B. was still quite jovial, and did not seem to care about anything as long as he could sing and talk.

Up to this time I had a difficulty in seeing into B.'s eyes. I now saw that his pupils were widely dilated, and I found that his pulse was rapid and small.

I left my patients in the care of a strong male nurse in the D.T. Ward. Next morning at 10:30 I called at the Infirmary, but found that my patients had left that excellent institution, the D.T. Ward, at 9:30 A.M., and had reached home in time for breakfast with their astonished and wondering sister, who had so peacefully slept through the previous night, in blissful ignorance of all that had occurred in the dining-room between the hours of 10 P.M. and 1 A.M.

The elder of the two patients, A.—the medical student—has written a description of his experiences, which I now append.

An Experience under Haschish, or "A Night Out."—With a view to experiencing the wonderful dreams said to be produced by haschish, or cannabis indica, my brother and I on three successive occasions took doses of that drug. On the first occasion we took twenty-five minims of the tincture. This produced no effect on my brother, but, on the other hand, I began to feel somewhat hysterical. Hoping that it would produce the desired effect, I went to bed. After about half an hour's sleep, I awoke trembling all over. I soon, however, went to sleep again, and there was no further result.

On the second occasion (a week later), we took over forty minims. My brother chose as a fitting subject to excite the dreamy, imaginative state of which we were in quest, De Quincey's famous "Confessions," from which he read aloud. I soon found myself totally unable to follow him, and was seized with uncontrollable convulsions of laughter, in which my brother joined, although he seemed to have more control over himself than I had. I soon went to bed. My brother followed two hours later in an extremely nervous condition, and frightened like a child in the dark. We neither of us experienced the dreams we had anticipated.

After a three weeks' interval, we tried a third time, taking on this occasion over ninety minims. My brother, taking the dose after me, drank in all probability a considerable amount of sediment, although there was still some of the drug left in the bottle when he had finished.

In about twenty minutes we both began to feel exhilarated, the dose, as before, having a greater effect upon me. I felt decidedly pleased with myself, and versatile. My brother failed to follow my erratic criticisms on some of Beardsley's weird drawings, at which we were looking. Then one of the figures before me began to nod and whirl round. Suddenly I felt myself carried away as it were by a whirlwind, and finally lose consciousness. Here I must quote my brother's account of what happened at this moment.

"Scarcely had my brother," he writes, "recovered from his hysterics when he sprang up with appalling suddenness, upsetting everything, and shouting exultingly, 'Hurrah! I'm off!' Almost instantaneously he became unnaturally serious, and began muttering, 'We've done a damned foolish thing, a damned foolish thing!' all the while stamping up and down the room, striking and kicking out with his arms and legs as if struggling with some invisible antagonist."

The next thing I remember after regaining consciousness was the room heaving up and down. I was standing, trembling from head to foot, clutching my brother. First it seemed I was towering above him; then he in his turn overtopped me. With each upheaval of the room I felt we were growing worse and worse. It was a nightmare in its most horrible phase—a feeling that we were drifting into an irrevocable madness. I felt as if I was at the mercy of some supernatural force, which was sweeping through my brain, keeping me in a breathless state of suspension. Everything—time, objects—seemed to be rushing past me. I was nerved to the extremest limit of excitement. Would this force suddenly break itself up and play havoc with my brain, urging me to the very verge of insanity? It was as if a mesmerist was compelling his unhappy victim to perform some act of hopeless madness. What was going to happen next? Should we indeed commit some senseless deed, which we were powerless to prevent? This growing sense of responsibility made me think of putting ourselves into the hands of a policeman; but before I could formulate such an idea into words, everything again became blank. When I again recovered consciousness, it gradually dawned upon me that possibly I alone was mad. It took some time to convince myself that this was really the case. My brother assured me that he was sane, and this gave me an immense relief. There was now somebody to look after me. I was in safe hands, in case I should attempt anything foolish. I now realised in a forcible yet dim sort of way the necessity of controlling myself. The importance of not arousing the inmates of the house was the predominant idea throughout my subsequent actions that night. I took an exultant pleasure in grinding my teeth, clenching my hands, striding up and down the room, in the endeavour to prevent the fit which every moment I was anticipating. Sometimes I would stand still, quivering from head to foot. Presently I heard my brother mention "mustard," which I must have unknowingly suggested to him, with the idea that a vomit would help matters. We failed to discover any. Then I remembered some morphine tabloids which I had upstairs with my hypodermic. This my brother went to fetch; but, feeling that I should be unable to control myself in his absence, I followed behind. I found the tabloids, and took them in my hand, and then again all was a blank. The next thing I remember was swallowing spoonfuls of salt, in the hope that this would make me vomit. Meanwhile my brother had awakened my youngest brother, and, on emerging from the pantry, I heard him giving him orders to fetch a doctor. In the middle of his directions he broke into an insane fit of laughter. This completely mystified my youngest brother, who had previously witnessed my own strange behaviour, and thought than in any case his other brother would be in his right senses.

At this juncture we returned to the dining-room. The sudden outburst of insane laughter on my brother's part somewhat sobered me. Was *he* also going mad? I realised now the increased horror of the situation. Every now and then he would burst out into laughter. It seemed to me an absolute necessity that, if he was going to abandon himself to the wiles of the drug, I should keep control over my actions. About this time I felt my limbs contracting. In my excitement I pictured myself assuming that posture of opisthotonos.

I rubbed my calves, stamped up and down the room, opened my pen-knife and dug it into my hand. My brother, however, in one of his intervals of sanity, not approving of my possessing a knife, endeavoured to take it from me; but before he could do so all again became a blank—this time for both of us. Strange and absurdly silly ideas now began to pass through our minds, one after the other. We related stories to each other, never failing to laugh at the conclusion of each, however much they might be lacking in wit. In fact we were immensely pleased with ourselves. There was a general feeling of cleverness in the air, exhilaration. Subsequently I noticed my brother getting more noisy, even pugnacious. I *had* to laugh now at his jokes, fearing there might be an unfriendly rupture between us if I did not. It was all-important that there should be no outbreak of hostilities between us. He now developed an insane desire to peep out of the windows, and see if people were watching us from the street. Then, imagining he heard whispers outside the room, he would rush off to the kitchen banisters and peer downstairs to see if the servants were listening to us. This irritated me intensely; I thought it quite unnecessary. Then he would begin marching round the dining-room table, waving his arms, striking absurd attitudes, and singing in a low voice.

Then perhaps there would be an interval of relative sanity. Thinking we heard steps outside, we would rush to the hall-door to see if the doctor had arrived; or else he would again go up to the window or peer down the kitchen stairs, returning eventually to the dining-room and resuming his march round the table. Now, instead of singing and preaching *sotto voce,* he would get louder and louder. In vain I imitated him in whispers, in the endeavour to make him follow my example, so as not to arouse the household. He could not control himself. At last the doctor arrived. I implored him to give us morphia; but, after deliberating for somme time, he decided to fetch our medical attendant. I besought him not to leave us alone, dreading that we might go totally mad during his absence. However, he decided to leave us.

The doctor once gone, my brother again returned to his

interminable march round the table. Sometimes he would get more boisterous and hit me about in a good-natured way. I meekly submitted to this, laughed, and pretended to enjoy it, knowing that it was best to humour him. Once or twice I was foolish enough not to fall in with his insane ideas, and then he would go for me in earnest. After that I disagreed with him no more, and he returned to his everlasting promenade. How many times we walked round that table I should not like to say. Of this period my brother writes: "I have an impression that throughout the evening we spoke to each other in husky whispers; and I can remember vividly how strangely our natural voices sounded when, on one or two occasions, we spoke aloud. The sound was as of voices coming from another and far-distant world."

The drug was now exerting a very different effect on me. I began to feel extremely depressed and weary. I felt as if some magnetic force was dragging me to the ground. My limbs were heavy and aching. I gazed in despair at my brother, who still, as idiotic as ever, was waving his arms, imagining himself at the head of some triumphal procession. How long this dreary comedy lasted I do not know—it seemed to me hours. I dared not now go to the door and look out, fearing my brother might stampede upstairs or out into the street. At last our medical attendant, Dr. Foulis, arrived. He immediately took in the situation. My brother took to him at once, shook hands, and probed him with good-natured jokes,— "Swinburne is the poet I like—Rossetti: now what do you think of Tennyson, doctor?"

It now dawned upon me that perhaps this escapade was going to end in death, and a most vivid picture presented itself to my mind. It was a picture showing Virgil and Dante standing on a rocky ridge overhanging a deep abyss, whence are issuing multitudes of lost souls on their way to Hades. I imagined myself standing on that ridge watching the unending and evermoving throng passing out of sight. Above me there seemed to be an irresistible force, dragging me most unwillingly from that spot. I told the doctor that I felt in the presence of death—that feeling described by patients who suffer from angina pectoris. The doctor assured that the drug seldom proved fatal. This annoyed me extremely. I felt a craving to linger over the scene of the picture, thinking that I might possibly participate in it. Eventually the doctor told me that he was going to take us off to the Hospital. While waiting for the cab, the doctor gave my brother a considerable dose of vin. ipecac., which, however, never acted. He subsequently examined his pupils and found them widely dilated; the pulse was rapid and full; mine was rapid, but weak. At last the cab arrived. My brother made but little difficulty about entering. "During the whole time," my brother says, "that I was under the influence of the drug, I felt nothing but merriment and elation. The only exception to this was on hearing that I was to be taken to the Infirmary, when I felt like a criminal being dragged off to prison, humiliated and fearful."

Once in the cab I experienced intense relief, the necessity for that rigid control having vanished, my brother could now give vent to his feelings without any disastrous consequences. In fact, he had somewhat quieted down. He seemed to have passed the most acute stage.

We entered the Hospital gates a little before one o'clock, i.e., two and a half hours after having taken the drug. It gave me rather a shock at first to know that I was to be an inmate of the famous D.T. Ward, but I soon entered into the novelty of the situation. I must say that I felt at first rather like a condemned criminal being conducted to his cell. Whilst waiting in the corridor outside the ward, my brother suddenly made a rush at me, and there we stood clasping each other's arms, gazing at each other half stupefied, and engaging in a half-hearted struggle—an exact reproduction of that characteristic picture of two drunkards struggling together, neither of them being any the worse for the encounter.

My brother was soon after taken off by the keeper and given a bath. Finding that the water sustained its normal tint, the attendant remarked cheerily, "You don't want much of a bath, *you* don't!" at which my brother was duly flattered. I was not even offered a bath. We were then handed over to the nurse. I am afraid she did not look upon us in a very favourable light, although I tried to impress upon her that it was an extremely interesting experience. Indeed, it was with difficulty that I could persuade anyone that we had not been taking the common drink. Lastly, our names and addresses were taken. My brother was under the impression that we ought to give false ones, but gave himself away by telling me so at the top of his voice. "Matthew," he said in answer to the nurse. "Nonsense," she replied. "Matthew Prior— Matthew, Mark, Luke, and John went"— In the end I had to answer for him.

Finally, thoroughly tired out, I sank into a doze. Sometimes I would hear my brother singing to himself, as pleased and contented as ever. I saw the resident pass round on his nightly round, and then succumbed to sleep.

The effect of the drug lasted for three or four days, during which time we were in an extremely unstable state of mind, and had to keep a constant guard over our actions. On the afternoon of the following day, my brother had another attack. "I became restless," he writes, "wandered about the house, and finally shut myself into the drawing-room, where I danced and sang for my own delectation in front of the looking-glass. Mixed with my merriment was a sinister vision of my brother coming back, raving mad, from a concert to which he had gone that afternoon. I pictured to myself the door being suddenly flung open, and my brother standing at the doorway with flaming eyes; and I knew if this happened I should rush at him with murderous intent."

The following is the account of his dreams, on falling to sleep at the Infirmary:—"Upon falling to sleep I experienced the most exquisite dreams. The sky was scintillating with delicate colours, rapidly succeeding one another. Then came shifting landscapes of unimaginable beauty, following fast upon each other, and all too quickly disappearing."

Such was the unexpected sequel brought about by a draught of that green liquid. I remember saying at the time how extremely suggestive it was—suggestive perhaps of some magic potion. I compared it to the crimson wine with which Circe intoxicated and beguiled away her unwary guests. Certainly, it seemed to me that there was some definite yet unfamiliar force which had taken temporary possession of my body, and was expending itself on my nervous mechanism, producing a state of molecular unrest which at any moment might culminate in a nerve storm. So real and persistent was this presence, that I should like to believe the drug to have acted in the following manner, that it so altered the relation of the molecules to one another in the nerve cells, by the increased influx of the blood to the brain, that they became capable of receiving waves of vibrations (thus producing the feeling described), which normally pass through the brain without exerting any influence over it. It was a most ludicrous and, under different circumstances, might have been a most enjoyable experience. The imperative necessity that ever weighed most heavily upon us—that of keeping ourselves under control—and the trouble we entailed on those who attended us, prevented this.

I think the following points to be of some considerable interest:—

First, the different ways in which the drug expended itself on my brother and myself. Our ages are respectively twenty and twenty-two. In my brother's case the onset of his period of excitement was postponed for some little time and was gradual in character. Also his lysis, if I might so call it, was more prolonged than mine. Then the occurrence of his outbreak on the following day. Lastly, his pupils remained dilated for at least four days after the taking of the drug. I think that all the above facts may be accounted for by the fact that his dose contained much of the resinous material undissolved, forming a sediment at the bottom of the bottle. His dose, therefore, took some time in being absorbed by the stomach, and some of the resin may even have remained undissolved until the day following, thus accounting for his second outbreak.

In comparing my own case with his, the onset was much sooner, and was almost instantaneous, reaching its climax at once. Later, this stage of excitement gave way to one of extreme mental depression. This state of mental depression stands out in striking contrast to that of my brother's, which was one of levity throughout the evening. I was able to experience the numbing effect of the drug whilst digging the knife into my hand. There were no dreams in my case. And, secondly, in neither of us did the drug produce its reputed aphrodisiac action.

CANNABIS, U. S. P. (American Cannabis):
   Fluid Extract No. 598......................(*Alcohol 80%*).. 5.00

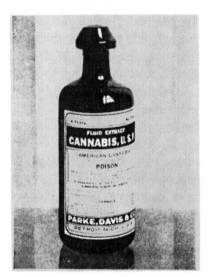

Fluid Extract Cannabis, in common with other of our products that cannot be accurately assayed by chemical means, is tested physiologically and made to conform to a standard that has been found to be, in practice, reliable. Every package is stamped with the date of manufacture. *Physiologic standardization was introduced by Parke, Davis & Co.*

This fluid extract is prepared from *Cannabis sativa* grown in America. Extensive pharmacological and clinical tests have shown that its medicinal action cannot be distinguished from that of the fluid made from imported East Indian cannabis. *Introduced to the medical profession by us.*

Average dose, 1½ mins. (0.1 cc). Narcotic, analgesic, sedative.

For quarter-pint bottles add 80c. per pint to the price given for pints.

[82]

Parke, Davis & Company 1929–1930 physicians' catalogue of the pharmaceutical and biological products.

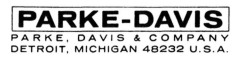

PARKE-DAVIS
PARKE, DAVIS & COMPANY
DETROIT, MICHIGAN 48232 U.S.A.

RESEARCH DIVISION
PRODUCT DEVELOPMENT DEPARTMENT

June 19, 1968

Dear Dr. Mikuriya:

Your letter of May 21 inquiring further into the role that Parke-Davis played in the early teens and twenties with respect to the stabilization of cannabis extracts is at hand. Fragmentary information has come to our attention by virtue of a recent visit to Detroit from his home in Florida of one of the individuals active on our staff at that time.

This individual informs us that Parke, Davis & Company and Eli Lilly Company did cooperate in the development of a standard cannabis preparation in the form of a fluid extract, a tincture, a solid extract, and a powdered extract. We originally used Cannabis Indica but later standardized on a strain of Cannabis Americana which we grew at our biological farm, Parkedale, near Rochester, Michigan.

Our retired employee gave us the following description, as best he could reconstruct it from memory, of the standardization procedure used in experimental animals at that time. The test method is as follows:

1. Select medium-sized, short haired dogs weighing less than 15 kilos, of fair degree of intelligence, preferably fox terriers. Do not feed for 12 hours prior to the test.

2. Determine susceptibility of the dogs by administration of minimum dose of standard preparation. The standard preparation is obtained from the Food & Drug Control Laboratory at Washington.

Published with the permission of the author.

3. *The dose of sample to be tested is determined by multiplication of the weight of the dog by the standard dose per unit weight.*

4. *Dose is administered in capsule.*

5. *The results of administration are apparent in about one hour. Muscular incoordination and drowsiness indicate activity.*

6. *The activity of the sample is dependent upon the degree of reaction and susceptibility of the dog. Do not use the dog oftener than once every three days.*

7. *The standard dose for various preparations is as follows:*

Drug (as a fluid extract)	*0.1 gm. per kilo gm.*
Fluid extract	*0.1 cc. per kilo gm.*
Tincture	*1.0 cc. per kilo gm.*
Solid extract	*4.0 mg. per kilo*
Powdered extract	*40.0 mg. per kilo*

8. *Retest the sample following adjustment on the basis of the first assay.*

Our interest in standardizing cannabis extracts was discontinued in 1938 when the "New" Drug Regulations called for the proof of safety of agents distributed for drug purposes. With this intermediate clarification of the description of drug, cannabis extracts fell into disuse by the medical profession since they provided no medical need that was not available in a more carefully standardized form from the more advanced work on natural alkaloids.

Since the current New Drug Regulations require both safety and efficacy to be clearly demonstrated in the hands of qualified investigators, it seems even more remote that cannabis might find a useful role in human medicine.

Sincerely yours,
L. M. Wheeler, Ph.D., Director
Department of Product Development

The Physiological Activity of Cannabis Sativa

BY H.C. HAMILTON, A.W. LESCOHIER,
& R.A. PERKINS

It has been claimed by various investigators that the common hemp (*Cannabis Sativa*) grown in the United States contains the same active constituent as is found in Cannabis Indica, the name of the official drug which is grown in India. Botanists do not distinguish between the two, the plant being identical wherever grown.

The fact that the Indian-grown drug was used in all the early accounts of its intoxicating action may have led to the belief that the peculiar climate of India is accountable for the presence of an active constituent not normally present in the plant.

No recorded data have been advanced, however, to substantiate the claim that drug grown elsewhere does not contain such constituents. On the other hand, Wood (Proc. Am. Phil. Soc., Vol. XI, p. 226), Houghton and Hamilton (Am. Journal of Pharmacy, January, 1908), True and Klug (Proc. A. Ph. A., 1909), True (Am. Journal of Pharmacy, January, 1912), and Hamilton (Am. Journal of Pharmacy, March, 1912), have submitted the drug to careful pharmacological tests, and report that extracts from American-grown drug are no less active than those obtained from India.

Dr. H. H. Rusby raised the question whether the test for activity on dogs can be accepted to prove its activity as a therapeutic agent.

Much of our knowledge of the action of drugs is obtained by observing their effects when administered to animals. The physiological action of almost every powerful drug is so characteristic as to be almost unmistakable to an experienced observer. Any one who has observed the characteristic effect

Reprinted from *Journal of the American Pharmaceutical Association*, vol. II, 1913, pp. 311–323.

of Cannabis Indica on susceptible dogs, symptoms which almost invariably appear in an hour after administering one to two grains of an active extract, and then has observed the same effect from an equal dose of an extract from the American drug, is inclined to accept it as proved that the two are identical.

The question raised by Rusby is, however, very pertinent and logically calls for proof of a different character. A series of experiments was therefore outlined which, it was hoped, would throw light on this much mooted question. To make a complete experiment it was decided that three persons would cooperate, each in turn, taking the same quantity of each lot of drug, while two would remain normal to observe its effect.

There is not much of interest in observing the effect of the drug on others, since its action is more mental than physical. One's own description, if it could be recorded at the time, would mean much more than that of others. The subject, however, is not in a condition at the time to record these observations, and if of a nervous disposition needs the presence of companions. Otherwise drowsiness is often the most characteristic effect of the drug.

The evening was taken for these experiments, partly to give opportunity for sleep immediately afterwards and partly to have everything quiet with no disturbing affairs going on to distract attention.

One of the three (Hamilton) had on a previous occasion taken two grains of an active extract Cannabis Indica and was, to that extent, familiar with its action. On that occasion there were developed some disagreeable symptoms but nothing serious.

Nausea and vomiting occurred, which were magnified by the imagination to an extent that was far from pleasant. Therefore, to duplicate conditions as nearly as possible the capsule containing two grains extract Cannabis Americana was taken at 5:30, followed by dinner at six o'clock.

Experiment I.   H. Relates his experience as follows:

About one hour after taking the drug a pleasurable sensation was experienced which can be described only as one of well-being and complete satisfaction. This was marred to an extent by the dread that the trip to the laboratory might not be entirely comfortable, and that in the street-car or on the street my behavior might be ridiculous without the cause being known. The walk to the car, the two-mile ride, and several blocks walk to the laboratory seemed interminable, although no unpleasant feelings were experienced during the trip. One other fact was observed, namely, the difficulty in holding my mind on one subject long enough to express my thoughts.

About two hours after taking the drug, an uncomfortable feeling was experienced, followed shortly by nausea and vomiting. Several ideas impressed me strongly; I had a morbid fear that some one other than my associates would observe me, also that the effect of the drug on me would deter the others from taking it. I was opposed to doing anything and wished most earnestly for a comfortable seat or bed. A feeling of constriction and dryness in my mouth and throat was observed. Later a feeling of depression and drowsiness followed and I appeared to sleep. Whether I did or not is uncertain, as I thought I remained conscious all the time. I knew that something in my condition was decidedly abnormal because of comments made by the observers, but I didn't know nor care what it was.

About four hours after taking the drug I felt much better and aroused entirely from my drowsy state. On the trip home I dozed off on several occasions, but for only a few minutes each time. A comfortable night's sleep followed and no unpleasant after effects could be noticed.

The result of this experience convinced me that no difference could be detected in the action of extracts from Indian and American hemp, for, although in the former experiment there were several phases which did not appear in this one, the general effect was identical in each case. On the former occasion all the peculiar sensations were more vivid, time dragged more slowly, the nausea was greater, even suggesting the fear of death, the constriction in the throat was so great as to suggest choking to death, there was a greater willingness to give free rein to my imagination and to relate experiences, and therefore greater difficulty in keeping the mind on one subject at a time. These differences were, however, in degree and not in kind and may be explained in part by my having become familiar with the drug and descriptions of its effect on others.

L.'s Observations on Subject H. Ex. I. About 6:30 H. began to manifest a certain amount of uneasiness and difficulty in concentrating his thoughts. Coming from down town to the laboratory it was observed that he seemed to be more or less worried and to lose, to a certain extent, sense of time, expressing the feeling that we had consumed an hour coming from down town, whereas the time for the trip was not more than ten or twelve minutes.

The laboratory was reached at 7:00 and H. expressed a strong desire to lie down or become ensconced in a comfortable chair. From 7:00 to 7:30 he appeared generally depressed and became irritating about seemingly trifling matters. At 7:40 pulse was taken and found to be 120, weak, irregular and easily compressible. Skin was cold and clammy and he expressed a belief that he was going to be nauseated. 7:50, pulse had dropped to 96, but was still weak and irregular.

8:00	Pulse	92	Severe vomiting
8:15	"	96	Vomited
8:30	"	88	
9:00	"	84	
9:30	"	86	
10:00	"	96	

The last record was taken after H. had been up walking around the room, which undoubtedly accounts for its increase over the one previously taken. It was observed throughout that when H. exercised, even to a slight extent, the heart action was markedly accelerated. In one instance the pulse rate was taken immediately after H. had been walking and was found to be 96. When taken less than a minute afterwards it was about 80, and was again increased to 96 by comparatively slight muscular movement. The pulse rate varied from 96 to 80 or 82 within a minute's time. Throughout it was soft and obliterated by slight pressure. During the whole evening his ideas seemed to be more or less confused, and it was apparently impossible for him to concentrate his thoughts on any particular subject. After beginning to make a remark, he would lose entirely his trend of thought, and be quite unable to complete it. At 10 P.M. the more marked effects of the drug had worn off.

P.'s Observations on Subject H. Exp. I. H. showed no symptoms whatever until about 6:30, when it became evident that he was worried and somewhat nervous. He said that the effect of the drug was coming on and expressed a desire to go to the laboratory as soon as possible. On the way he worried and fretted, at times fearing that he would be unable to walk and would make a spectacle of himself before reaching the laboratory. However, nothing of particular interest happened during the trip except an evident lapse of memory and evidence of nervousness. On arriving at the laboratory he expressed a desire for a comfortable chair or a bed and complained of feeling sick at his stomach. He was pale and his skin was cold and moist. Before long he vomited freely. This was repeated after a few minutes, but did not seem to relieve him greatly. He complained of a dryness in his throat and was continually wetting his lips. His pulse rate was almost alarming, varying greatly in rate from 84 to 120 within a minute, but for the most part being very fast and weak. His skin was cold and clammy and respiration somewhat shallow.

For over two hours he lay back in his chair in a sort of stupor, seeming to be asleep, but easily aroused. He had no disposition to attempt anything, not even to talk. During the early part of the evening he was evidently much worried, fearing that his condition would deter his colleagues from taking the drug. He also seemed to have a dread that some one other than those associated with him in the experiment would see him. He was asked to write, but firmly refused even to attempt it. When asked if he were having beautiful dreams and visions, his only reply was, "I wish I could tell you." He remained in this semi-conscious condition until about ten o'clock, when suddenly he aroused himself, said he felt all right and was ready to go home.

He dozed off momentarily twice in the car, and felt all right the next day except for a very faint headache.

L.'s Personal Experience. A two-grain dose of solid extract **Experiment II.** Cannabis Americana was taken upon an empty stomach. For two hours no symptoms of any kind were experienced. Then there was a peculiar unnatural sensation. The initial manifestation is difficult, in fact, impossible of description. No distress was evidenced nor was the feeling exceptionally pleasant. It was simply a recognition of the fact that I was not quite myself. Following this period there shortly developed a feeling of great elation, and a sense of well being. With no particular reason for being so, I felt inexpressibly happy. There was a twitching and drawing of the corners of my mouth and an uncontrollable desire to laugh, although I could not laugh aloud. Everything pleased me and I felt that my happiness was absolutely complete. The only tinge of regret that I experienced was that my colleagues were not having the same delightful experience. The more marked effects of the drug appeared to come in waves, although the general sense of elation was never lost. An occasional undulation would sweep over me and I would feel as though my body was swaying, and there was an inclination to strike the table with my hands in an exuberance of delight. At times I had great trouble in coordinating my thoughts, although between the paroxysms which have been described, my mind seemed reasonably clear. I felt that I was acting in an exceedingly foolish manner, but had no power to control myself and in fact did not care to. As it grew late in the evening the stimulating effects of the drug decreased and I became somewhat irritable and touchy about trifling matters. At ten o'clock the greater part of the effects had worn off, although I did not feel entirely normal. After a light lunch I retired and slept very soundly. No after effects of any kind were experienced on the following day.

H.'s Observations on Exp. II. L.'s experience was almost entirely one of enjoyment. There was no nausea and no evident discomfort, although he once remarked that the earlier effects were much the more pleasant. There was unquestionably the same well-being, expressed by his repeatedly saying, "I feel so good." Hearty laughter for which there was no evident reason was explained in this way. At no time was there any desire to carry on conversation more than to answer any questions addressed to him. This would account for there being no noticeable difficulty in keeping his thoughts collected.

Later a sensation of drowsiness was evident and with it expressions of irritation when anything of a disturbing nature was said or done. The effect of the drug was long delayed in appearing, nothing being noticed either by himself or the others until nearly two hours after its administration. This probably explains why its effect was so persistent, intoxication being very evident fully six hours after the drug was taken.

P.'s Observations on Exp. II. No effect was noticed for about two hours, when a slight twitching of the corners of the mouth was observed and a tendency to smile. When asked why he smiled he said he didn't know, just felt good but could not define the sensation, it was simply one of enjoyment. He said that he felt sorry for us, as he was the only one enjoying himself. Presently he broke out into a restrained but hearty laugh. When questioned, he said it was simply because he couldn't help laughing. He admitted that he was making a fool of himself, but said he couldn't help it and didn't care anyway. At one time he pointed at an article of furniture in the room and had another laughing spell. When asked the reason he merely said that it was funny. He answered all questions put to him, but showed no tendency to be talkative, most of his answers being short.

These spells would last for probably a minute or two and then there would intervene a normal period of ten to twenty minutes. He said he was simply "happy" drunk, and he looked and acted that way. Later in the evening he showed a decided disposition to be annoyed by talking or answering questions and remarked that the earlier effects of the drug were much the more pleasant. At ten o'clock the action of the drug had worn off sufficiently so that he felt inclined to go home. He was somewhat irritable on the walk from the laboratory and said afterwards that he was very drunk on the way home. He ate lunch before retiring and enjoyed a comfortable night's sleep and felt fine the next day, with no bad effects whatever. Observations were taken of the blood pressure (systolic) and of the pulse rate at intervals during the evening, but nothing abnormal was noticed. The pulse was full and steady and the rate averaged about 80, not varying more than six beats at any time. The blood pressure was 130 mm. of mercury throughout the evening.

Experiment III. P. relates his own experience as follows: At 4:30 I took a capsule containing two grains S.E. Cannabis Americana on an empty stomach. About one hour later, while talking to my colleagues about the best time for them to go out for a lunch, they asked me if I didn't feel anything; I answered, "No," and truthfully I did not, but no sooner had I spoken than I experienced a peculiar sensation. The corners of my mouth commenced to draw and I could not refrain from laughing; I laughed so heartily that I was tired afterwards, although nothing seemed particularly amusing. This spell lasted for probably half a minute, although it seemed much longer to me.

Then my associates left me, and I was alone in the laboratory. At this time I felt most exhilarated. Everything seemed so enjoyable and I was extremely comfortable. I walked up and down the corridor, swinging lightly along, seeming to walk on air or feathers. My feet weighed nothing. It was no effort to walk; it was more like floating along. My sense of proportion was lost, my feet seemed miles away from me, my arms were long and big. The corridor was miles long; I walked or rather floated up and down apparently for hours, waving my hands and arms, marking time to imaginary music. All this while I was smiling and enjoying myself immensely. All my faculties were not impaired, however, because to test myself I read part of a typewritten notice on the bulletin board. I was standing there when a person who knew nothing of the experiment passed by. We greeted each other, and evidently he noticed nothing peculiar in my appearance nor actions. I was suprised at this, for it seemed to me that he must see how silly I looked and how I swayed when I walked, but especially he should have noticed my voice, which sounded to me like the deepest bass. It seemed to me to be musical and full toned and I liked to hear myself talk. My colleagues, however, did not seem to notice it, nor did they appreciate that I felt so good toward them and myself.

After what seemed hours of walking I sat down to await their return from lunch. Several waves swept over me during this time and also later on, which are very difficult to describe adequately. The feeling was one of well being and perfect satisfaction, beginning with a sort of numbness or fullness in the extremities, a feeling of unreality in the surroundings. I knew that my hands were normal in appearance, but when not observing them, they seemed to be detached and not a part of me. We played a game of cards, and in playing a card I seemed to be throwing some enormous but very light article over a great distance. These spells usually started by smiling and ended in laughing rather hysterically, pounding the table with my fist. But I could not laugh aloud because of the peculiar drawing and contriction about my face and neck previously noted. As the effect began to wear off these paroxysms became less frequent but no less irresistible. I felt no unpleasant symptoms at any time. About ten o'clock I was hungry and ate some sandwiches with great relish before going home. I reached home without any difficulty, not feeling drowsy and without any change in my feeling of enjoyment. Upon arriving home I retired immediately because I felt that I was not entirely normal. Before going to sleep, however, I experienced another wave.

I awoke early next morning very much refreshed and none the worse for my experience.

H.'s Observations on Exp. III. The experience of P. was practically a duplicate of L.'s. The effect appeared one hour after taking the drug, and except for an occasional lapse his normal condition was regained five hours afterwards. There was more uncontrollable laughter in his case, no irritability and no apparent discomfort at any time. He seemed to give himself up more completely to the enjoyment of his sensations than the others. At times he seemed to be addressing an imaginary audience, pacing back and forth, gesturing and appearing to talk to himself.

We were inclined to question whether some of his actions were not assumed and voluntary; but he assured us that he was acting just as he felt.

L.'s Observations on Exp. III. P. began to feel the effect about an hour after the administration of the drug. He seemed to be possessed of a desire to move about, paced up and down the corridors, declaring he felt as though he weighed not more than fifteen pounds. He was apparently very much pleased with himself, and bubbling over with happiness. At times he would be seized by fits of uncontrollable laughter, which in some cases was spontaneous and without apparent cause, but usually it was incited by the others laughing at or with him. Between these paroxysms of laughter P.'s condition was practically normal, he could talk rationally, and his mind, as far as indications could be depended upon, was clear. At no time did there seem to be a loss of coordination. It was observed that the action of the drug was apparently produced in waves, while between these seizures one's condition would be practically normal.

During the three experiments recorded above, the one under observation felt a certain restraint, knowing that the others were watching for every abnormal action. For this reason it was decided to vary the conditions in the further experiment and have all three under the influence of the drug at the same time. It was hoped in this way to eliminate the restraint evident in each of the individual experiments and perhaps observe some new features in the action of the drug.

Experiment IV. In this experiment H. took Extract of Cannabis Americana again, while L. and P. took extract Cannabis Indica. This gave an opportunity for L. and P. to compare the effect of the two varieties, both on themselves and on the others, while H. took this opportunity to repeat the experiment with all the conditions the same, except that he ate no dinner until the effect was practically gone. All three took the drug at 4:30 on empty stomachs, the dose in each case being two grains.

The last experiment, while not developing any new features, was in other respects successful. H. had no unpleasant experience and the evening was one of unalloyed pleasure, proving that all the discomfort was directly traceable to the nausea from having food in the stomach. L. considered the effect to be much less intense and of shorter duration in this experiment than that from the American drug, while P. took the opposite view in his case.

H.'s account of the experiment is as follows: L. was the first to note the characteristic effect of the drug, while P. and I remained unaffected for fully two hours after it was taken.

The same feeling of well-being and complete satisfaction was experienced by all, this being as evident to the observers as to the subject himself. Uncontrollable laughter was more frequent and longer continued than in the individual cases, probably because during a cannabis intoxication so little is necessary to excite it, and when one started the others joined in the hilarity. No one felt inclined toward any activity, but only to give himself complete relaxation. Each of the three was emphatic in stating that he knew when he was making himself more or less ridiculous, but could not control the impulse nor did he wish to restrain himself.

About six hours after taking the drug, at the end of a quiet card game, without any comment, each of the three assumed as comfortable a position as possible and fell into a doze. It was apparently not sleep in any case, as each was fully conscious of noises in the building and annoyed by them.

This lasted not more than ten minutes, at the end of which we all felt fully aroused and ready for something to eat. This ended the experiment as outlined in advance. The only variation from the original plan was, as noted, for all three to experience the effects at the same time. No point was lost because of this, since the subject is at all times acutely conscious of everything occurring.

L.'s Account of Experiment IV. My personal experience with Indian Cannabis was very much the same as those already narrated as occurring with the Cannabis Americana, although the effects were developed somewhat more promptly, and were not quite so pronounced or lasting. P.'s feeling seemed also to duplicate very closely those which he had had from the Cannabis Americana, but contrary to my own were somewhat more pronounced. H. did not have any of the nausea or any of the other uncomfortable features which occurred during the first experiment, indicating very clearly that these symptoms were due to the hearty dinner which he had eaten, and were not to be construed as characteristic of Cannabis. The drug in this last experiment was taken at half-past four, and the greater part of the effects were felt from about half past six to eight o'clock. After that time the more exhilarating action had worn off, and I experienced only a drowsiness. For a half or three-quarters of an hour after I had ceased to feel any more marked effects of the drug H. and P. continued to be very much exhilarated. About nine o'clock all three of us became drowsy, and as if by mutual consent laid our heads on the table in a sort of doze, although none of us really went to sleep. This condition continued about ten to fifteen minutes, after which we felt much refreshed.

P.'s Account of Experiment IV. L. was the first one to show any symptoms from the effect of the drug. He had practically the same experience as on the previous occasion. H. and I did not feel any effect for fully an hour later than L., but finally went under the full influence of the drug very suddenly, there being no premonitory symptoms whatever. At times one of the three would have a paroxysm of laughter alone, but usually one would start laughing and the others join him at once. It was observed, however, that L. was getting over his intoxication early, and he sat there seemingly rather bored and provoked at the others for being so happy. The effect on myself was apparently more intense than that of the previous test, and more so than was experienced by the others, laughing spells being more frequent and inclined to be hysterical. No unpleasant symptoms were experienced by any one of the three during the evening. After several hours playing cards and talking a peculiar thing happened. Suddenly and without a word from any one we stopped the game, lay back in our chairs and dozed. It seems to me that I slept for a long time, although it was in reality only about ten minutes. It probably was not really sleep, as I remember hearing the watchman on his rounds, and wondering whether he would come into the room where we were. As suddenly and spontaneously as we had dozed, we aroused and, having practically recovered from the effects of the drug, prepared to go home.

Conclusions. It may be stated with certainty that the physical and mental condition of the human subject at the time of administering this drug influences its effects both in degree and kind. For that reason no two persons can be expected to exhibit the same symptoms as a result of ingesting equal quantities of the same drug, and no person can be depended upon to react in exactly the same manner from the same drug on different occasions. With these facts in mind the differences in the three personal experiences above related are readily explainable, and there is no reasonable ground for doubting that Cannabis Sativa grown in India and America contains the same active constituent.

The method of assaying extracts of Cannabis Sativa described in detail by Houghton and Hamilton (Am. Jour. of Pharm., January, 1908) makes use of dogs for exhibiting the characteristic effect of the drug. Attention is called in this article to the fact that the animals must have been specially selected for the purpose. They must not only be susceptible to the drug but their behavior under its influence must have been determined by preliminary observation. We may thus avoid errors due to their individual idiosyncrasies. There are, apparently, no such marked differences in the character of the reaction in dogs as are observed in human subjects, nor are they so variable at different times if they have been carefully selected as described above.

When proper precautions are observed the activity of an extract Cannabis Sativa relative to a standard extract may be determined with reasonable accuracy. Twelve years' experience in observing tests of Cannabis Sativa obtained from different countries, Africa, India, Germany, Greece and various localities in North America, has supplied data to prove that they all contain the same active constituent.

Description of the Hashish Experience

BY R.P. WALTON, M.D. Ph.D.

At about the same period as the more imaginative descriptions by the French voluptuaries and the American adventurers were composed, various members of the medical profession and otherwise scientifically trained people observed and reported the effects of hashish on themselves, their friends and their patients. This general display of interest was occasioned by the sudden prominence of Indian hemp as a medicinal agent. The therapeutic applicability of this drug had been advocated by Aubert-Roche in 1839, by O'Shaughnessy in 1843 and by Moreau de Tours in 1845. Each of these physicians contributed descriptions of the pharmacologic and what might be called the psychopharmacologic effects.

Moreau de Tours made numerous experiments on himself, normal individuals and patients. He reported that with smaller doses of dawamesc, a person does not feel particularly different and only experiences a mild feeling of expansion. With larger doses there is a marked euphoria, slight pressure in the temples and upper cranium, retarded breathing, slightly accelerated pulse, a feeling of warmth over the whole body with the exception of the feet which are usually cold and a heaviness and numbness of the hands and arms. With still larger doses, there are choreic movements, ringing in the ears, and a feeling of oppression in the region of the heart. Subjectively there is no such effect. There is a development of tonic spasms, particularly of the flexors, all with short or long intermissions. There are numerous psychologic phenomena such as a feeling of lust without sexual excitation, an indescribable feeling of peace, happiness and delight, a

Reprinted from R. P. Walton, *Marihuana: America's New Drug Problem* (J. B. Lippincott, 1938), pp. 86–114.

distorted, a powerfully heightened effect of music, fixed ideas and delusional convictions which change rapidly, irresistible impulses and illusions and hallucinations which are closely allied to insanity.

Rech, in 1847, reported the effects of hashish administered to a number of young interns. Three main types of effects were obtained: (1) a disturbance of digestive functions; (2) purely nervous effects; and (3) confusion of mental faculties. The first manifested itself as a loss in appetite, dryness of the mouth, burning thirst, pain in the epigastrium and inclination to vomit with sometimes outright vomiting. These effects pass off rapidly and are of subordinate importance with respect to another symptom, namely, a coldness in the extremities. The second group of effects includes involuntary contractions, a disturbance of locomotion, a feeling of paralysis and a convulsive laughter, which is sometimes disagreeable but more often is pleasant. In one case the lower extremities seemed to be as heavy as lead and nailed to the floor, another felt a heaviness in all extremities and felt as if he were walking in snow. The purely mental effects lasted longer and were most prominent. The subjects could not converse rationally, ideas displaced one another without relationship, memory and the sense of passing time were extinguished. Imagination was intensely stimulated; the most brilliant ideas flashed by; some had hallucinations and thought they were transformed. A deep torpor gradually set in. Of all the intellectual capacities, the power of comprehension remained in the most normal state.

Donovan took large doses of extracts made from hemp plants grown near Dublin. No effects were obtained. However, ten drops of the tincture of *Cannabis indica* from Calcutta caused marked effects. The walls of the room seemed to move in on him. His thoughts came more slowly and finally were extinguished. This condition lasted for two hours after which he recovered and manifested a strong appetite.

Clarke had substituted cannabis for morphine in a case of mania. The first dose from a renewed supply produced marked depression with cyanosis. Some of the same sample was taken by the author who had a typical hashish experience, also accompanied by cyanosis and by partial paralysis of the left arm.

De Luca was prompted by curiosity to swallow two to three grains of a sugary paste containing hashish recently brought from the Orient. Effects began in a quarter of an hour and prevented him from continuing work. Movements seemed to progress from without to the interior of the body. There was a sensation of things entering through the fingers and proceeding directly to the brain. These sensations were not unpleasant and did not seem to derange intellectual faculties. Space seemed greatly exaggerated, there were sensations of walking on air and of great superiority to other people. Ideas passed with great rapidity and seemed to be very clear and exact. The effect lasted about four hours. Ideas then began to come more slowly, distances diminished, nervous movements disappeared and finally the only thing noticeable was that the lips were not as moist as usual.

H. C. Wood, Jr., of Philadelphia, was chiefly interested in determining if there was any activity in American grown cannabis. He made an alcoholic extract from male plants grown for fiber purposes in Lexington, Kentucky. An estimated twenty to thirty grains of this extract were ingested at 4:30 P.M. Apparently forgetting or disregarding this fact, he went on a professional call and at 7:00 P.M., while attending a patient, the effects suddenly became evident. By 7:30 the feeling of hilarity had rapidly increased.

It was not a sensuous feeling, in the ordinary meaning of the term . . . It did not come from without; it was not connected with any passion or sense. It was simply a feeling of inner joyousness; the heart seemed bouyant beyond all trouble; the whole system felt as though all sense of fatigue were forever banished; the mind gladly ran riot, free constantly to leap from one idea to another, apparently unbound from its ordinary laws. I was disposed to laugh; to make comic gestures . . . There was nothing like wild delirium, nor any hallucinations that I can remember . . . I think it was about eight o'clock, when I began to have a feeling of numbness in my limbs, also a sense of general uneasiness and unrest, and a fear lest I had taken an overdose. I now constantly walked about the house, my skin to myself was warm, in fact my whole surface felt flushed; my mouth and throat were very dry; my legs put on a strange, foreign feeling, as though they were not part of my body. I counted my pulse and found it 120, quite full and strong . . . My legs felt as though they were waxen pillars underneath me . . . I began to have marked "spells," periods when all connection seemed to be severed between the external world and myself . . . The duration of these to me were very great, although they really lasted but from a few seconds to a minute or two . . . The periods of unconsciousness became at once longer and more frequent, and during their absence intellection was more imperfect, although when thoroughly roused, I thought I reasoned and judged clearly. The oppressive feeling of impending death became more intense . . . Under the influence of an emetic I vomited freely without nausea and without much relief . . . When I awoke early in the morning, my mind was at first clear, but in a few minutes the paroxysms, similar to those of the evening, came on again, and recurred at more or less brief intervals until late in the afternoon. All of the day there was marked anesthesia of the skin. At no time was there any marked aphrodisiac feelings produced. There was a marked increase of the urinary secretion. There were no after-effects, such as nausea, headache or constipation.

A Dr. Thomas, who was called, reported that zinc sulphate produced free emesis in fifteen minutes and after that the pulse rate fell from 136 to 104 and the warmth of the skin was restored. The mental state was not affected by the emetic.

Another, and evidently more potent, extract was subsequently prepared from the same Kentucky hemp. Three-quarters of a grain of this resin produced effects but of a much milder sort than the original experience. There were no marked periods of unconsciousness but only a feeling of hilarity, a prolongation of time and a total inability to fix the attention except for short periods. A friend took one grain of this same resin and experienced approximately the same effects. In addition, however, he became ravenously hungry, ate excessively and experienced a marked degree of sexual excitement which lasted several days.

Kuykendall had administered cannabis frequently in neuralgia and obtained only the exhilarating effects. However, in an experimental trial on himself, terrifying sensations were experienced. The intoxication reached its greatest intensity in about one and a half hours and lasted about six hours.

Wiltshire had a patient who expressed reluctance at taking any further doses of cannabis because the first produced peculiar sensations. In order to reassure her of the innocence of this drug, he took fifteen drops of the fluid extract and was surprised to be affected by the typical hashish sensations.

> I remember perfectly well all the phenomena that were produced; even when I was engrossed with the idea that death was at my door . . . Felt much intoxicated, body growing larger; indescribable sounds came to my ears; imagined that the blasts of old winter were lashing at my windows and walls. Reason good; memory heightened . . . A feeling of aphrodisia possessed me; fast upon this comes a feeling of alarm and restlessness . . . My heart now began to beat fearfully, thought it would leave its walls. Moments seemed hours . . . Head now felt as though it would burst. Consciousness of my corporeal existence had somewhat left me, though I could see, and feel with my hand my lower extremities, as in perfect health, but expressed to my physician that I had better not go to sleep, for fear I would not awake . . . At one time I could feel a sense of tremor passing over my body . . . I began to improve and walked around the room with a feeling of delightful calmness, and with thoughts so pleasant that I remarked to my friends, "this is true ecstasy."

The writings of Bayard Taylor prompted Duncan to try cannabis on his patients. Since no effects were obtained, the preparation was considered worthless and, to establish this more certainly, he took three teaspoonsful of the tincture. Four hours later, typical effects were manifested.

> I was so giddy that I could not stand still, and the damned in the infernal regions could have felt no more agonizing terrors. My skin was burning up with heat, pulse so fast that I could hardly count it, and a general paralysis taking possession of my whole person, more

especially my stomach . . . The most intense headache
accompanying the other symptoms. I was in this condition about three hours, having several times concluded
I was dying, with not altogether the most comfortable
feelings, being decidedly in doubt as to my final destiny,
disposed rather to view myself as lost. At the expiration
of three hours, the pulse became normal, the skin cool
and moist, and the paralysis gradually wore off. Then of
all the happy mortals that ever existed, I was the most
supremely so. I saw the most beatific visions, the most
beautiful women, angelic in their mental and physical
configurations. If all the gold of Solomon's Temple had
been offered me, I would not then have relinquished my
perfect happiness and mutual repose counterbalancing
the exciting experience of the previous three hours.
These mental hallucinations lasted, I suppose, four to
five hours. Then came the reactionary feeling, dull,
heavy headache for forty-eight hours; uncertain in gait,
and terrible mental confusion . . . Whilst I would not be
without the experience gained, relative to its action, I
would not for the same length of time undergo similar
doubts and feats, to say nothing of the unpleasant after
effects.

An English physician, who preferred to remain anonymous, reported some self-experiments in which he took
doses of one-fourth to two grains of the extract without
effect. Likewise, a dose of one dram of the tincture produced
no effect. Some months later, a fresh specimen of tincture
was obtained and one dram of this was taken.

The effect this time was quick and alarming. In
fifteen minutes I was unable to walk, shook all over, and
felt my mind in a whirl with fast-flowing, grand, or
grotesque ideas of a more or less constantly unpleasant
nature, and all tinctured by an undercurrent of restlessness and anxiety; occasionally, for a brief interval, I
would suddenly drop, so to speak, into my normal state,
and be able to think clearly about my condition, only to
soon relapse into the same condition of wild and more
or less painfully vague and intense perverted mental
action. This condition lasted two or three hours and

then gradually passed into a deep sleep, from which I awoke the next morning feeling none the worse for my somewhat rash experiment.

Von Mering made a number of experiments with an extract of charas resin and described, in summary, the condition which is ordinarily produced. According to him the extremities are heavy and without sensation, there are muscle tremors, ringing in the ears, difficulty in hearing, defective perception, a feeling of heat or cold in the head, vertigo, flashes before the eyes, dryness of the mouth and a feeling of oppression and anxiety. After this a very pleasant phase of the effects develops. The subject becomes hilarious, laughs very loudly, phantasies move rapidly; sensory delusions are manifested and visions come and go in quick succession. Consciousness is retained. Illusions are present if the eyes are closed; but disappear when they are opened. In this state most individuals sleep for hours. Side actions of headache and vertigo are infrequent. Bowel movements are not affected; appetite is distinctly increased. The pulse is usually accelerated in the beginning. The pupils are dilated during the hashish effects. With some individuals there is a muscular rigidity.

The observations which Marshall carried out on himself were unique in one particular, i.e., he was the first to use the vacuum distilled product termed "cannabinol." "With doses of twenty mgm., the first symptom was usually loss of power for mental work. A typical condition of mental exhaustion set in. Sentences could not be conceived except by powerful efforts, and these were not often forthcoming ... After intermediate doses (fifty mgm.) the ability to work was lost altogether ... Pleasurable tingling in the limbs, very slight ataxia and other symptoms similar to those obtained after larger doses were present. Time passed quickly. Sleepiness was sometimes but not always present. As an early symptom, a peculiar indistinctness of the periphery of the visual field occurred, and later it was found that the point of regard was made to travel with difficulty, as along the line of a page. Depression usually continued throughout the following day ... After a large dose of cannabinol my own pulse increased in frequency. Constipation was rarely present. Salivation was not usually observed, dryness of the mouth being a more constant symptom . . . A most interesting condition, after large doses, is the occurrence, alternately, of loss of control and lucid intervals. The crude drug seemed to produce more excitment than pure cannabinol." This latter is attributed possibly to the associated terpenes in the crude drug.

Binet-Sanglé, along with a companion and in the presence of an observer, swallowed 0.2 grams of a pill of extract of hashish. The effects became manifest in about half an hour. There was intense thirst, the saliva had a peculiar taste, the head seemed full and there was a peculiar restlessness. Voluntary movements were uncertain and almost ataxic. On the other hand, tactile sensibility seemed to be more acute. Objects, when viewed directly seemed enormously exaggerated, but in the peripheral field of vision they were of normal dimensions, i.e., there was a sort of "macropsie centrale." The perception of space was also distorted. Sounds were extraordinarily intensified and caused painful sensations. Suggestive ideas became so vivid they amounted almost to hallucinations. There were spells of laughter usually preceded by ecstatic emotions. Fatigue and confused mental processes persisted into the next day. The companion experienced marked respiratory depression, congestion in the face, transitory muscular incoordination, visual hallucinations and intermittent spasms of laughter.

Robinson tried the fluid extract on himself and his friends and recounted the effects with special emphasis on the ludicrous aspects of the experiences. Manifestations particularly noted were uncontrollable laughter, the revival of previous ideas, a lost sense of time, euphoria, erotic sensations, occasional nausea, a double sense of consciousness, alternating sensations of lightness and heaviness and, most prominently, a feeling of immense geniality and mirth, accompanied by sentiments of the most expansive good will. One of the subjects awoke the next morning with a ravenous appetite which was attributed as much to the great expenditure of energy in laughing as to any direct effects of the drug.

Burr has recorded the experiences which he and a fellow interne had when under the influence of hashish. At 7:30 P.M. he took sixty minims of Parke-Davis' tincture of *Cannabis indica* after having eaten an hour and a half previously. At

10:00 he noticed that he couldn't tell the difference between an ace and a club and couldn't see to read because his eyes were so widely dilated. His mouth became dry; he became intensely thirsty and drank three quarts of water during the evening. At 10:30 he suffered a general convulsion which lasted three minutes. He felt well; his speech was not affected. The convulsion resembled an attack of hysteria. He had a pronounced feeling of well-being and was supremely happy in a quiet, mentally unexcited way. He was not boisterous or noisy and was able to describe his sensations clearly. There was no increase in intellectual power. Sex ideas were entirely absent and he said that Venus herself couldn't have tempted him. After the first convulsion he became very hungry and ate a whole cold chicken, a large loaf of bread and some butter. He had six convulsions in four hours; they were all like the first and ended abruptly. The convulsions appeared willful in that he willed to convulse; he knew that he was throwing his arms about, that he was writhing like a snake, acting like a clown, making silly grimaces. But he could not will to do otherwise. He could restrain a convulsion for a few minutes, but soon the will to convulse overcame the will to inhibit. At 11:00 P.M. ideas of time became prolonged. One minute seemed like twenty. This distortion wasn't due to a rapidity of ideas; it wasn't due to ennui. He had some feeling of space enlargement and also had ideas of double consciousness. He was himself, yet was somebody else, sitting in a boat floating through the sky amid pink clouds. This was his only hallucination; it occurred about six times, and lasted about a minute each time. At 4:00 A.M. he became drowsy and went to bed. He got up five hours later and went to work. Throughout the day he felt comfortably tired. He was dreamy, had a sense of unreality, and was unable to keep his attention concentrated on any long conversation. During the experiment there was no change in respiratory rate. His pulse was 100. He passed large quantities of dilute urine. There was no tactile anesthesia, no paresthesia and no loss of power in the limbs.

Four days later his friend took the same dose of the same drug from the same bottle. His symptoms were quite different. Two hours after swallowing the drug he was suddenly seized with a sense of death by suffocation. This hallucination lasted for four minutes. Similar seizures came on every

twenty minutes for about three hours. There was no disturbance of the pulse or the respiration. Even when he thought
he was suffocating, his breathing was quiet and regular. He
had no other symptoms and went to sleep three hours later.

Schneider took three cc. of the fluid extract of *Cann.
indica* experienced mental effects in ten to twenty minutes
and intense apprehension in thirty minutes. After one hour,

> quite suddenly there is developed an indescribable feel-
> ing of exaltation and of grandeur. The words "fine,"
> "superfine" and "grand" come to my mind as being
> applicable to the feeling. This indescribable feeling is
> purely subjective. Self-consciousness is completely an-
> nihilated for the time being. The concepts time, place
> and space have vanished. The confines of my room are
> no longer existent. I say to myself, "If this drug can
> produce such marvellous effects, I will certainly take it
> often!"

The feeling of exaltation came in waves. The mouth and
lips were dry. An hour and a half after taking the drug:

> I am capable of anything and everything. No task
> would be too great, no problem too difficult. The
> exalted feeling is wholly indescribable and appears to be
> general and all-inclusive. [During the next three hours]
> the feeling of supreme exaltation and grandeur con-
> tinues for varying degrees. The idea of oneness with all
> nature and with the entire universe seems to take hold.
> There is no material body or personality . . . The skin is
> now moist but the mouth continues dry. I have momen-
> tary visions or glimpses of vast beautiful landscapes,
> showing wonderful color effects . . . I do not visualize
> persons nor do persons play any part in the mental
> imagery . . . There is a marvellous color imagery, blue,
> purples and old gold predominating with most delicate
> shading effects . . . Beautiful gardens filled with flowers
> appear. Again, grotesque monsters of ever-varying forms
> and without producing any terrifying effects . . . I regret
> that others cannot share with me this feeling of well-
> being . . . Evidently sleep gradually set in and continued
> undisturbed until the usual rising time. No special

sensation on rising. Feeling, if anything, more than usually refreshed. All of the sensations recorded above have completely vanished. The recollections of the experiences are however very clear and vivid. Mouth continued dry until morning. No after effects of any kind. The action of the kidneys is increased but no effects as to the intestinal tract.

Six days later, a second dose was taken which did not produce any distinct mental exaltation or feeling of grandeur. Color and form imagery were poorly developed as compared to the first test. Months later, a third dose which was identical with the first, did not produce any feeling of exaltation and grandeur. The color imagery, though, was specially marked. The next day there was a slight feeling of nausea.

One month later, eight cc. of the original fluid extract were taken. The idea of a dual nature and the color imagery were not as marked as before and there were none of the feelings of exaltation and grandeur.

Probably for a period of not less than six hours I suffer from nightmare. I am convinced that the end has arrived and that I cannot recover.

Dizziness and nausea develop and some nausea persists into the next day.

Among others who have similarly experienced and described the hashish episode may be mentioned Ragsky, Judée, Hamburg, Bell, Owen, Campbell, von Schroff, Polli, Richet, Beane, Renz, Williams, and Lange.

The therapeutic exploitation of Indian hemp in Europe and America, which dates from about 1840, correspondingly resulted in a great many instances of individuals suffering a hashish experience which was wholly unexpected and often undesired. There are several general factors responsible for the high degree of variability in cannabis effects—and these are further augmented when the drug is given to invalids. The patient's condition itself is subject to more than ordinary variations. We have repeatedly seen that animals in poor condition are more severely affected by this type of drug than healthy animals and this parallel is hardly needed in order to emphasize the fact that debilitated patients are much more likely to respond unfavorably than normal individuals. The collection of descriptions which follows is characterized by a high proportion of cases in which there was marked motor and sensory depression. The effects on consciousness were predominantly the agonizing sort rather than the euphoric. The case of a patient receiving an unexpected overdose represents one of the least favorable conditions of mental preparation, and it is generally recognized that the state of mental preparation for a hashish episode is an important determining factor in the character of the resulting cerebral effects.

The dosages taken by these individuals usually are given in specific terms but these have only a casual bearing on the actual dosage of active material. Bioassays of any degree of reliability were not introduced before 1900 and satisfactory chemical assays have not yet been introduced. Accordingly, the dosages which were administered have only an approximate significance in terms of any standardized activity.

One of the first to describe a case of this sort was Brown. He was called to see a druggist's clerk who had taken six grains of the solid extract in installments. About three and one-half hours after the first dose he became nervous and dizzy, felt an irresistible inclination to run, a great desire to urinate, great thirst. Spasms supervened, during which, at times the flexors and extensors, at times the abductors and adductors of the whole body were thrown into violent alternate action. The spasms increased in severity and frequency for half an hour and then gradually diminished after emesis had been induced. The spasms were unaccompanied by pain but did produce a sense of weariness. At no time was there delirium or loss of consciousness. The symptoms lasted in severity about an hour, then gradually diminished. Twenty-four hours later the desire for constant motion and occasional slight spasm persisted but soon passed away.

Kelly administered thirty mg. of the extract to a woman of sixty who had severe rheumatic pains. She experienced a marked reaction, her fingers became icy cold and benumbed. She heard noises and had visions of objects before her eyes. The phenomena passed away in a few hours. The dose was later repeated with the same result.

Strange was called to see a phthisical patient who had

accidentally been given an overdose of the extract. Three hours after taking the extract, the patient had suffered such a marked reaction that he was thought to be dying.

> There was complete superficial anesthesia, the patient declaring that he could touch nothing. He felt as if dead; could scarcely recognize anything. He had intense dread of death; a frightened countenance; the pupils were dilated, but contracted slightly to light. Vomiting, which was not present, was induced by mustard and water, and the green extract came up with the mucus of the stomach. During the whole time, I was cheered by the fact that the pulse did not fail, nor was there any clammy perspiration.

The patient fell asleep after two hours and next morning ate a ravenous breakfast.

Mary Hungerford had been taking small doses of Indian hemp without any appreciable effects. A very large dose was then taken which produced near unconsciousness in a short time. There was a much exaggerated appreciation of sight, motion and sound.

> It was not only death I feared with a wild, unreasoning terror, but there was a fearful expectation of judgment, which must, I think, be like the torture of lost souls ... In place of my lost senses I had a marvelously keen sixth sense or power, which I can only describe as an intense superhuman consciousness that in some way embraced all the fine and went immeasurably beyond ... As time went on, and my dropping through space continued, I became filled with the most profound loneliness.

These effects persisted for a considerable length of time.

Sticker administered Cannabinon in about thirty cases with no particular after effects except in the instance of a young man who took 0.1 gram of the drug. Effects began in one-half hour. There was intense anxiety and depression with a tonic-clonic twitching of muscles of the extremities. Shortly after that there was complete paralysis of the motility of the extremities. During the next few hours there were several long periods of psychic exaltation. He went to work the next morning but there were minor residual effects for some time. Using this same preparation, "Cannabinon," Richter, Buchwald, and Pusinelli have similarly observed cases in which the ordinary doses of 0.1 to 0.3 grams caused alarming symptoms.

Seifert reported the case of a patient who took 0.1 grams "Balsamum Cann. Indica" and became violently delirious with residual effects which lasted several days.

Hamaker was called in to see a young physician who had taken forty-one drops of Squibb's fluid extract of *Cann. indica* with the idea of testing the quality of the medicine. He was walking on the floor excitedly, laughing and talking continuously, but not incoherently. At times he would cry, and then suddenly change to laughing. He was abnormally irritable and said he felt as if he were "rattling around among the centuries." There were redness of the eyes and profuse lachrymation, with a fast pulse. He subsequently became drowsy and afterwards reported that during the beginning of the experience he had a feeling of dread of danger which had passed off quickly.

Prentiss reported the case of a dentist suffering from an irritable cough who took five drops of a Parke Davis "liquid preparation" in installments. The effects became manifest in two hours. He became oblivious to all surroundings, excessively happy and, after potassium bromide was administered, eventually fell asleep. The next morning he reported that all the sensations were agreeable and in no way accompanied by unpleasant emotions. The effect came on in waves until he lost himself.

> He was moving through space with lightning speed, and in his path were clouds of the most beautiful, ever-changing colors, and when he touched them each one played a beautiful tune.

Windscheid observed a twenty-eight-year-old healthy male who took about three grams of extract of *Cann. indica* within a period of two and one-quarter hours. After two and one-half hours, he was suddenly seized with a feeling of apprehension, intense excitement with exalted ideas and hallucinations. An hour and a half later he became apathetic and extremely thirsty. Windscheid found him with dilated pupils, hyperesthesia and tremors, particularly in the extremities. The pulse of 172 was weak but regular. On the following day, only mild hallucinations were experienced, the pulse was 120, he was hyperesthetic and had heightened skin and patellar reflexes and reactive pupils. After an apathetic period of eight days he was about normal. This was considered a case of special resistance to an enormous dose.

Winter reported a case of poisoning in a fifty-seven-year-old woman who was healthy but of weak constitution. The patient had taken increasing doses (20 to 300 mg.) of the extract to combat the pain of trigeminal neuralgia. Then for several weeks she had taken three doses each day of 0.3 grams each, without any disturbing effects. On stopping the medication for two days and starting again on the third with one dose of 0.3 grams, marked depression set in after a few hours. The patient became weak and somnolent, did not respond to questioning, reflexes were absent and pupils were dilated. After an hour, the patient recovered to some extent but later relapsed to an excitable, delirious state followed by despondency and weeping. After two hours of such condition she fell into a deep sleep and awoke the next morning with only a little dullness and very slight recollection of the experience.

Geiser reported that seven minims of a fluid preparation of cannabis produced severe effects in an elderly woman suffering from malarial cachexia. There were none of the usual hallucinations but there was a marked exhibition of deafness, labored breathing, weak pulse and alternating loss of consciousness. The drug had been given to relieve migraine.

Fischlowitz was called to attend a physician who had taken one teaspoonful of the fluid extract of *Cannabis indica* in order to relieve a troublesome cystitis. He had fallen asleep but awoke with unpleasant dreams one-half hour after taking the drug. He thought he had slept for hours, and had a feeling of tingling all over his body, especially around the angles of his jaws and in the region of his stomach. He soon developed a happy frame of mind and became quite garrulous. He complained of the tingling and uneasiness in his limbs, said his legs were as heavy as lead and that when walking he felt as if wading through feathers. His throat felt parched, the conjunctivae were reddened, the pulse ranged from 100 to

118 and the respiration was very rapid. Four hours after taking the drug he fell asleep and awoke the next day with no residue other than a frontal headache.

Minter reports an instance of a prescription containing Indian hemp which was taken regularly for about a month with no symptoms other than drowsiness after the first three doses. On taking the last dose, however, the patient had severe effects which began in a few minutes. The impressions and hallucinations were of an unpleasant sort. After a restless night, the patient awoke with a very vivid recollection of his experience.

Sawtelle administered twenty-five drops of fluid extract of *Cannabis indica* in installments to a well-developed, middle-aged man suffering from a severe occipital neuralgia. On visiting him that night, he found the neuralgia was relieved but that the patient was in a state of increased mental and motor activity, which was soon followed by partial delirium and hallucinations. The pupils were dilated. The hallucinations were of a jovial character. The patient talked freely and pleasantly, and when relating some incident he would burst into laughter. He first thought the ceiling was falling and placed himself in position for protection by extending his arms and calling loudly for help. He then moved his bed to the opposite side of the ward and imagined he saw pieces of timber floating in space about him. He left his bed and went to a corner of the ward where he became intensely excited over what he took to be a fight between a large and a small dog. After watching the imaginary fight for a few moments, he returned to the bed and remarked that the large dog had torn the small one into pieces and expressed sympathy for the small dog. At first he attempted to leave the room through a window and it was necessary to restrain him. Symptoms continued for three days. From the first the pulse was full and strong, respiration normal; during the night he was troubled with erection of the penis. There was slight anesthesia of the lower extremities and the patient complained of weakness of the legs for several days after the other effects of the drug had passed off.

Atlee prescribed ten minim doses of tincture of *Cann. indica* for a twelve-year-old boy, suffering from headache. He took one dose of the prescription and, in a few minutes, said he felt a burning pain in the pit of his stomach and soon became strange in his manner saying that his legs were humping about, that he heard a ticking like a watch, that he saw the room on fire, saw pictures falling down, etc. Examination showed a weak pulse with a rate of 120 and dilated pupils which reacted sluggishly to light. He was given two drams of brandy and ten grains of citric acid in syrup of lemon. A blister was applied to the nape of the neck. He soon began to revive, his color improved and, in about two hours and a half had recovered, his headache was gone and he was able to walk home. The same dose of tincture was given to another child the same morning with no ill effects.

Baxter-Tyrie was called in to see a young lady who had first taken three half-grain pills of Indian hemp for the relief of headache. When these had caused no apparent effect she had concluded that the preparation was a "fraud" and, to demonstrate her conviction, had proceeded to swallow nine more of the same pills. When observed four hours later, she was in a state in which fits of laughter and incoherent ravings alternated with comparatively lucid intervals. She complained of various hallucinations and delusions, chief of which were a complete perversion of the relations of time and a loss of identity. She was now herself, now again a different individual, and the modifications of her behaviour in relation to her dual personality were grotesque. Coffee and strychnine were administered and she was entirely normal the following day.

Bicknell reports a case in which three grains of an English extract produced effects which were most distinguished by convulsive movements and opisthotonos. The opisthotonos was later relieved only by violent friction over the affected parts. At no time was there fear or foreboding of a fatal result.

Benedict reports having seen about twenty cases of intoxication attributable to variations in susceptibility, voluntary increase or repetition of dose by patients.

The sole symptom of intoxication has been anxiety and subjective feeling of danger from the drug.

Downer was called in to see a young girl who had introduced tobacco dust into her nose after the manner of taking snuff. (The tobacco was subsequently shown to contain *Cannabis indica*.) The girl became frankly intoxicated, talked incoherently and giggled in a fatuous manner. She could not move her lower limbs, the feet and lower legs being completely anesthetic and there was a general paresthesia. She was oblivious to her surroundings unless well shaken, when she took some notice and would answer questions. After the administration of an emetic and coffee she slowly improved.

Baker-Bates has recently reported an instance from England in which a young man grew hemp in his garden and several times smoked the dried leaves and tops. He experienced mild symptoms which included loss of sense of time and space, vivid dreams or hallucinations and subsequent drowsiness.

Incredulous about his experiences, his fiancée, aged twenty-two, smoked—and to some extent inhaled—about two-thirds of a cigarette, made from the top of a fruiting plant. This was at about 10:10 P.M.. Soon afterwards she fell asleep and a few minutes later, on being disturbed, she awoke with a start and exhibited apprehension. The eyes were bright, the hands were twitching, and she appeared intoxicated; she asked where she was—probably deceived by hallucinations— but seemed happy. At about 10:25 P.M. she was taken for a short walk, which was interrupted by outbursts of laughter and of affection; her speech became slurred from dryness of the mouth and her gait increasingly unsteady. At 10:30 P.M. she was taken to a doctor and the history explained; he recorded that she was pale, but able to stand and walk although feeling dizzy; she was very excited and talkative and made stiff purposeless movements with her hands; her state was highly emotional, even amorous, towards her companion; at one moment gay, she was next anxious and said she felt "enclosed"; she exaggerated the passage of time and was confused about spatial dimensions; her tongue and mouth felt parched and words were pronounced with difficulty, while sentences lapsed into incoherencies; the eyelids were half closed; the pupils dilated, but reacted to light; the pulse was rapid, but strong. She was transferred by police ambulance to the casualty department of the Liverpool Stanley Hospital where she arrived at 11 P.M. in a collapsed condition. Her symptoms at that time were loss of power in the legs and inability to stand; dizziness, dryness of the mouth, and palpitation; and lengthened estimation of the passage of time. She believed her condition had lasted many hours and, although fully conscious of her existence, she imagined she was "outside her own body," enclosed in a small space, and surrounded by a mist from which she could not escape. This imaginary mist did not impair her vision for distant objects. On further examination speech was found to be confused, rambling, and often inarticulate. She was unable to stand steadily or without support, and showed great incoordination in the movements of the hands. There was tachycardia (140 per minute) and also marked inspiratory dyspnoea. No other abnormality was found. Following general treatment for shock the patient recovered in nine hours and there were no sequelae except severe headache.

Approximately forty more case reports of this type are listed in the indexes of the Surgeon General's Office and of Schmidt's *Jahrbücher*. Most of these appeared at fairly regular intervals during the period 1840 to 1900 and, in this respect, closely paralleled the therapeutic popularity of the drug.

Within the last decade the hashish episode has been subjected to extensive analyses in several of the most prominent psychiatric clinics. This series of studies has included a sort of merging of the ancient "hashish" and the current "marihuana." While both are essentially the same, there are differences of degree which at times seem to make almost qualitative differences in the resulting picture. "Marihuana" consists of the dried tops and leaves of American *Cannabis*, which ordinarily is not so rich in active resin as the same plant grown in Asia and Africa. "Anascha" is the term applied to the drug in *Asia Minor* and, more recently, in Russia and, apparently, is quantitatively of about the same degree of activity as marihuana. The manner of use in both cases is almost exclusively by smoking in the form of cigarettes. The ancient "hashish" on the other hand was usually swallowed

Psychiatric descriptions of the Hashish experience.

or, when smoked, was not smoked in cigarettes. Recently "hashish" smoking in the cigarette form has become prevalent in Greece, and in this case the term seems to include both the plant and the resinous exudate.

Of the modern psychiatric studies, the earliest were from clinical groups in Utrecht, Munich and Heidelberg, each of which used an orally ingested form of the drug. The later studies in Russia, Greece and the United States were directly concerned with the more current preparations which are smoked in cigarettes. An additional distinction of these later studies is that the chronic effects were investigated in considerable detail.

Fraenkel and Joël made numerous experiments with normal individuals, their dosages being one hundred mg. of the extract of *Cann. indica* (Parke Davis). Their observations and conclusions may be summarized as follows:

One of the first indications that the drug has begun to act is an oppressive foreboding and feeling of apprehension; something strange and inescapable seems to approach. Activities cease, the feeling of impotence and anxiety becomes overpowering.

When the intoxicated subject surrenders to this new authority, he soon comes to feel even more imprisoned and oppressed by conceptions, ideas, words, actions, emotions and outbursts which no longer seem to belong to him. Images and series of images, long-buried recollections appear, whole scenes and situations project into the present. They excite first interest, sometimes pleasure, finally, since they cannot be controlled or stopped, torture and exhaustion. The subject is astounded and overwhelmed by all that takes place and by what he says and thinks. His laughter, all his expressions happen to him like happenings from the outside world. He passes through experiences which seem to amount to supernatural revelations. All these oppressive forces cannot be dispelled by simply saying "This is not reality it is only the effects of a drug." The character of the delusions, for example, cannot be evolved at will; one recognizes that they are hashish phenomena, yet they remain unaltered. These delusions are mostly illusionary transformations of the outer world, which at first had become very strange and singular. The room widens itself, the floor slopes precipitously, atmospheric sensations develop; vapors and fogginess cloud the air;

colors become brighter and more luminous; objects become more attractive or, again, they may become grotesque and menacing. Tormenting doubts of the reality of things assert themselves. It is remarkable what variations take place in all animate things; they assume expressions of mask-like fixity and lifelessness. Physiognomies turn to gypsum, wax, and ivory. True hallucinations are rarely experienced. In the haptic sphere there often develops a disintegration of the feeling of the body's coherence. There are also dynamic sensations such as that of being hurled through space as by a powerful centrifugal force. All this is accomplished not as a continuous development but rather as a continuous change between the dreaming and waking state, a lasting, finally exhausting alternation between completely different regions of consciousness; this sinking or this emerging can take place in the middle of a sentence. For the comprehension of the intoxification-episode, this precipitous change is of great significance. The dream-like phases have an influence on the often grotesque over-evaluation of periods of time, which likewise is a characteristic hashish phenomenon. The mood and affectivity vary according to the consciousness of compulsion, the restriction of activity and the frequently resulting feeling of defencelessness and dependence. Or there may develop a simple feeling of well-being, which can increase to a state of blissful euphoria and ecstatic rapture. An agonising combination of incompatibles, which often exists in the way of thoughts and opinions, can also dominate the affectivity and introduce moods of affective perplexity and disintegration. The intoxicated subject usually reports in a form which varies considerably from the normal. The associations become difficult because of the frequent sharp separation of each recollection from that which preceded. Conceptions cannot be expressed well in words, the situation can become so dominated by an irrepressible mirth that the hashish-eater for minutes at a time is capable of nothing but laughter. Even his other types of expression, facial appearance, gestures, and his whole motor behavior are changed. Contracture states alternate with periods of increased motility, bizarre movements and sudden outbursts. The recollection of the intoxication is particularly clear. Among the bodily symptoms may be mentioned, dry throat, coughing, occasionally increased blood pressure. Fatigue in the usual sense does not develop.

Frequently there is a marked feeling of hunger, and considerable quantities of food are consumed with a pleasure not ordinarily experienced, in spite of the tongue being coated and dry. Objective sensibility is not disturbed. That hashish does not cause any local anesthesia is considered to have been previously emphasized. Aphrodisiac effects are lacking.

At the suggestion of Professor Straub, Kant and Krapf in the Psychiatric Clinic at Munich made a series of self-observations with hashish. Doses corresponding to three to nine grams of "Herba Cannabis Indica" were used in the experiments. This medication was prepared by Gayer who extracted the crude drug and then absorbed the potent extract on chocolate powder. The activity of this preparation was previously defined in terms of the amount producing corneal anesthesia in a rabbit. The lowest orally administered dose of the crude drug producing this effect in rabbits corresponded to three grams per kilo. This dose of three grams was also found to be the smallest dose producing recognizable effects in human subjects. Some chocolate tablets containing no drug were used in these human experiments as a control against auto-suggestion. In general, neurologic disturbances were not observed nor was there any depression of surface sensibilities as might have been expected from preceding descriptions. Further, aphrodisiac effects were not experienced. With large doses there was fatigue, thirst, vomiting, vertigo and collapse phenomena with a soft and arrhythmic pulse. Taking hashish stimulated the appetite but never produced intense hunger.

In one person, recognizable effects usually began in thirty to forty-five minutes, while a distinct clouding of the consciousness did not begin until fifty to seventy-five minutes. With the other subject, initial effects were recognized in eighty-five to one hundred five minutes and the first change in the state of consciousness in ninety to one hundred eighty-five minutes. Effects appeared more quickly with the larger doses. Disturbances of consciousness were manifested by a feeling of "the superficiality of things," "a stupid feeling," "a slowing of thoughts." The subject declared "things go away from me, they are taken from me," "I must speak rapidly else I will forget what I mean to say," "a veil of smoke is drawn over the brain," "I can't remove myself from this condition without forcing my will," "I forget everything except the last sentence." There was a subjective feeling of obliviousness. With some exceptions the mood was one of pronounced euphoria. The subjects felt very well disposed to things in general and had an expanded sense of self-appreciation. Between spells of laughter, the subjects sometimes became sensitive and seemed to dread the recurrence of the laughing spell. With large doses the feeling of intoxication expressed itself in an agonizing fear of death.

The inclination to motor activity was much increased. "It felt as if all joints of the body were freshly lubricated." The subjects mimicked common movements such as riding or dancing. The capacities of critical perception were dulled. There was a marked over-estimation of the passage of time. Impressions of light and sound seemed extraordinarily exaggerated. The light from a table lamp blinded the eyes and ordinary noises, such as the ticking of a clock, resounded loudly. An inconclusive but suggestive experiment indicated that the actual threshhold of sound stimuli was lowered; steps in an adjoining room, which were imperceptible to other people, were heard and counted correctly.

Illusionary misconceptions developed. "I see now that you have become much more square. Now you have a very sharp-pointed chin." The flow of imagination at the height of the experiment was slowed. "I have the feeling that ideas can come very rapidly, however, they do not come at all."

There were crawling sensations in the legs, which seemed to become alternately light and heavy. Sensations of heat coursed in waves from the feet to the head or seemed to locate in specific organs. These sensations along with a slight feeling of numbness were the first subjective symptoms of drug action. These elementary phenomena, which are purely body sensations, produce a much more complex effect when they become multiplied. These body sensations constitute the primary basis of the experience.

Taste sensations were experienced by only one of the subjects and then only with the larger nine-gram dose. Sweet, salty and metallic tastes were experienced. Visual phenomena were also experienced. In some cases the subject became suspicious, irritable and easily provoked to a dangerous degree of aggressiveness. One of the subjects attacked his colleague with a knife and had to be locked up for a time.

Straub, in describing the typical hashish effects, used one

of the experiments by this group as an example. In this case, the experimenter had taken a dose corresponding to six grams of the crude drug. The first effects were felt in forty-five minutes. The eyes became moist, the lids heavy and there was an uncomfortable sort of fatigue. He broke out in spells of uncontrollable laughter. The extremities seemed to have no weight and to be of exaggerated length. Corresponding to the increasing euphoria, the personality seemed to divide into individuals, one critically rational and the other of a fantastic spiritual character. The senses seemed more acute. Scientific problems seemed to be solved instantly in front of his eyes. Visions in bright, harmonious colors moved before him. This rapturous state seemed to last for many hours. In spite of this condition, there also existed, at times, an almost normal degree of rational consciousness. After four hours there was marked hunger and food was taken. During the remainder of the day there was some mental confusion. The following day there was not the slightest after-effect.

Kant subsequently extended his observations with these preparations to nine manic-depressives and ten schizophrenic women. The drug produced tachycardia, dryness of the mouth, heaviness of the limbs, a feeling of warmth and paresthesias. The effects only varied in degree from those he had observed in himself.

Meggendorfer about the same time also contributed a discussion of cannabis psychoses.

The series of studies from the Utrecht and Munich clinics were followed shortly afterward by a similar series from the Heidelberg clinic. The dosages in this latter series were considered much higher and, correspondingly, the degree of narcosis and psychopathological phenomena were more intense. "Cannabinol," prepared by a commercial firm, was used in oral doses of one hundred mg. in about thirty "selbstversuchen." This dose, according to Marx, contained forty of the "corneal units" defined by Gayer. According to this comparison, the dose of one hundred mg. of "Cannabinol" represented forty times as much activity as that which gives a human subject clearly recognizable effects, and this would clearly be a tremendous dose. The possibility of such an extraordinarily large dose actually acting on the nervous system, is opposed by various other considerations. For instance, the highly purified preparation may possibly undergo more destruction in the alimentary canal than an equally active crude preparation; there is no very convincing evidence that the "Cannabinol" made by commercial houses at this date was to be considered so much more potent than the "Cannabinol" of Wood, Spivey and Easterfield. Marshall working with this latter preparation, found that twenty mg. was the minimal oral dose producing recognizable effects in man. Accordingly, the doses of the Heidelberg group may be considered as large doses but possibly not so large as the comparative figures would imply. Relatively severe effects were obtained, such as pronounced states of apprehension, somnolence and collapse. Metabolic studies made at the same time indicated "fundamental functional disturbances" which were considered to be a new observation in this type of study.

Disturbances of thought caused by the drug were classified by Beringer according to three general types: (1) a disturbance within the higher complex processes which are responsible for integrated conception as a whole; (2) a disturbance of the ability to retain memories; (3) a disturbance of the flow of thought, or disconnection of thought ("Gedankenabreissen"). The hashish phenomena were compared with various psychotic states and with mescalin intoxication.

V. Bayer proposed and explained a schematic division of the motor phenomena. Three main types were recognizable in these experiments: (1) movements similar to normal expressive movements, representing elation, ecstasy or apprehension, frequently with excessive exaggeration; (2) movements which originate in a primary change of the motor apparatus, that is, an impulse excess or an inhibition of the motor apparatus—and they are only later filled with meaning and expression; (3) movements which were actuated at more peripheral points and were not associated with the higher center of consciousness. Typical of this group, are myoclonic movements which take place in special sets of muscles, choreiform restlessness, and also, the pseudo-cataleptic effects in the limbs. This latter uncomfortable condition was produced in three of the thirty hashish experiments.

Marx made numerous observations of body changes. One group of symptoms, suggesting a febrile syndrome, included a rise in body temperature and pulse frequency. Circulation velocity and venous pressures were frequently increased.

Dryness of the mouth and throat simulated atropine effects. The eyes were characteristically glazed as in febrile patients and there was a marked injection of the conjunctival vessels. This latter is referred to as a recognized symptom in the Orient. The hands and feet were cold and moist. Blood concentration took place, hemoglobin values sometimes rising as high as 50 percent. The fact that this often accompanied a marked diuresis was considered very unusual. Hydrogen-ion concentration and carbon dioxide combining power of the plasma did not show any remarkable variations. Significant hypoglycemic changes were described.

Stringaris, also of the Heidelberg clinic, had occasion to study a large number of persons in Greece who were addicted to the smoking of hashish. Skliar and Iwanow, at the Psychiatric Clinic in Astrachan, Russia, have similarly studied cases of "Anascha" smoking in Russia.

Stringaris reported that the acute intoxication is characterized by euphoria, increased motor activity, excitability, talkativeness, laughter and appetite. Hallucinatory and delusional experiences were frequent. Occasionally, especially in persons who suffer from chronic addiction, depression instead of euphoria occurred. A considerable number of the addicts declared that the drug is a sexual stimulant. Libido is increased both during the action of the drug and during the intervals between doses.

Skliar and Iwanow carefully studied the intoxication phenomena after administering the drug to fifty-two cases, most of whom were chronic "Anaschisten." The number of individuals showing the individual typical symptoms has been recorded. For instance, fifteen noticed a lightness in the head at the beginning; six noticed tinnitus and nausea; four, clouding of vision; four, thirst; two, heaviness in the legs and arms; five, palpitation; seventeen, increased appetite; thirty-four, a calm and pleasant euphoria; thirty-two, laughed; seven, a depressed, anxious condition; six, moderate motor phenomena; twenty-two, inclination to reveries; four, disturbance of personality-consciousness, etc. True hallucinations of the special senses, such as vision, hearing taste and smell were not common. There was macropsy in twelve cases, micropsy in two cases. Functions of the sense organs in several cases were intensified and in other cases diminished.

In eight cases, there was excitement which passed over into sleep. This is more usual with the neophytes than with chronic users. Other distinctions between the neophyte and the experienced user were noted. The neophyte usually is ecstatically euphoric, laughs loudly and has an increased appetite and thirst. A subject, who has taken it for, say two years, is much more repressed in his laughter and general boisterousness.

Objective symptoms were glazed eyes, red eyelids, hyperemic conjunctivae, tremors of the tongue and extended fingers, increased patellar reflexes, marked palpitation, and accelerated pulse. These observations were considered to resemble in general the classic descriptions of Baudelaire, Gautier, Moreau de Tours, Joël and Fraenkel, Schroff and Freusberg, but certain differences were pointed out. The hashish effects are considered more pronounced than those with anascha. With hashish the laughter is more violent and unrestrained. Consciousness is much more affected with hashish and the fantastic illusions and pseudo-hallucinations are more frequent and vivid. Also with hashish there are true hallucinations of sight and hearing, which are lacking altogether with anascha. The disturbance of time sense is considerably greater with hashish. Particularly distinctive with hashish is the disintegration of personality and the resolving of the individual into the environment and all nature at large, which phenomena are infrequent or very slight with anascha.

These distinctions are considered only quantitative rather than qualitative. Anascha is obviously a mild form of hashish (and smoking is a means of ingestion permitting smaller systemic dosage). Also, the mentality and character of these subjects varied considerably from that of the writers and scientists who were the subjects for the classic descriptions. Further, the age range of these subjects was low, seven to twenty-five years! When larger doses of anascha were given the effects resembled in intensity the hashish effects.

Dontas and Zis also made careful observations of the immediate effects of hashish smoking. The hashish they used evidently corresponded to the resinous exudate rather than the crude plant. Their studies were primarily concerned with the physiologic changes and included good comparisons of the effects on normal individuals and on those habituated to the use of the drug. Medical students in the University of

Athens were used as normal subjects. After several minutes
they experienced a dryness of the mouth and pharynx and
were seized with a violent cough which at times became
spasmodic. The face became red and there was a feeling of
warmth. Very often there was a bitter taste and the saliva
became thick. The respiratory movements became irregular,
the pulse was accelerated and increased ten to fifty pulsations
per minute. Blood pressure was usually diminished. Often
there was vertigo, nausea, and vomiting. The subjects always
felt a general weakness and numbness in the extremities.
Sometimes there was a general or partial muscular trembling
with a rapid rhythm which was periodically accelerated; at
other times the trembling was myoclonic. Almost always
there was a marked increase of the tendinous reflexes.
Throughout the experience, the intelligence remained clear.
If the person continued to smoke, psychic phenomena
appeared. Frequently there were cataleptic phenomena. In
the beginning, the smokers experienced a muscular relaxation
and a pleasant torpor. They avoided all movement, fixed
their eyes, had the air of thinking profoundly and experienced hallucinations which for the most part were agreeable
and which rendered them happy and gay. Later if the subject
continued to smoke, the psychic phenomena were accentuated, the hallucinations and paresthesias took on a general
character. One of the students thought that he was flying in
space, another thought his feet had become very large while
at the same time his pipe had become microscopic. Another
thought that the wall of a nearby house was a lake surrounded with trees. Suddenly thinking he was being mocked
he attacked the assistants. Such symptoms were always very
transitory. Several minutes after the subject had ceased to
smoke, the psychic phenomena disappeared, the other
symptoms disappeared later and in the course of several
hours they were no longer recognizable.

When smoking a stronger preparation from Serbia, one student, among other usual symptoms, was seized with a general
muscular trembling followed by a tonic contraction of the
extensor muscles of the fingers of both hands. His fingers
remained in extension for five minutes.

Another series of experiments was made on subjects who
had smoked hashish for one to four years. All of them
showed an augmentation of reflexes, pallor, fixity of expres-

sion, nervousness and variability of moods. Deprived of hashish they became nervous and despondent and their attitude belligerent. After smoking, they became gay and talkative. These individuals smoked hashish almost every day, sometimes by cigarettes but most frequently by narghile.*

When studying such cases in the laboratory and comparing them with subjects unaccustomed to hashish, it was noted that the nervous phenomena were less marked although there was a distinct augmentation of reflexes.

Dreury recently described an instance of marihuana psychosis with sexual stimulation and marked schizophrenic coloring.

Marihuana smoking as a social problem and as a subject for psychiatric analysis has been similarly studied by Bromberg, a psychiatrist at Bellevue Hospital. According to him, the chief effect of smoking is an intoxication of transitory nature and relatively uniform symptomatology. A period of anxiety is developed in ten to thirty minutes and is associated with restlessness and hyperactivity. A few minutes of this and the subject begins to feel more calm, develops a definite euphoria, becomes talkative, exhilarated and filled with a vivid sense of happiness.

Walking becomes effortless. The paresthesias and changes in bodily sensations help to give an astounding feeling of lightness to the limbs and body. Elation continues: he laughs uncontrollably and explosively for brief periods of time without at times the slightest provocation: if there is a reason it quickly fades, the point of the joke is lost immediately. Speech is rapid, flighty, the subject has the impression that his conversation is witty, brilliant; ideas flow quickly. Conclusions to questions seem to appear ready-formed and surprising in their clarity. The feeling of clarity is, of course, spurious: it is merely a subjective feeling. When the user wishes to explain what he has thought, there is only confusion. The rapid flow of ideas gives the impression of brilliance of thought and observation. The flighty ideas are not deep enough to form an engram that can be recollected—hence the confusion on trying to remem-

* waterpipe

ber what was thought. The smoker is seized with the desire to impart his experiences to others; he wishes in some way to transmit the glory and the thrill. Activities speed up tremendously and time is slow in passing: there is a feeling of changed reality. Sex excitement consists in the fact that the sexual objects in his environment become extraordinarily desirable. At the stage (about twenty to thirty minutes after starting) he may begin to have visual hallucinations which may start as misinterpretations and illusions. Characteristically there are at first flashes of light of amorphous forms of vivid color which evolve and develop into geometric figures, shapes, human faces, and pictures of great complexity. The depth of the color and its unusually arresting tone strike the subject. After a longer or shorter time, lasting up to two hours, the smoker becomes drowsy, falls into a dreamless sleep and awakens with no physiologic after-effects and with a clear memory of what had happened during the intoxication.

Bromberg himself smoked two marihuana cigarettes within forty minutes and experienced a pronounced lightness in the head immediately after the second. In general, the sensations experienced were typical.

New thoughts seem to come from the background with a startling clarity and speed. The imagery I have is so luminously clear it stands out in the background like sharply cut figures in a frieze.

The uniform symptomatology of cannabis links up the psychotic states, the experimental findings and the effects obtained by the casual user. From a clinical view point the importance of this symptomatology is that when it occurs in a mental picture (such as a schizophrenia with toxic features) it can be recognized as such because of its almost specific distortion of the clinical picture. The relationship of the personality reaction to the physiological changes due to the drug in the resulting clinical picture becomes obvious in studying mental reactions where marihuana is a factor.

The cases of intoxication are considered to fall into three clinical categories as follows: (1) Intoxications illustrating any or all of the characteristic symptoms; (2) reactive states to these features of the intoxication; (3) toxic psychoses which seem usually to be the admixture of the toxic effects of the drug to a basic cyclothymic (manic-depressive) or schizophrenic reaction.

Eleven illustrative cases are given in considerable detail. The first group consisted of three negroes who had been smoking "reefers." Two of them had appealed to the police when they became alarmed at their peculiar sensations; the third had been taken in custody by police after he was seen following women in the park. Excitement, disorientation, visual hallucinations and sexual excitement characterized these cases. All were discharged in one to several days with no evidence of psychosis. A second group of two cases illustrated mental reactions to the changed somatic sensations which the patient experienced. Suicidal impulses and homosexual tendencies characterized both cases. The third group comprised cases of psychotic conditions in which marihuana intoxication provided a characteristic coloring to the mental picture.

Fraenkel studied the hashish intoxication according to a scheme of psychiatric analysis based on the Rorschach test. This test involves the interpretation of ink spots and is considered to show the particular direction of the variations of emotion. For instance, in some cases sexual emotivity is manifested, in other cases the maternal instincts. Subjects under the influence of hashish, in interpreting images, attribute an abnormally significant importance to details. The detail tends to break its boundaries, it tends to emancipation. Accordingly, it ceases to be a detail. Interpretations of detail are collectively reduced and, in turn, changed in character. It no longer simply stimulates affectivity, it becomes epic in character.

of his lungs. After this, deep sleep ensues, lasting for many hours, even as many as fourteen or fifteen, without intervals of wakefulness. One of the most constant and marked symptoms in poisoning in man is the sensation of prolongation of time, so that minutes seem like hours, and, in addition to this, a peculiar separation of the mental powers occurs, during which both hemispheres of the brain seem to think differently on the same subject. If the dose be very large, the respirations are slowed very considerably, but no death from the use of cannabis by man is on record, and enormous amounts have been given to the lower animals without causing a lethal effect.[1] Applied to a mucous membrane, it acts as a severe irritant, and then as a local anesthetic, but the primary effect is so powerful as to prevent its application to mucous membranes for the relief of pain.

Therapeutics.—Cannabis is one of the best additions to cough mixtures that we possess, as it quiets that *tickling in the throat*, and yet does not constipate nor depress the system as does morphine. In advanced *phthisis* it is justifiable to keep the patient constantly in a state of quiet comfort by its use. For the relief of *pain*, particularly that depending on nerve disturbance, hemp is very valuable. Before the introduction of antipyrine and its congeners, tincture of gelsemium and the tincture or extract of cannabis were our best remedies in the treatment of *migraine*. The gelsemium in such cases should be given in full dose, 20 drops (1.3) of the tincture, and be followed by 10 to 20 drops (0.6–1.3) of the fluidextract of cannabis, it being known that the sample about to be used is active. After this dose of gelsemium the patient should be carefully watched, lest he suffer from an excessive influence of the drug, as such an amount may produce great depression in susceptible persons. In true *migraine* with hemianopsia this treatment is often most effectual in aborting the attack. The prevention of further attacks is to be attained by the use of smaller amounts of the cannabis during the intervals, the gelsemium only being used at the onset of the symptoms. In *paralysis agitans* cannabis may be used to quiet the tremors, and in *spasm of the bladder*, due to cystitis or nervousness, it often gives great relief. In *sexual impotence*, not dependent upon organic disease, it is said to be of value combined with strychnine or nux vomica and ergot. It acts as a nervous sedative in *exophthalmic goiter*.

In *headaches* at the *menopause* cannabis is useful, and if the headaches are associated with constipation and anemia, iron and aloes should be given simultaneously. Where headaches are due to *retinal asthenopia* a very useful prescription, according to de Schweinitz, is as follows:

R—Tincturæ nucis vomicæ . . . . f ℥ij (8.0)
Tincturæ cannabis . . . . f ℥ij (8.0).—M.
S.—15 drops (1.0), in water, twice or thrice a day.

[1] The author has injected as much as 5 drams of a fluidextract, active in the does of 10 minims to man, into the jugular vein of a small dog without producing death.

From Hobart Amory Hare, M.D., Practical Therapeutics, *Philadelphia, 1922.*

III

THERAPEUTIC EXCURSIONS

Western medicine having few effective sedatives and analgesics before the latter part of the 1800s relied heavily on opiates and cannabis products. These drugs were used mostly for purposes of sedation and analgesia.

The introduction of parenteral techniques of administration made the water-soluble opiates vastly more popular than the alcohol- or fat-soluble cannabis preparations. Although the opiates were stronger and more reliable, they were, unfortunately, physically addicting and tolerance-producing.

The advent of synthetic sedative and analgesic drugs, while having more specific actions, unfortunately increased the liabilities of toxic reactions or abuse. The allure of the new, but toxic, pre-empted the safe but occasionally erratic marijuana products.

Cannabis products, while possibly habituating, are comparatively innocuous, non-toxic, and minimally tolerance-producing. Further clinical therapeutic study of cannabis products is needed to evaluate their efficacy in the treatment and palliation of various ailments.

The progression of papers demonstrates the slow progress and growth of sophistication of uses and observations. Walton climactically summarizes the therapeutic applications before medicine and science dropped into a generation of ignorance as a result of the 1937 tax act.

The comprehensiveness and knowledge then declines through a study of synthetic homologs with five institutionalized epileptic children, and ends in a dialogue between a psychiatrist and his patient who clandestinely obtains crude, illicit marijuana to substitute it for her alcoholic habit.

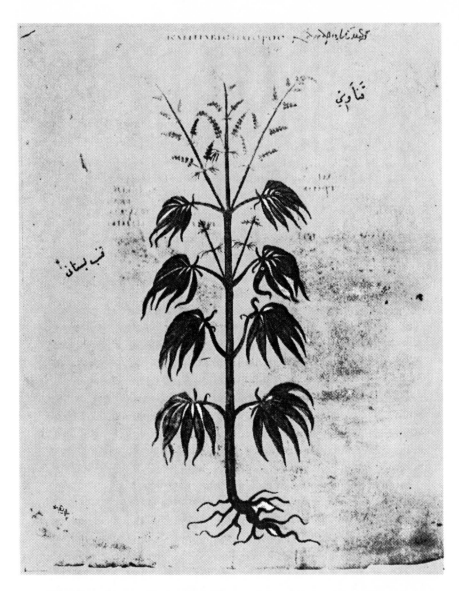

The first known botanical illustration of Cannabis sativa, *dating from the first century A.D. From a manuscript of Dioscorides'* Constantinopolitanus *in the British Museum.*

Report of the Ohio State Medical Committee on Cannabis Indica

BY R.R. McMEENS, M.D.

As chairman of the committee, appointed at the last session of the Ohio State Medical Society, to report upon Cannabis Indica, I have to say that no extended or adequate efforts have been made, either by myself or the other members of the committee, in soliciting the concurrence of the profession at large, with the view of ascertaining and collaborating the opinions entertained, or practical results observed, from the use of this remarkable and renowned exotic, and accordingly can offer but a partial and imperfect report at this time.

However, as the medicinal properties and therapeutical value of this abnegated and nearly obsolete agent has engaged much of my attention and inquiry for several years, and been somewhat frequently administered and attested by me, I feel too great an interest in the subject to allow so favorable an opportunity to pass without endeavoring to enlist a more general interest and co-operation in the further investigation of this peculiar, potent and misapprehended article.

I shall therefore only attempt to submit a brief historical sketch of the plant, with an abstract of its physiological effects, modes of preparation, therapeutical applications, reports of cases, and personal experience, derived from the very limited sources of information placed at my command, with the object of fulfilling my obligations to the Society, and adding whatever of consequence or certainty I can to the progress and perfection of the medical armamentarium.

Reprinted from the *Transactions of the Fifteenth Annual Meeting of the Ohio State Medical Society at Ohio White Sulphur Springs, June 12 to 14, 1860*, pp. 75-100.

History.   The Cannabis Indica, or Indian Hemp, is alleged to be one
of the most ancient medicinal substances and Oriental luxuries on record, and was resorted to by the voluptuary for the
production of pleasure, and by the valetudinarian for the
palliation of pain. "Herodotus mentions the hemp plant, and
states that the Scythians, who cultivated it, made themselves
garments of it. He also adds, that they threw the seeds on
red-hot stones, and used the perfumed vapor thereby obtained as a bath, which excited them to excess of exaltation.
This is supposed to be produced by the intoxicating properties of its smoke." *(Pereira on Cannabis Indica.)* Dr. Royle
mentions that the hemp might have been used as the assuager
of grief, of which Homer speaks. Dr. Simpson says the
anodyne, ecstatic and anaesthetic effects of Indian hemp, and
the various preparations made from it, have long been known
in Africa and Asia. He states that "Sir Joseph Banks says it is
always taken in Barbary, when it can be procured, by
criminals condemned to suffer amputation; and it is said to
enable those wretches to bear the rough operations of an
unfeeling executioner better than we Europeans can the keen
knife of our most skillful surgeons." M. Julien lately pointed
out to the French Academy an old Chinese work, proving
that, 1500 years ago, a preparation of hemp was employed
medicinally in China to annul the pain attendant upon
cauterization and surgical operations. The wonderful power
of endurance of the Hindu devotees, appears to have been
sometimes produced by the influence of this powerful drug.
Some high Biblical commentators maintain that the gall and
vinegar, or myrrhed wine, offered to our Saviour immediately
before his crucifixion, was in all probability a preparation of
hemp, and even speak of its earlier use. *(Obstetric works.)* It
is also alleged that during the Crusades it was frequently used
by the Saracen warriors to stimulate them to the work of
slaughter.

The botanical relations of the plant appear to have been
somewhat involved in a confusion of the several varieties of
its class; but it is at present conceded by most, if not all,
distinguished botanists, to be identical with the Cannabis
Sativa of Linnaeus. Pereira believes the differences to depend
upon locality and cultivation, and cannot be considered
specific. Dr. Wood remarks, in his work on Pharmacology,
that the plant is a native of the interior of Asia, but

cultivated in many parts of the world, and to a considerable extent in our own Western States, but that it is only the product of the plant grown in the East Indies that is used medicinally; while Dr. Dunglison states that the use of Cannabis Indica is unknown in Western Europe, and it is questionable whether the hemp of that region, or of this country, be possessed of the same properties. Dr. O'Shaughnessy, who has had the most ample opportunities of observation, from a long residence in this Indies, asserts that the extraordinary symptoms produced by the Oriental plant, depend upon a resinous secretion with which it abounds, and which seems to be wholly absent in the European plant. This absence of the resinous secretion, and consequent want of narcotic power, is ascribed to difference of climate. Messrs. Smith, of Edinburgh, satisfied themselves that the resin contained in itself the whole properties of the plant. Dr. Fronmueller says, the external appearances of Indian and European hemp are the same, as are their botanical characters. The differences described by many authors, are probably due to local causes only. The only real difference is the quantity of narcotic resin which is secreted by particular glands, like the lupulin in the hop plant. This resin is called in India, *churrus.* Its quantity increases with the southern direction.

Mr. Donovan made numerous experiments with hemp cultivated by himself, and was satisfied that the domestic hemp is quite destitute of the principle which renders the Indian plant so desirable to the voluptuous people of the East. To the impurity of the hemp, is to be attributed the diversity of opinion as to its operation and benefit in disease. An English author remarks that very little, if any, genuine hemp can be found in Europe; and the same fact will undoubtedly apply to this country. The active principles, according to Dr. Wood, consist in a volatile oil, and a peculiar resin called *cannabin.* "That the former has narcotic properties, is to be inferred from the effects of the odor of the plant. The latter is a neuter substance, having a somewhat fragrant odor, especially when heated, and a warm, bitterish subacrid and balsamic taste. It is insoluble in water, but soluble in alcohol and ether, and from its alcoholic solution is precipitated white by water."

Physiological Effects. Dr. John Bell, of New Hampshire, published an able and somewhat elaborate article in the Boston *Medical and Surgical Journal,* of the effects of the drug, experimentally produced upon himself, by taking a moderately large dose of Tilden & Co.'s extract, and can consequently be cited as a reliable exposition of personal and professional experience.*

Dr. Fronmueller states that physiological experiments on healthy persons, instituted by Lanslerer, Beron, Rech, Wolff, Indee, Schroff, and himself and others, show more or less a disturbance in the digestive tract, affection of the nervous system, with convulsive movements and sudden shocks, congestions of the brain, confused ideas, excited imagination, with frequently changing pictures, torpor and sleep, the cerebral symptoms being more constant, while the others vary to a great extent, sometimes nothing being mentioned but a few confused ideas, followed by sleep.

Bayard Taylor, the ubiquitous traveler and popular writer, in a work entitled "The Lands of the Saracen," gives a highly ornate and exquisite delineation of the physical sensations and mental phantasmagoria produced by an extreme dose of the Oriental preparation of the drug. The experiment was made by himself and two friends, while sojourning at Damascus. He had, on a previous occasion, in Egypt, subjected himself to a very moderate influence of the same article, which, he states, after "provoking a wonderfully keen perception of the ludicrous in the most simple and familiar objects," as gradually subsided as it came, overcoming the senses with a soft and pleasant drowsiness, eventuating in deep and refreshing sleep. The description of his second trial is too poetically and elaborately depicted to be introduced in a report of this character, but a summary of the prominent phenomena will serve to show the striking analogy, as portrayed in the account given by Drs. Bell and Fronmueller, already referred to. The same rapid scintillations of thought, brilliant coruscations of light, shifting adumbrations of scenery, and transient flashes of lucid intervals, eddying through the brain in inextricable confusion, are observed and illustrated in both cases. He states, they commenced by taking a teaspoonful each of the mixture, procured by a servant. As this was about the quantity taken in Egypt, and the effect then had been so slight, they had no fears of its being an overdose. He says, "The strength of the drug, however, must have been far greater in this instance, for whereas I could in the former case distinguish no flavor but that of sugar and rose-leaves, I now found the taste intensely bitter and repulsive to the palate. We allowed the paste to dissolve slowly on our tongues, and sat sometime quietly waiting the result. But, having been taken on a full stomach, its operation was hindered, and after the lapse of nearly an hour, we could not detect the least change in our feelings. My friends loudly expressed their conviction of the humbug of hasheesh, but I, unwilling to give up the experiment at this point, proposed that we should take an additional half spoonful, and follow it with a cup of hot tea, which, if there were really any virtue in the preparation, could not fail to call it into action. This was done, though not without some misgivings, as we were all ignorant of the precise quantity which constituted a dose, and the limits within which the drug could be taken with safety." This last portion was taken at ten o'clock at night. Soon after he became sensible of its operation by experiencing a nervous thrill suddenly shooting through the system, accompanied with a burning sensation at the pit of the stomach. Among the many and remarkable illusions and sensations he so vividly and minutely describes, the following striking condition of the perceptive faculties is worthy of notice and consideration: He says, "I was conscious of two distinct conditions of being in the same moment; yet, singular as it may seem, neither conflicted with the other. My enjoyment of the visions was complete and absolute—undisturbed by the faintest doubt of their reality; while in some other chamber of my brain, Reason sat coolly watching them, and heaping the liveliest ridicule on their fantastic features—one set of nerves was thrilled with the bliss of the gods, while another was convulsed with unquenchable laughter at that very bliss." About midnight, the influence of the drug had reached the acme of its power; and about three o'clock in the morning, he sank into stupor—rather more than five hours after the hasheesh began to take effect. He lay thus all the following day and night, only once arousing sufficiently to drink two cups of coffee and making an attempt to dress himself, of which he did not retain the least knowledge. On the morning of the second day, after a sleep of thirty hours, he awoke, as he remarks, "with a system utterly prostrate and unstrung, and a brain clouded with the

lingering images of my visions." He states that he subsequently learned that he had taken a sufficient quantity for
six men. One of his companions, as soon as the drug took
effect, was suddenly metamorphosed into a locomotive;
which impression continued, and kept him in a violent state
of imitative exertion, until overcome by the somniferic or
stupefactive influences of the narcotic. This circumstance and
singular vagary, I shall have cause to refer to hereafter, when
treating of its therapeutical application. The other individual,
an Englishman, retired, on the first intimation of its action,
immediately to his room, where he remained, in company
with his wife, during its operation, and refused ever after to
make any disclosure of his conduct; in consequence of which
it might be inferred, from the reputed properties of the drug,
to have been of an aphrodisiacal character.

Dr. O'Shaughnessy, to whom is entitled the honor of
having first brought the article before the notice of the
profession as a remedy, in the various experiments made
upon himself and upon animals, observes that the general
effects on man are, usually, alleviation of pain, remarkable
augmentation of appetite, aphrodisia, and great mental cheerfulness.

Modes of   The defective pharmaceutic processes employed by the
Preparation. inhabitants of its native countries, render its preparations of
very different strength, and admixtures of various foreign
substances make its effects uncertain. A specimen obtained
from Damascus, contained about twenty-five percent of
opium, a considerable quantity of camphor and spices, and
nearly half was a mixture of rancid butter and extract of
hemp. The substance widely known in in this country under
the Arabic name of *Hasheesh,* is obtained by boiling the
leaves and flowers of the plant with butter, and when pure
and carefully prepared, is said to be a very active preparation.
The extracts prepared in this country from the Indian plant,
contain all the properties of the hasheesh, and are every way
preferable to it. The U.S. Pharmacopeia recognizes only an
alcoholic extract, under the name of Extract of Hemp, or
Extractum Cannabis. The Tincture of Hemp may be made by
dissolving six drachms of the extract in a pint of officinal
alcohol (sp. gr. 0.835). The dose equivalent to one grain of
extract is about 20 minims, or 40 drops. Dr. O'Shaughnessy

gave 10 drops of the tincture every half hour in cholera, and a fl. drachm as often in tetanus, until effects were produced (Wood). Tilden & Co.'s Fluid Extract is probably most frequently used in this country at the present time, but so far as my experience extends, it has proved ineffective, if not entirely inutile, in almost any quantity. I have ever preferred, in my own practice, the alcoholic extract (Herring's), and have never been disappointed in obtaining its peculiar effects. The best forms of preparation or combination I consider to be that of the tincture, or pills of the extract, rolled in a powder of the hemp. Sometimes I have dissolved it in ether and water, or chloroform. In cases of children, I have incorporated it in simple syrup, or the aromatic Syrup Rhei, or Syrup Aurantii. In this affection, three grains of the extract, dissolved in one ounce of proof spirits, one drachm of which is to be given every half hour, until the patient be brought under its influence. For its beneficial effects upon this direful disease, he refers to fourteen cases, nine of which recovered.

Professor Miller, of Edinburgh, says, "My own experience speaks loudly in favor of the hemp in tetanus." He believes it valueless as an anodyne, as well as hypnotic, in ordinary circumstances, but thinks its virtues consist in a power of controlling inordinate muscular spasm.

Dr. Duncan says he used the hemp in 1846, in the Royal Infirmary in Edinburgh, as a calmative and hypnotic. The object was in general obtained, and no evil results followed. Hemp was given in other wards of the Infirmary for a like purpose, and with like results.

Mr. Donovan was convinced of the beneficial effects of hemp, particularly in neuralgia, in his own case as well as in that of others.

Dr. Christison has administered hemp in many instances, and has observed that it produces sleep, and that its power over uterine contraction is very marked and powerful in many instances.

Dr. Simpson states that he had been induced to try hemp, in consequence of Dr. Churchill stating that it possessed powers similar to those of ergot of rye, in arresting hemorrhage from the uterus. In the few cases of labor in which he tried it, parturient action seemed to be very marked and distinctly increased.

Dr. Gregor gave the hemp in sixteen cases of labor, in seven of which it succeeded well.

Dr. West says the hemp is extremely serviceable in controlling neuralgic pain, and recommends it, combined with camphor, in dysmenorrhoea and in flexions of the uterus, when there is excessive menstruation, in connection with pain. Its power in checking uterine hemorrhage is favorably spoken of by many, and in some cases in which it would not do to give the ergot of rye.

Dr. J. P. Willis, of Royalston, from whose communication, in the Boston *Medical and Surgical Journal,* the foregoing therapeutical facts are chiefly abstracted, says, "I have used the Indian hemp for some time and in many diseases, especially in those connected with the womb, in neuralgic dysmenorrhoea, in menorrhagia, in cessation of menstruation, where the red discharge alternates with uterine leucorrhoea of long continuance, in repeated attacks of uterine hemorrhage, in all cases of nervous excitability, and in tedious labor, where there is restlessness of the patient, with ineffectual propulsive action of the uterus." He further remarks, "Authors generally attribute puerperal convulsions to some irritation caused by the uterus, coming on during gestation or after delivery. From these statements, I was led to the use of hemp in puerperal convulsions, having also seen its beneficial effects in convulsions in general, after all the common remedies had been tried without relief. I made use of it in chorea, more particularly in that form connected with hysteria, or partaking of the character of both; in delirium tremens, both in the period of excitement and after the delirium subsides, and where long-continued watchfulness and great mental excitement continue; in mania, where there is watchfulness and excitement; in shaking palsy; in whooping-cough, and all coughs of a spasmodic character. In phthisis, and other lung diseases, it may be given, especially where opium has ceased to procure sleep."

The late Dr. E. Dresbach, of Tiffin, made use of the article as early as 1847, and was the first to administer it in practice, so far as I am able to ascertain, in this region of country; and as I remember from familiar converse with him, was favorably impressed with its curative powers, especially in diseases of a nervous character. My first experience with the remedy was its recommendation by him in an inveterate case of infantile convulsions, in which he was consulted, and where it acted most promptly and effectively, after everything else had failed to afford any relief. This interesting case, together with three others of a similar nature, in which it had proved equally successful, were communicated by me and published in the June number of the *Western Lancet* (Vol. xvii., 1856). Dr. Dresbach, at this time, expressed an undoubted confidence in its efficacy in general nervous disorders, particularly of a persistent or paroxysmal character. However, Dr. J. A. McFarland, of the same place, and for many years his immediate confrere and intimate friend, in reply to inquiries made by me in February last, says, "My experience with the article is confined to a single case (nervous irritability), in which it was suggested by our old friend, Dr. Dresbach, but in which its effects were not very decided. It was for a time frequently employed by Dr. Dresbach, especially in derangements of the nervous system, and I am not sure that his confidence in the remedy was increased in proportion to his experience. My impression is that the contrary is true."

Dr. C. E. Buckingham reports, in the Boston *Medical and Surgical Journal* (Vol. lviii. March number, 1858), a case of acute rheumatism, in which he had experimentally used the medicine. In the discussion that ensued before the Boston Society for Medical Observation, the following facts were elicited: Dr. B. stated that he had been making numerous experiments of late with this drug, as to its powers of relieving pain, and it had answered so well in other cases that he wished to use it in this. He thought that opium might perhaps have relieved the pain more quickly, but having bad results in other cases with opium, he felt disinclined to use it. As to Cannabis Indica, Dr. Buckingham said that he thought the activity of the medicine depended very much upon the parcel from which it was taken. When used in five-grain doses, he thought it a good substitute for opium. He was first led to use it from results obtained by Dr. Jno. C. Dalton, Jr., who took it in doses, commencing at 20 drops of the tincture, three times daily, increasing the amount to 100 drops three times daily. The use of it in the latter dose induced a peculiar, prolonged and agreeable sleep.

Dr. Cabot said that he had employed it, and never saw any result obtained from less than three-grain doses.

Reports of Cases.

Dr. Clarke asked if any peculiar mental effect was produced. Dr. Buckingham had not seen any; he had never given
the medicine in over five-grain doses at a time. He commonly
orders one or two grains every hour, till the pain is relieved.
The apothecaries commonly consider three grains as the
maximum dose. He had not found it to produce any peculiar
effect on the skin, nor to act as a diuretic.

Dr. Clarke said that of late the Cannabis Indica was much
used in the treatment of the insane, and that it had been
found to be exceedingly variable in its effects.

Dr. Buckingham remarked, that as prepared by one or two
London chemists, the drug was very even and powerful;
generally it was not so. The best of it only dissolves in
chloroform, ether, or the strongest alcohol. The best way of
making a mixture, was to dissolve the drug in chloroform,
and then add to its simple syrup. In about twenty-four hours
it will settle to the bottom, but it may readily be shaken up
again.

Dr. H. J. Donahoo, of Sandusky, Ohio, read a paper on the
use of Cannabis Indica before the Eric County Medical
Society, in August, 1857, in which he details a full history of
two interesting cases, where he had used the medicine with
decided effect and complete success. The following is a copy
of his paper, as read:

> "B.O., a bookbinder, says he has been troubled with
> an obscure affection of the stomach for the past year,
> and had submitted to almost every kind of treatment,
> without any marked improvement in his general health.
> Morphine had given him more relief than anything else,
> and he was fast getting into the habit of keeping himself
> under its influence. The case seemed to me to be one of
> gastrodynia. I accordingly ordered anodynes and anti-
> spasmodics, with very little relief. Finally this attack
> subsided, and he enjoyed a respite of some ten days
> from the attack of his enemy. He usually had warning of
> an attack some hours before it became fully developed.
> Damp, rainy weather scarcely ever failed to bring with it
> an attack of his disease. Being conscious of an approach-
> ing attack, he sent for me. I advised him to abandon the
> use of morphia; for, as I stated before, he was not only
> contracting the habit of using it constantly, but it was

deranging the entire economy, by locking up the secretions of the liver and producing a jaundiced condition, with constipation. I prescribed a laxative, combined with extract of cicuta and hyosciamus, and instructed him to procure some charcoal, and take a dessert-spoonful, in case he should have an attack, and to repeat it, if necessary.

"As anticipated, he was seized with a most terrible attack. I was sent for in the night, and found my patient suffering as much, one would think, as mortal flesh could bear. His friends said they would much rather see him die than be compelled to witness a continuance of such agony. I administered chloroform by inhalation, until he was brought fully under its influence, but he soon came out of its anaesthetic influence. It was repeated, but the effect soon subsided. I instructed his nurse how to administer it, and left the patient. Next morning, much to my surprise, I found he had suffered so much that he had been kept almost constantly under the influence of the chloroform. His countenance looked care-worn and haggard, his pulse was feeble, and the heat of the body was below the normal standard. As a kind of dernier resort, I prescribed the 'Tincture of Cannabis Indica;' dose twenty drops every three hours. In one hour after the first dose was taken, his pains grew easy, and before the time arrived for him to take the second dose, he was almost entirely free from pain. He took the second dose, however, but did not find it necessary to take any more. I instructed him to take a dose of the Cannabis, in case he should have any premonitions of a return of his trouble. He remained here some six weeks after his last attack, and had succeeded in preventing a recurrence of his disease by following the above course. The action of his bowels became regular, and his general health improved as rapidly as himself, his friends, or his physician could have desired.

"On Sept. 24th, 1857, I was requested to visit Col. McK., in consultation with Dr. Austin, the attending physician. He was suffering very severely from an attack of spasmodic asthma. We prescribed the smoking of stramonium, but this, contrary to our expectations, gave no relief. We then ordered equal quantities of Hoffman's anodyne and comp. tinct. opii, dose one teaspoonful every hour. This gave him much relief, but it soon lost its magic power; and we found that something else must be tried. I advised the use of the Cannabis Indica; the doctor acquiesced, and we accordingly gave one grain of the extract every three hours. Its effects were almost magical; the patient became quiet, breathed easily, and assured us, next morning, that he had never been so happy, the same length of time, as while under the influence of the Cannabis; to use his own words, 'he was in Heaven all night.' With a view to excite expectoration and correct existing hepatic derangement, we ordered a pill composed of submur-hydrarg, Doveri and ipecac. This prescription relieved him somewhat, produced nausea and vomiting, and finally acted upon the bowels. Towards evening he grew restless, and was ordered to resume the use of the Cannabis, in connection with the above pills. With these instructions, we left the patient for the night. About one o'clock in the morning, I was sent for in great haste. I found the patient suffering from a most terrible spasm. His features wore a sharp, pinched and cadaverous appearance. The inquiry was made, with much alarm, if I could relieve him. I responded in the affirmative, and immediately pro-ceeded to administer a pill of the extract Cannabis Indica (one grain to the pill); repeated the pill in one hour. This relieved the spasms, and by giving one of the pills every two hours, I succeeded in keeping up the effect, so that he not only breathed well, but slept tranquilly until morning. He afterwards occasionally took a pill of the Cannabis, but, with the exception of a little comp. tinct. opii, to relieve some pain of the bowels, caused by a slight bilious diarrhoea, he required no further treatment. I am not aware of the Cannabis having before been used in asthma, having in vain searched for authority for using it in his disease. If the Cannabis proves as useful in other hands as it has in mine, asthmatics will bless the hand that administered it. I have likewise frequently prescribed the hemp in cases of hysteria, and have always been pleased with its effects.

Dr. Robert Andrews, of North New Salem, communicates the history of an interesting case to Dr. J. P. Willis, in which the latter had recommended the use of the hemp, with evident success, and was published by him in the Boston *Medical and Surgical Journal* of Sept., 1859. The case was one of placenta praevia, and after a great loss of blood by hemorrhage, was delivered by a resort to podalic version, and the hemorrhage subsequently controlled by the use of a swathe and compress, cold applications, rest, etc. On the third day after delivery, he found her doing well, and dismissed her. Ten days afterwards, he remarks as follows:

I was again called, July 28th, and found her with headache and nervous excitement, which I thought were caused by her having taken cold, and permitting her milk to dry up too soon. I gave her a cathartic and some powders of camphor, nitre and valerian. I heard no more from her till August 2d, when I was called to visit her in the night, and found her delirious, crying 'fire,' 'murder,' etc. From this time to August 19th, I saw her every second or third day, and used the ordinary remedies in such cases, with little if any mitigation of her symptoms. August 20th she was moved from Freysville to her father's, in Orange. I there saw her almost every day till August 27th, when you were called in consultation. You undoubtedly recollect the peculiar, restless condition in which you and D. C. found her at that time. She had actually worn the flesh from her elbows and hips by the constant rubbing of them together. She had gnawed her finger nails and the ends of her fingers till they bled. She refused to take anything which she suspected was medicine, or from any one whom she thought was a doctor. Her bowels were torpid. Under these circumstances, the 'hemp' which you prescribed, had a wonderful effect in quieting the nervous system, and the dose was so small that we succeeded in getting it down in her food. The torpid condition of the liver and bowels was removed by small doses of podophyllin, administered daily in the same manner as the hemp. The hemp was given in doses sufficient to keep her quiet. Some days one dose was sufficient; other days it would be necessary to repeat the dose once or twice. Under the above treatment she gradually improved till Sept. 12th, when she was dismissed permanently cured.

Dr. M. D. Mooney, of Georgia, reports that he has used the following prescription in four cases of gonorrhoea, and was successful in every case in from five to seven days:

> R Sugar of milk, ... ℥ ss.
> Extr. Cannabis Indica, ... xx grs.
> Mix well and divide in 60 powders.
> One to be taken every three or four hours.

This prescription, he says, will relieve the most obstinate cases in a short time.

Dr. O. C. Kendricks, Superintendent of the Northern Lunatic Asylum, in the fifth annual report of that institution, says: "We have made brief trial of the Cannabis Indica (Herring's Extract), in the cases to which it seemed applicable, but as yet with indifferent success."

The following case of hysterical insanity, which came under my care in February, 1859, I introduce as being one in which the patient was under no medical influences whatever, and on which the hemp acted with almost magical power, and with complete success.

Daniel Van F——, an unsophisticated and eccentric nondescript of the genus "homo," became infatuated, at a rather mature age, with the idea that he possessed extraordinary talents and ingenuity as a mechanician. He accordingly abandoned his trade of carpenter and joiner, and concentrated all the energies of his mind in designing the model of an invention of his, to supersede the popular patterns in use at the time, as planning-machines. After long and arduous labor, and repeated failures, to satisfactorily consummate his project, he subsequently irretrievably involved his property and impoverished his family, by the expenses incurred in obtaining a patent-right for what he conceived to be the most important discovery of the day, while the golden dreams that filled his imagination knew no bounds. But, after many sore and heart-sickening disappointments and overwhelming misfortunes, together with the upbraidings and bitter taunts of an unsympathizing family and unfeeling public, his already overtaxed intellect began to stagger, and his spirits to sink under the weight of his heavy sorrows. At this time he was seized with symptoms of pneumonic inflammation, which his wife had treated with considerable skill and success. But becoming alarmed from the debility that ensued, and an unusual display of irascibility of temper and incoherency of language, I was requested to visit him.

I found him a good deal prostrated, pulse soft and excited, expectoration free and favorable, tongue somewhat coated, surface moist and pliable, respiration as full, easy and unobstructed as would be anticipated. His mind was morbidly active, occasionally inconsistent, and evidently, from his manner and expressions that escaped him, impressed with suspicions of nefarious designs on the part of his family. He had been, for several nights, unable to sleep and extremely restless. I prescribed Dover's powder and hyosciamus in combination, to meet the above indications, and decoction of senega to facilitate expectoration. I was then formally dismissed, and assured that I would be duly notified if further assistance should be required. I did not again hear from him for ten days, when his wife waited upon me, and informed me that his cough had about disappeared, but that his mental disquietude had constantly increased, and at present he appeared to be wholly insane. He remained resolutely in bed, persisted in covering his head and face with the bedclothes, and obstinately refused to see me or any other physician, asserting that we were all in league with the rest of community to encompass his death—that the Lord had visited him in person, and warned him of the conspiracy. He refused to take any nourishment, and but rarely a drink of water. He had sent for a Methodist exhorter, of about his own calibre and character, to read the Bible; while they both sang hymns and prayed without ceasing. I accompanied her home. He received me coolly but not unkindly, and watched me closely but furtively. All my efforts at flattery and familiarity failed to secure his confidence, to persuade him to partake of food, or to convince him of the fallacy of his fears. The influence of his spiritual adviser and the importunities of his wife had no avail. I then attempted a variety of subterfuges, to secure the introduction of a saline cathartic, as he had become very constipated, but without success; and, as a dernier resort, assumed a determined and dictatorial manner, threatened and even exercised some force; but he maintained the same stoical, silent and imperturbable indifference. After the lapse of near forty-eight hours, he became so exhausted and feeble that some fluids were forced down him, together with a mixture of senna and salts, after the operation of which, I succeeded in administering a drachm of laudanum, with an equal quantity of tinct. valerian in brandy. This failed to procure sleep or have any other beneficial effect, but only produced a dull unnatural expression of the countenance. I then attempted to bring him under the influence of chloroform; but he so stoutly resisted its application, and avoided its inhalation, that no decided impression could be obtained. His features began to assume a haggard, contracted, and sallow hue, his hands affected with tremor, his eyes injected and their nictation spasmodic, and his whole frame greatly emaciated. He now imagined himself to be a steam-engine, and began to work both his upper and lower extremities alternately and constantly, in imitation of his fancied congener. This he continued almost without a moment's cessation for one whole night, and without a particle of sustenance. We then resorted to a concerted deception, by all present feeling his pulse and declaring the water in his boiler to be about exhausted, and expressing great fears of an approaching explosion. This, to our gratification, had the desired effect; and he blew off steam with loud and forcible expirations, and came to a stand-still, his whole body bathed in a profuse perspiration, while great drops of sweat beaded and rolled from his brow. I was prepared with one drachm of the tinct. of Cannabis Indica, which was administered in a cup of diluted coffee. He then gradually let on steam, and resumed his locomotive operations. I then left and returned in about three hours, and found him perfectly quiescent, with a relaxed and placid countenance, dilated pupils and a fixed, dreamy expression of the eye. He was obviously in a state of complete inebriation, and I remained to watch its further developments. He made no movement whatever, but would smile with his eyes fixed on vacancy, and subsequently broke out in sudden exclamations of suprise, then laugh loud and immoderately. After some hours, he sank into a deep and sonorous slumber. He awoke from an interrupted rest of six hours quite rational, but somewhat confused and extremely exhausted. A milk and brandy punch was given, and he again slept; afterwards chicken broth, some simple tonic, and he recovered without any relapse or further remedies.

Upon reading the effects of hasheesh, as described by Bayard Taylor, in which his friend was affected with a similar hallucination, as heretofore stated, I was agreeably surprised with the striking analogy of the two cases, produced by the hemp in one, and induced by disease in the other.

The *modus operandi* of the hemp in the above case, would appear to be that of substitution, the existing disorders of the cerebral and nervous centres being displaced or extinguished by the powerful and persistent impression made by the medicine upon the sentient economy of the same system. I have also derived decided benefit from the use of the hemp in a case of laryngismus stridulus, which was reported by me and published in the *Cincinnati Lancet and Observer* (Vol. ii. No. 8, August, 1859).

In a variety of forms of nervous rheumatism, I have also been very successful with the following combination of the hemp, first recommended, I believe, by Dr. Atlee of Philadelphia, and find it preferable in many cases to the preparations of opium, especially where constipated habits contraindicated their use:

R Etherial Tinct. Guiacum . . . . fl ℥j.
Etherial Tinct. Colchicum . . . . fl ʒvj.
Etherial Tinct. Cannab. Indica . . . . fl ʒij.
M—Dose 25 to 30 drops every 3 to 4 hours on
sugar.

In all forms of bronchitis, I have frequently found it one of the best adjuvants, in combination with any of the ordinary expectorant mixtures, used in that affection.

Dr. A. P. Dutcher, of Enon Valley, Pa., reports an interesting case in the *Cincinnati Lancet and Observer* (Vol. ii. No. 5, May, 1859). The patient had been afflicted with bronchitis for five years; had at this time but recovered from an aggravation of the disease, complicated with a degree of pneumonic inflammation; after the subsidence of which, he states, "that the cough and expectoration were now about the same as they had been for the last five years— troublesome and unmanageable. As she had taken every therapeutical agent known to have any power in the cure of bronchitis, and been the rounds of quackdom, I concluded, as a last resort, to try the following:

℞ Extr. Cannabis Indica . . . . fl. ℥ ss.
Alcohol . . . . fl. ℥ iv.

"A teaspoonful of the above was to be taken, three times a day, in a wine-glassful of simple syrup. From this time she recovered rapidly, and in six weeks her cough disappeared entirely, and up to the present time (Feb. 26th, 1859), a period of nine months, there has been no return, and her general health is better than it has been for six years." He concludes the article as follows: "The happy result, in this case, by the use of Cannabis, I regard as a little remarkable; for it is not often that bronchitis is cured after it has run so long, particularly in a person as old as my patient (60 years). From the trials that I have made with the article, in chronic pulmonary affections, I am favorably impressed with its virtues. It may be given in all cases to allay cough and produce sleep, as a substitute for opium, especially where this latter is contraindicated by its effects upon the brain, and by its property of checking mucous secretion."

Dr. Fronmueller, of Fuerth, makes the following remarks as the sum of his experience with the hemp:

I have used hemp many hundred times to relieve local pains of an inflammatory as well as neuralgic nature, and judging from these experiments, I have to assign to the Indian hemp a place among the so called hypnotic medicines next to opium; its effects are less intense, and the secretions are not so much suppressed by it. Digestion is not disturbed; the appetite rather increased; sickness of the stomach seldom induced; congestion never. Hemp may consequently be employed in inflammatory conditions. It disturbs the expectoration far less than opium; the nervous system is also not so much affected. The whole effect of hemp being less violent, and producing a more natural sleep, without interfering with the actions of the internal organs, it is certainly often preferable to opium, although it is not equal to that drug in strength and reliability. An alternating course of opium and Indian hemp seems particularly adapted to those cases where opium alone fails in producing the desired effect. The best form is small pills, made from the spirituous extract, with a little of the powdered leaves. The smallest dose may be set down at eight grains; a rapid increase is frequently required.

I would here introduce and direct attention to the interesting report furnished me by Dr. W. P. Kincaid, of Neville, associated with me on this subject, and whose experience with the medicine has been of a most direct and practical character. (See report of Dr. Kincaid.)

In conclusion, I would state as the result of my own experience and observation, in addition to the cases already reported and referred to, that I am fully convinced of the peculiar efficacy and pertinency of the remedy to certain pathological conditions, occupying or involving the nervous system. In those mixed and indefinable paroxysms of an hysterical nature, I have found no remedy to control or curtail them with equal promptness and permanency. In the protean and painful conditions connected with uterine disorder, I have ever found it an admirable adjuvant in their treatment, as an anodyne ingredient, in a variety of combinations. In sleeplessness, where opium is contraindicated, it is an excellent substitute. In two cases of nervous spasmodic cough, it proved efficacious, where a number of antispasmodics failed to afford any relief. In a violent case of puerperal mania, it acted most happily and beneficially in controlling the fury of the patient and in securing sleep. As a calmative and hypnotic, in all forms of nervous inquietude and cerebral excitement, it will be found an invaluable agent, as it produces none of those functional derangements or sequences that render many of the more customary remedies objectionable.

Neville, Ohio, Feb. 21, 1860

Report of
W. P. Kincaid, M.I

R. R. McMeens, M.D., Chairman Committee on Can. Ind.:

Dear Sir:

Yours of the 5th has just come to hand, and as you are now engaged in making up your report, I will, without delay, very briefly give you some of my observations upon the action of Cannabis Indica.

My attention was first directed to this medicinal agent by yourself, at the meeting of the Ohio State Medical Society, held at Sandusky, in June, 1857.

Since that time, while engaged in the practice of medicine,

I have embraced every opportunity to test its virtues in such cases as I thought it applicable.

The diseases in which I have prescribed it, and to which my observations have especially been directed, are, laryngismus stridulus, epilepsy, tetanus, hysteria and mania-a-potu.

By laryngismus stridulus, I mean spasm of the glottis, recurring at irregular intervals of from a few minutes to any period of time, either in children or adults.

My design in the use of this article has been to test its effects, separate and apart from any other medicine, given at the same time, as far as it was consistent to rely only upon one remedy.

In several instances where the symptoms were imminent, I used chloroform in conjunction with the hemp, and in those cases am unable to say whether the effects produced were the combined action of the two, or of one or the other separately, but am inclined to the opinion that they were the result of the two acting in harmony.

In one case of laryngismus stridulus, infant, aged seven and a half months (case published in the Transactions of the Oh. St. Med. Soc. of 1858), I gave the two combined for the first twenty-four hours, with marked improvement; then discontinued the chloroform, and increased the quantity of hemp, with entire cessation of the spasms after the second dose. The spasms in this case had recurred at intervals of 10 or 15 minutes for 95 days.

On the 9th of the present month, I was called some distance back into Kentucky, to see a Miss Conly, aged 18 years, of sanguine temperament, unmarried, a patient of Dr. Boner's of that State. Found her laboring under spasm of the glottis, with slight spasm of fingers and toes. These paroxysms recurred at intervals of five or six minutes, and were, in duration, from three quarters of a minute to a minute and a half. There was entire suspension of respiration during the spasm. Her pulse was very small, moderately frequent and irregular, and, while in the paroxysm, imperceptible. Extremities cold, surface pallid, pupils dilated to double their normal size, voice entirely extinct.

Her friends had encircled her bed for the previous twelve hours, momentarily expecting her exit.

The physician assured me the symptoms *now*, and frequency of the paroxysms, were about the same as they had been for the past twelve hours.

Her mother informed me, she had formerly enjoyed as good health as other girls in the neighborhood, except that she suffered rather more than usual at her catamenial periods, and about that time was very nervous.

She had taken nothing in the way of medicine or nourishment during these twelve hours, owing perhaps to the fact that all were of the impression that an effort to swallow brought on the spasms.

I suggested to Dr. Boner that this was a choice case in which to test the Can. Ind., but when I came to examine my saddle-bags, to my great disappointment and chagrin, I had none with me, and was at a distance of six or eight miles from where it could be procured.

It being a case of emergency, I could not, with prudence, wait until a messenger could go that distance and return with the hemp. I therefore put her upon chloroform and com. tinct. opii, aa 3ss, to be repeated every two hours until the Can. Ind. was obtained. Directed sinapisms to the extremities, and epispastics to the cervical and dorsal spine.

I am reliably informed there was slight improvement, the spasms being rather less frequent before the medicine arrived. On the return of the messenger, she took tinct. of the ext. 3ss, to be repeated every three hours.

After she had taken the third portion of hemp, and one additional portion of chloroform (given through a misunderstanding), the spasms ceased, and she slept well for nine hours.

When she roused up, she was again in possession of her voice, and having, from joy, talked too much, the spasms returned, but in a milder form, and soon yielded to the same prescription.

The spasms recurred, at two or three irregular periods, within the next four or five days, but soon yielded under the action of the Can. Ind., given as before.

This lady is now convalescent, it being twelve days since I first saw her, and owes, most likely, her present existence to the action of Can. Ind., or the combined effects of it and chloroform.

I have treated four cases of epilepsy with the hemp; two were permanently benefited (at least to the present time); one temporarily, and one not at all.

I will give one case in detail, and compare the others with it, for the sake of brevity, being fully satisfied that your report will be full and comprehensive within itself.

Case 1. Mr. J. K., aged 40 years; unmarried; of lymphatic temperament, and rather feeble constitution; had been subject to epilepsy for twenty years; called upon me in July, 1858, to treat him for, as he said, those "falling spells' he was subject to. He informed me they came on him at irregular intervals. Sometimes he would not have any for two or three weeks; then he would have one or two a day, or every alternate or third day, for a week or two. He was so much afflicted with them he was unable to attend to ordinary business, or go from home alone.

I put him on the tinct. Can. Ind. ʒss twice a day for two weeks, then three times a day for two weeks, when it was suspended for one week.

During the first week of treatment he had two fits, one in the second, and none in the third or fourth.

About the last of the fifth week, he had another fit, when he was again put on the hemp twice a day for five weeks; then reduced to once a day for five weeks. In these ten weeks he had no "falling spell," neither did he have any for a month after that, although he was taking nothing the last four weeks.

In December, 1858, they returned on him; and as I was not engaged in the practice of my profession that winter, I lost sight of his case until May, 1859.

He informed me, on my return to professional duties in the spring of 1859, that he had had a few of his "old spells" during the winter, but nothing like so frequent as before he took the hemp. He has only been taking the medicine occasionally the past season, as he had become tired taking it, and not having a fit more than once in three months, which did not greatly interfere with his ordinary engagements, he concluded to rest for a time, unless his "spells" got worse on him.

Case 2. Male; aged 46 years; of sanguine or bilious temperament; rather plethoric habit; married; has been subject to epilepsy for five years, recurring at intervals of about four weeks. Sometimes he had only one fit at the recurring period, and at others from two to seven.

He was put on the use of the Can. Ind. in September,

1858; given the same as in case 1, with even better results.

He has had but one fit in the past nine months; has taken no hemp for four or five months; considers himself cured. Whether he permanently cured or not, the future only will demonstrate.

Case 3. Male; aged 35 years; married; of nervous temperament; subject to fits for 17 years.

He has sometimes two or three fits a day; then will miss three or four days, and again recur upon him.

I am informed by his wife that for the past five years he has had, on an average, about fifty per year.

He took the hemp for three months without any marked improvement, when it was discontinued.

Case 4 Male; aged 38 years; married; of nervous temperament; subject to epilepsy for ten years, recurring at intervals of four or five weeks.

Treated as cases 1 and 2, with slight improvement. This patient has been taking the hemp for two and a half months, and is still under treatment.

I have given the Can. Ind. in two cases of tetanus: one idiopathic, the other traumatic. In the former I gave ʒss every three hours for six hours; then every two hours, with chloroform, for eight or ten hours, but could produce no impression upon the disease. Patient died.

In the traumatic case, its beneficial effects were very visible. The frequency and force of the paroxysms were lessened just in proportion to its constitutional effects upon the patient.

This lady took half a drachm (tinct.) every three hours, until there was dilatation of the pupils, and that peculiar expression of countenance attending the exhilarating effects of stimulus, when the spasms ceased. They returned at two or three irregular periods before convalescence, but were each time controlled by the hemp.

This was a case in which the tetanic spasms continued after the amputation of the diseased limb. The hemp was not given before the amputation. Tetanus was the result of mortification of the hand.

I have given the Can. Ind. in a few cases of hysteria, and am much pleased with its action, especially in those cases of a spasmodic character.

I have not had an opportunity of testing its effects in

delirium tremens to the extent I had desired, but so far as my observations were carried, it did not meet my expectations. It seemed to exalt the nervous excitement already present, rather than calm it; but such is the case in many instances, even with morphine.

As to its action in chorea, I have had no good opportunity of testing it, but should anticipate good results from the persevering use of it in that disease.

In conclusion, I would remark, that I regard the hemp as an excellent nervous stimulant, applicable in all diseases of a *purely* nervous character.

Yours, very respectfully,

W. P. Kincaid

The Use of Indian Hemp in the Treatment of Chronic Chloral and Chronic Opium Poisoning

BY E.A. BIRCH, M.D.

In 1887, at Calcutta, at nearly the same time, I met with two cases, both of them distressing and interesting. The first was that of a European gentleman, who I remembered to have met some two years previously, when he brought his wife from a distant district with a view to placing her under a physician in consequence of her habits as a confirmed chloral drinker. At that time I discovered that she was also a sufferer from valvular cardiac disease; but I need allude no further to her than to state that no power of persuasion or fear of consequences produced any effect. She made no real effort to overcome her vice. When denied her regular dose on two occasions, she became so outrageous, and, in her husband's opinion, so alarmingly ill, that she remained but a few days in town. Her husband then states that his wife had continued her habit, and that she ultimately died. The object of his visit was, he stated, to consult me about his heart. A very careful examination of that organ enabled me to assure him that it was healthy, though it certainly was in an irritable condition. Thus encouraged, he went on, to my amazement, to tell me that he had followed in his wife's footsteps, that he could not live without chloral, that he was utterly miserable, and that he took about forty grains daily. His depression of spirits he described as being terrible; he had frequently contemplated suicide; insomnia was almost complete, no sleep whatever being obtained without the aid of chloral, and then but little. He could take scarcely any food. The patient was a fresh, healthy-looking man, whose occupation was out-door and health-giving. He neither drank nor smoked. Change of air and scene had proved useless, but then he had never been able to release himself from his habit. I could not ascertain,

Reprinted from *Lancet*, vol. I, March 30, 1889, p. 625.

with any certainty, how long he had been addicted to chloral, but I suspected he commenced it long before his wife's death, though that event was the excuse he offered in extenuation. His organs were healthy, and worked healthily, except the functionally deranged heart.

I prescribed a sea trip, a mixture containing tinct. cannabis indica (ten minims), tinct. strophanth., and tinct. chlorof. co., with a bitter infusion, and appealed to him in the strongest language to abandon his vice. Six weeks later he returned, in much the same state, and reported that at first he had improved, but soon became intermittent in the use of his medicine, and he had not given up his chloral. He now agreed voluntarily to place himself under circumstances which admitted of surveillance and restraint. His chloral was peremptorily stopped, and he was prescribed a pill containing half a grain of ext. cannabis ind. with a few grains of the compound colocynth pill, to be taken three times a day. The result was an *immediate* improvement. The craving for the chloral had almost vanished in twenty-four hours, natural sleep returned after a few days, and he began to enjoy his food. Eventually he returned to his home and work, a happy man; but much disappointed because the name of the drug used was not communicated to him.

The second case was briefly this: I was requested by his friends to see a young Eurasian gentleman, whom I found to be a most miserable object, aged about twenty-four years, yellow, intensely anaemic, and extremely emaciated—an "exhumed corpse," in fact, lying upon a couch, suffering acute agony in every limb. His liver and spleen were both materially enlarged. His history was shortly this. Occupying a position of considerable responsibility, and compelled to reside in one of the most desolate and depressing regions of Bengal, he became a confirmed and very excessive spirit drinker till, fearing the consequences, he resolved to conquer the habit, and he did so most thoroughly, but with the frightful assistance of opium. Laudanum was the form selected, and for at all events four months prior to his coming under my notice he admitted having consumed not less than two ounces daily. His friends, who had only just rescued him from his isolated position, were quite hopeless of the possibility of recovery. Here there was the well-known train of symptoms—insomnia, anorexia, disordered bowels, conscious delusions, though there was no confusion of ideas in conversation, and so forth. Again I resorted to cannabis, commencing with only a quarter of a grain of the extract, gradually increasing it to half a grain, one grain, and one grain and a half three times a day, with the happiest result. Ability to take food and retain it soon returned, and after a time an appetite appeared; he began to sleep well; his pulse, which could not be counted at first, exhibited some volume; flesh rapidly accumulated; and after three weeks he was able to take a turn upon the verandah with the aid of a stick. After the lapse of six weeks he spoke of returning to his post, and I never saw him again.

I have never before or since had such typical cases of this class to deal with, but I have lost no opportunity of testing the cannabis in the direction indicated as far as possible, and I am satisfied of its immense value. The chief point that struck me was the *immediate* action of the drug in appeasing the appetite for the chloral or opium, and in restoring the ability to appreciate food. It seems to supply the place of the poison, to stimulate the appetite, to increase the heart's power, and thus to procure sleep indirectly, as well as directly, by its own sedative effect. Moreover, I am convinced that it is a diuretic, and that this action helped in the above cases. I prescribed the cannabis simply with a view to utilising a well-known remedy for insomnia, but it did much more than procure sleep. I think it will be found that there need be no fear of peremptorily withdrawing the deleterious drug, if hemp be employed. I know that the mere withdrawal of chloral will effect a cure, but at the expense of an interval of suffering which need not be incurred; and the same in a different degree holds true of opium. Upon one point I would insist—the necessity of concealing the name of the remedial drug from the patient, lest in his endeavour to escape from one form of vice he should fall into another, which can be indulged with facility in any Indian bazaar in the forms of gunjah (the dried flowering tops), churrus (the resinous exudation), bang or subzee (the larger leaves and capsules), or majoon (a compound of bang, butter, and flour). Hence the prescription should be made as complex as possible, and at the earliest moment the dose of the extract should be diminished gradually till eventually it is withdrawn altogether from the prescription.

TOXIC EFFECTS OF CANNABIS INDICA.

To the Editors of THE LANCET.

SIRS,—The following short account of symptoms experienced in my own person may be of interest to some of your readers. Not long ago, whilst suffering severely from neuralgia, I was induced by a medical man, to whom I was then acting as assistant, to take forty drops of the tincture of cannabis indica, which I did, he himself having on previous occasions done the same, with relief from neuralgia and with no unpleasant symptoms following. The neuralgia was soon forgotten, and in about an hour's time I began to feel giddy, full in the head, and very faint, and soon experienced a sensation of heaviness and numbness in the feet and legs, followed by partial anæsthesia, gradually extending upwards to the knees. My feet and legs felt as if enormously swollen and thickly covered over with wool. Soon the loss of sensation became complete as far as the knees; walking was then impossible and even standing a difficulty. Shortly similar symptoms appeared in the upper extremities, commencing at the finger tips and extending as far as the elbows. The anæsthesia was not so complete as in the lower extremities. During this time there was great anxiety and fear of death through cardiac paralysis, which seemed almost imminent. The heart's action was tumultuous and irregular. On the return of sensation to the extremities, I was possessed with an almost irresistible desire to commit suicide, by rushing into the adjoining canal or cutting my throat with the knives on the table close by, though no attempt was made at doing so. Shortly upon this I was seized with fits of alternate laughter and crying, without any apparent cause. When the symptoms were subsiding, my appetite became ravenous, accompanied by great thirst scarcely to be appeased, and then sleep intervened. The following morning I awoke, after a very sound sleep and a good night's rest, determined never again to take cannabis indica, and be most careful in prescribing it for others. I may state that I experienced no pleasurable intoxication or feeling of happiness, but the very reverse. It is well known that cannabis indica does not affect all persons similarly; some are particularly susceptible to its action, whilst others are not so. I have known a female to take forty drops of the tincture without any bad after-effects, besides a little merriment and laughter, which soon subsided.

I am, Sirs, yours faithfully,

W. W.

March, 1890.

The letter of W. W. From the Lancet *of March 15, 1890.*

Therapeutical Uses and Toxic Effects of Cannabis Indica

BY J. RUSSELL REYNOLDS, M.D.,F.R.S.

The letter of "W.W.," in *The Lancet* of March 15th, induces me to submit this communication on the therapeutical value of Indian hemp and the circumstances which have led to its having obtained a somewhat questionable character in our Pharmacopoeia.

In 1848, Dr. C. J. B. Williams, in his lectures on medicine in University College, spoke of this drug as one from which he, after using it in many cases, had expected much, but it was so uncertain in its action, and its exhibition was sometimes accompanied by such distressing toxic effects that he had discontinued its use, and advised his pupils to do the same. Some seven years after this Mr. Peter Squire, the most distinguished pharmaceutist of the time, informed me that for at least three years he had been unable to obtain a good specimen of any preparation of the drug from India, or even to obtain the plant; strange things had been sent him, and other plants, but the former were bad, and the plants were not even of the same genus. However, he had recently been successful in obtaining the plant and in making an alcoholic extract and a tincture, with which he hoped I would make experiments. To this request I very readily acceded, and have made very numerous observations of its action from that time until now; and with this general result, that Indian hemp, when pure and administered carefully, is one of the most valuable medicines we possess.

In order to furnish the results to which I have been led by more than thirty years' experience of the drug, it will be well to arrange the maladies in which it has been either useful, or

Reprinted from *Lancet*, vol. I, March 22, 1890, pp. 637–638.

useless in the order to be followed in this paper; then to speak of its "uncertainty" of action, and of the methods to be adopted in order to avoid its toxic effects.

First, some of its most markedly valuable results are to be found in curious conditions of mind:—

1. *Mental.*—In senile insomnia, with wandering; where an elderly person probably with brain-softening, in the "delirium form" (Durand-Fardel) is fidgety at night, goes to bed, gets up again, and fusses over his clothes and his drawers; thinks that he has some appointment to keep, and must dress himself and go out to keep it; but may be quite rational during the day, with its stimuli and real occupations. In this class of case I have found nothing comparable in utility to a moderate dose of Indian hemp—viz., one-quarter to one-third of a grain of the extract, given at bedtime. It has been absolutely successful for months, and indeed years, without any increase of the dose. In alcoholic delirium it is very uncertain; but has very occasionally been useful. In melancholia it is sometimes of service in converting the depression into exaltation; but I have long since discontinued its use, except when the case has merged into that of senile degeneration. In mania I have found it worse than useless, whether that malady has been chronic or acute. In the occasional night restlessness of patients with "general paralysis," and in those of "temper disease" (Marshall Hall), whether in children or adults, it has proved of eminent utility.

2. *Sensorial.*—In almost all painful maladies I have found Indian hemp by far the most useful of drugs; and it is especially so in those cases which are, to the present time, relegated to the "functional" order. Neuralgia, periodic or not, has often yielded to cannabis indica—pure and simple, no other treatment being given,—after ten, fifteen, or twenty years' duration. This result has been obtained most frequently in facial pain. In one case (University College Hospital) a man, with neuralgia of the lower branches of the nerve, had lost two stone* in weight during four years, from inability to take food, except by fits and starts; his pain had been present for eighteen years, and had resisted every kind of treatment that had been adopted, but was relieved completely after two days of hemp treatment, and the trouble never returned. Very many cases, of varying duration, have been found equally amenable to treatment. Neuritis: Indian hemp here is

*One stone weight equals 14 lbs. or 6.3 kilograms.

only useful in conjunction with other treatment, but it is a most valuable adjunct to mercury, iodine, or other drugs; as it is in neuralgia when given together with, when required, arsenic, quinine, or iron. Migraine: Very many victims of this malady have for years kept their sufferings in abeyance by taking hemp at the moment of threatening, or onset of the attack.

I have found Indian hemp almost useless in sciatica, and in myodynia, whether in the neck, the thorax (pleurodynia), or the back (lumbago, sacralgia). The pains that occur only on movement do not, so far as my experience extends, receive any relief from its administration; and I say this after having tried it in full doses in very many cases and during many years. Again, it has proved, in my experience, useless in cases of gastrodynia, enteralgia, tinnitus aurium, muscae volitantes, and almost all the other so-called "hysteric pains"; whereas, on the other hand, it has relieved the lightning pains of the ataxic patient, and also the multiform miseries of tingling, formication, numbness, and other paraesthesiae so common in the limbs of gouty people.

3. *Muscular.*—In clonic spasms, whether of epileptoid or choreoid type, I have found hemp very useful. For example, in the eclampsia of children, or of adults, whether from worms, teething—first or second dentition, or the cutting of the wisdom teeth—in a very large number of cases I have relied, and successfully, upon it alone. In true, chronic epilepsy I have found it absolutely useless, and this as the result of very extensive experience. There are many cases of so-called epilepsy in adults, but which, in my opinion, are either eclamptic, or the result of organic disease of a gross character in the nervous centres, in which Indian hemp is the most useful agent with which I am acquainted. Such cases, for instance, as attacks of violent convulsions (epileptoid in every actually present symptom) in an overfed man, who has had a heavy supper, and is attacked two or three hours afterwards while asleep, and whose attacks may recur two or three times in the hour, for a day or two, in spite of "clearing the *primae viae,*" bromine, and other drugs, but whose fits may be stopped at once by a full dose of hemp.

Again, there are cases of brain tumour or other malady in the course of which there occur a series of epileptiform convulsions, followed by coma, and coma by delirium, at first quiet and then violent, the delirium time after time passing into a renewed convulsion and repetition of events; and this may go on for hours, or even days, in spite of any other treatment, and yet yield at once to Indian hemp. Further, with regard to genuine epilepsy and allied affections, I have found this, that Indian hemp has been, on the one hand, useful only in those cases where the diagnosis has led me away from a belief in the presence of the really classical disease, to the suspicion of organic lesion or of eccentric irritation; and on the other hand, entirely useless, when there is no doubt of the nature of the malady. In many cases of genuine epilepsy, where attacks of petit mal are exclusively present and very frequent, and have been so for years, I have given Indian hemp in gradually increasing doses until some slight toxic effect is produced; but have never found it to reduce either the frequency or severity of the seizures, or to materially affect their character. In tonic spasm, such as torticollis and the like, in writer's cramp, in general chorea, in paralysis agitans, in the jerking movements of spinal sclerosis, in trismus, and in tetanus, Indian hemp has proved in my experience absolutely useless; but at the same time it is a most valuable medicine in the nocturnal cramps of old and gouty people; it in some cases relieves spasmodic asthma, and is of great service in cases of simple spasmodic dysmenorrhoea.

Second, in explaining the occasional toxic effects of Indian hemp, two things must be remembered:—

1. That the drug is one which, by its nature and the forms of its administration, is liable to great variations in strength. For practical purposes, its active principle has not been separated, and extracts, as well as tinctures made from the extract or from the plant, cannot be made uniform; because the hemp grown during different seasons, and in different places, varies in the amount that it contains of the therapeutic agent. It is desirable, therefore, that it should always be obtained from the same source, and that a minimum dose should be given to begin with, and that the dose should be very gradually and cautiously increased.

2. That individuals differ widely in their relations to many medicines and articles of diet, and perhaps to none more widely than to those vegetable in origin—such as tea, coffee, ipecacuanha, digitalis, nux vomica, and the like; and there

fore, in addition to securing purity of drug, the possibility of idiosyncrasy should be borne in mind, to emphasise the need of caution, in the first administration of Indian hemp. By habituation and gradual increase of the dose, two, three, or even four grains of the extract may be taken not only with impunity, but with advantage; but such a dose as one grain would, so far as my experience goes, be attended with toxic effects in the majority of healthy adults. I have seen them in mild form from one-third of a grain, and very rarely from one-fourth, but have never known them arise from one-fifth. Therefore, for an adult I always give one-fifth or less to commence with, and for a child one-tenth. The best, because most convenient, form for administration is the tincture. Pills often become hard and insoluble, and their strength cannot be so readily and so gradually increased. The tincture, if suspended by mucilage, is apt to separate in the mixture that contains it, and thus the doses become uneven. Therefore, during many years I have given it with instructions that the dose required should be taken in drops on a small piece of sugar or bread. The tincture of the Pharmacopoeia contains one grain in about twenty minims, and this is convenient for use with children; but for the adult, where a gradually increasing dose is required, a tincture with a strength of one grain in ten drops is more useful. The dose should be given in minimum quantity, repeated in not less than four or six hours, and gradually increased by one drop every third or fourth day, until either relief is obtained, or the drug is proved, in such case, to be useless. With these precautions I have never met with any toxic effects, and have rarely failed to find, after a comparatively short time, either the value or the uselessness of the drug.

It is no surprise to me that "W.W." should have suffered as he did, and which, he so accurately and graphically describes, from the dose that he had taken; nor does it astonish me that his friend, possessed of a different idiosyncrasy, could have taken it with impunity; and the object of this communication will be attained if, by giving my experience of the great value of Indian hemp, my brethren may be deterred from abandoning its use by any dread of its causing "toxic effects," unless it be given in a "toxic" dose.

Cannabis Indica
as an Anodyne and Hypnotic

BY J.B. MATTISON, M.D.

Indian hemp is not a poison. This statement is made, just here, because the writer thinks a fear of its toxic power is one reason why this drug is not more largely used. This mistaken idea lessens its value, because it is not pushed to the point of securing a full therapeutic effect. This is a fact. One of the best pharmacologists in this country not long since expressed a very touching solicitude lest the writer's advocating robust doses of this valued drug might cause a decrease in the census that would seriously imperil his professional good repute.

There is not on record any well-attested case of death from cannabis indica. Potter says: "Death has never been produced." Hare asserts: "No case of death from its use in man is on record." Bartholow affirms: "Cases of acute poisoning have never been reported." Stillé states: "We are not acquainted with any instance of death." Wood declares: "Hemp is not a dangerous drug, even the largest doses do not compromise life. No acute fatal poisoning has been reported." A prolonged personal experience, compassing the history of many cases—men and women—and hundreds of doses ranging from thirty to sixty minims of the fluid extract, has never brought any anxiety along toxic lines.

Having thus brushed aside this bugbear, we may note, *en passant*, the statement, on high authority—Potter—that "cannabis was formerly much employed as an anodyne and hypnotic. It is now somewhat out of fashion." Why this early repute has not been continued, is due to a cause cited, coupled with non-reliable products, and doubtless, the coming of other analgesic-soporifics. The first cause need no

Reprinted from *The St. Louis Medical and Surgical Journal*, vol. LVI, no. 5, November 1891, pp. 265–271.

longer obtain; the second can be removed by careful choosing
and trial; while the last should not preclude the use of a drug
that has a special value in some morbid conditions, and the
intrinsic merit and superior safety of which entitle it to the
place it once held in therapeutics. Digitalis, for a time, was in
disuse. So, too, codeine, which my experience has proved a
valued anodyne—one worthy a wider use than it has had, and
which I think it will surely get—and impelled me to present
the American Medical Association, at its last meeting, with a
paper thereon, that I trust you have done me the honor to
read.

There is a consensus of opinion among writers on therapeutics as to the anti-agrypnic, analgesic and anaesthetic
power of Indian hemp. For the latter it was used prior to
ether. Wood, testing it in himself, asserted "marked anaes-
thesia of the skin all day." Stillé says: "Its anaesthetic virtue
is shown in allaying the intense itching of eczema, so as to
permit sleep." And that a similar seemingly trivial disorder
may have a serious outcome is proven by the fact that a
well-marked case of triple addiction, under my care last
year—a medical man who took daily fifteen grains morphine
with thirty-five grains cocaine, subcutaneously, and fourteen
ounces of rum—had its rise in a morphia hypodermic taken to
relieve urticaria.

Stillé says: "Its curative powers are unquestionable in
spasmodic and painful affections." Noting the latter in detail,
its most important use is in that opprobrium of the healing
art—migraine. In a paper by the writer, eight years ago,
"Opium Addiction Among Medical Men,"—*Medical Record,*
June 9, 1883—in reviewing the causes, this was asserted the
most frequent. Enlarged experience has not changed that
opinion. A case from such cause, woman, ten years morphia
taking, thirty grains, by mouth, daily, is now under my care.
A sister, so situated, from the same cause, awaits similar
service; and the mother took morphia for headache till death
ended her need.

Ringer says: "No single drug have I found so useful in
migraine." He thinks it acts well in all forms, but seems most
useful in preventing rather than arresting. He deems it
specially effective in attacks due to fatigue, anxiety, or
climacteric change. Dr. E. C. Seguin, in 1877, commended it
highly.

Dr. Wharton Sinkler, in a paper on migraine, gives first place to cannabis, and thinks it of more value in this form of headache than any other. Richard Green, who first commended it in this complaint, thinks it not only relieves, but cures; in nearly all cases giving lasting relief.

In the *Brit. Med. Jour.*, July 4, 1891, Dr. Suckling, Prof. of Medicine, Queen's College, Birmingham, writes: "I have during the last few years been accustomed to prescribe Indian hemp in many conditions, and this drug seems to me to deserve a better repute than it has obtained." He calls it "almost a specific" in a form of insanity peculiar to women, caused by mental worry or moral shock, in which it clearly acts as a psychic anodyne—"seems to remove the mental distress and unrest." After commending it in melancholia and mania he says: "In migraine the drug is of great value; a pill containing one-half grain of the extract, with or without one-quarter grain of phosphate of zinc, will often immediately check an attack, and if the pill be given twice a day continuously, the severity and frequency of the attacks are often much diminished. I have met with patients who have been incapacitated for work from the frequency of the attacks, and who have been enabled by the use of Indian hemp to resume their employment." In a personal note from the doctor he wrote: "I have used Indian hemp as an anodyne and hypnotic, and find it most useful in both ways. I have never seen any ill results."

Anstie commends it in migraine and the pains of chronic chloral and alcohol taking. In his work on neuralgia—the best ever written, and one which I advise every one to read—he says: "From one-quarter to one-half grain of *good extract* of cannabis, repeated in two hours, if it has not produced sleep, is an excellent remedy in migraine of the young. It is very important in this disease that the *habit of long neuralgic paroxysms should not be set up.*"

Russell Reynolds thinks that in neuralgia, migraine and neuritis even of long standing, it is by far the best of drugs. Mackenzie has used it with success in constant all-day headache, not dependent on anaemia or peripheral irritation. Bastian and Reynolds commend it in the delirium of cerebral softening, and the latter says it calms the head pain and unrest of epileptics. In cardiac tumult, in senile insomnia and delirium, and the night unrest of general paresis, it acts well.

In some diseases common to women, hemp works well. Graily Hewitt says, that in many cases of uterine cancer it allays or prevents pain. Ringer asserts it sometimes signally useful in dysmenorrhoea. West commends it here. Potter states that its anodyne power is marked in chronic metritis and dysmenorrhoea; and Hare thinks it of great value in chronic uterine irritation, and nervous and spasmodic dysmenorrheoa. Donavan and Fuller claim it of value in migraine and chronic rheumatism; and Mackenzie in hay fever and hay asthma.

In genito-urinary disorders it often acts kindly—the renal pain of Bright's disease; in vesical spasm; retention of urine, and chordee; and it calms the pain of clap equal to sandal or copavia, and is less unpleasant. The distress of gastric ulcer and gastrodynia are eased by it, and in other and varied neuralgias it serves one well. In some cases of phthisis and other cureless disease it will bring euthanasia by allaying pain and unrest.

My experience with hemp covers more than a decade, many cases and several pounds of fluid extract. It is proper to state that these cases have been solely habitués or ex-habitués of opium, chloral or cocaine. In these, often, it has proved an efficient substitute for the poppy. Its power, in this regard, has sometimes surprised me. Both sexes took it, and with some no other drug anodyne was used. One of these—a naval surgeon, nine years a ten-grains daily subcutaneous morphia taker—recovered with less than a dozen doses. My oldest female patient—sixty-four—found its service complete. Its action has varied, as some cases respond more fully. This during the early abstinence time. Later it has done good in the post-poppy neuralgia, especially the cranial kind, and it has calmed mental pain and unrest.

As a hypnotic, Fronmueller gave hemp in 1,000 cases. Success, 530; partial success, 215; no success, 253. As such in delirium tremens, Potter declares it "the best." Anstie thought it better than opium when the pulse is feeble. Phillips asserts it "one of the most useful." Tyrrell and Beddoe say the same. Suckling's opinion has been given. McConnell commends it in the insomnia of chronic cardiac and renal disease. Oxley lauds it in the insomnia of severe chorea, especially in children; the tincture "more effectual than any other hypnotic."

My own results prove it a satisfactory soporific, even oftener than as an anodyne. And this, too, under conditions that test thoroughly the power of any drug in this regard, for the insomnia of ex-poppy habitués finds its equal only in the agrypnia of the insane. With many, no other hypnotic was used. The sleep has been sound and refreshing. Many cases showed a notable influence to it as regards time—somewhat akin to sulfonal. Two hours sufficed. The first, pleasant stimulation; the second, increasing drowsiness, ending in sleep.

Again, I admit my special cases may involve a condition making them more easily subject to hemp hypnosis, but these do not preclude the wisdom of its trial with other patients in whom it may act equally well.

Writers on cannabis refer to certain peculiar effects— which, in our thinking, are more often peculiar to the patient—that may here be noted. One is a mild intoxication. I say "mild," because the hashish, assassin-like, running-a-muck form is less fact than fancy. ·It is said temperament largely determines the mental effect whether it be grave or gay, merry or mad. Most of my cases—when such—have been in a merry mood. Of the hundreds of times given, only once did it excite to violence. That was a young physician, six years ago, in which it came close to a personal assault on the writer that was warded off only by superior strength. The patient afterward avowed no knowledge of such a situation, was profuse in apology, and stated that once, after taking hemp simply to note results, he routed every one out of the house, including his own grandmother!

Catalepsy is a rare sequence. We have seen it once. A woman, twenty-three, brunette, small but active, took, in early evening, forty minims Squibb's fluid extract as a soporific. After playing cards half an hour, she began to be very jolly, and it was suggested she retire. Visiting her later, she was found completely cataleptic. It soon subsided, sleep followed, and no after ill-effect.

Failure with hemp is largely due to inferior preparations, and this has had much to do with its limited use. It should never be called inert till full trial with an active product proved it.

Wood thinks the English extracts best. I have used, mainly, Squibb's fluid extract. To a small extent, Parke, Davis & Co.'s

Normal Liquid. They are reliable. Hare commends the solid extract made by the latter, and by McKesson & Robbins.

Merck has produced two elegant and efficient extracts—cannabine tannati and cannabinone. They are essentially hypnotic. The former has been found by Prior, Vogelsgesang, Mendel and others, a satisfactory soporific. Prior gave it one hundred times to thirty-five persons—the most with success. In hysteric cases not calmed by chloral or opium, it acts specially well. In the small dose of one grain it has brought sleep when one-third grain morphia failed.

Another cause of failure is too timid giving. I am convinced that the dose of books is, often too small. The only true way is, once a good extract, push it to full effect. My doses have been large—forty to sixty minims of the fluid extract—overlarge for the nonnarcotic habitué; but, as we years ago asserted, habitual poppy taking begets a peculiar tolerance of other nervines, and they must be more robustly given. Both sexes have taken them—women frequently—with no other effect than quiet and sleep. I think, for many, small doses are stimulant and exciting; large ones, sedative and quieting. They are the outcome of an experience with smaller doses that failed of effect desired. They prove hemp harmless, and they add proof to the opinion of most neurologists that, once a nervine needed, it is often better to give one full dose than several small.

The tincture—three grains to the drachm—may be given in doses of twenty to sixty minims. The fluid extract, five to twenty minims. The solid extract, one half to two grains. Tannate of cannabin, five to fifteen grains. Cannabinone, one half to one and one half grains. Cannabinone with milk sugar, five to fifteen grains, and each repeated or increased till a full effect is secured. It is said that in women cannabinone acts twice as strongly as in men. In headache, periodical or long continued, one half to two grains solid extract may be given each hour or two till the attack is arrested, and then continued in a similar dose, morning and night, for weeks or months. It is important not to quit the drug during a respite from pain.

I close this paper by again asking attention to the need of giving hemp in migraine. Were its use limited to this alone, its worth, direct and indirect, would be greater than most imagine. Bear in mind the bane of American women is headache. Recollect that hemp eases pain without disturbing stomach and secretions so often as opium, and that competent men think it not only calmative, but curative. Above all remember the close genetic relation of migraine relieved by opium, to a disease that spares neither sex, state nor condition.

Dr. Suckling wrote me: "The young men rarely prescribe it." To them I specially commend it. With a wish for speedy effect, it is so easy to use that modern mischief-maker, hypodermic morphia, that they are prone to forget remote results of incautious opiate giving.

Would that the wisdom which has come to their professional fathers through, it maybe, a hapless experience, might serve them to steer clear of narcotic shoals on which many a patient has gone awreck.

Indian hemp is not here lauded as a specific. It will, at times, fail. So do other drugs. But the many cases in which it acts well, entitle it to a large and lasting confidence.

My experience warrants this statement: cannabis indica is, often, a safe and successful anodyne and hypnotic.

Marijuana:
Therapeutic Application

BY R.P. WALTON, M.D., Ph.D.

The therapeutic application of Cannabis is more a matter of history than of present-day practice. Synthetic analgesics and hypnotics have almost entirely displaced these preparations from their original field of application. The newer synthetics are more effective and reliable and, in addition, have been more intensively exploited by commercial interests. Cannabis preparations have come to occupy so minor a place among modern medicinals that it has been suggested that they be abandoned altogether, this latter point of view being based on the assumption that they represent a menace from the standpoint of the hashish habit. Such an action would certainly be too drastic in view of the circumstances. For one thing, the therapeutic use of cannabis and the hashish habit are almost entirely unrelated. The drug has been readily available in this country for almost a century without developing more than a very occasional, isolated instance of hashish abuse. The marihuana habit came into this country by other channels, although it is true that once established as a practice, some few individuals have made use of the "drug store" preparations. The 1937 Federal legislative acts should be wholly effective in making these preparations completely unavailable for any further abuse of this sort. More stringent regulations making the drug unavailable for medical and scientific purposes would be unwise, since other uses may be developed for the drug which will completely overshadow its disadvantages. The drug has certain remarkable properties and if its chemical structure were determined and synthetic variations developed, some of these might

Reprinted from R. P. Walton, *Marijuana: America's New Drug Problem* (J. B. Lippincott, 1938), pp. 151–157.

prove to be particularly valuable, both as therapeutic agents and as experimental tools.

Essentially the same general opinion has been expressed recently be the committee on legislative activities of the American Medical Association. They concluded that

> there is positively no evidence to indicate the abuse of cannabis as a medicinal agent or to show that its medicinal use is leading to the development of cannabis addiction. Cannabis at the present time is slightly used for medicinal purposes, but it would seem worthwhile to maintain its status as a medicinal agent for such purposes as it now has. There is a possibility that a re-study of the drug by modern means may show other advantages to be derived from its medicinal use.

Although hemp preparations may have been used by the ancients to produce anesthesia, these drugs were not introduced generally into medicine until about 1840. At this time O'Shaughnessy, Aubert-Roche, and Moreau de Tours observed its use in India and Egypt and proceeded to experiment with its therapeutic possibilities. After using it in different sorts of conditions, they were each enthusiastic in representing it as a valuable therapeutic agent. Their activities resulted in a very widespread and general use of the drug both in Europe and America. During the period 1840–1900 there were something over a hundred articles published which recommended Cannabis for one disorder or another.

The popularity of the hemp drugs can be attributed partly to the fact that they were introduced before the synthetic hypnotics and analgesics. Chloral hydrate was not introduced until 1869 and was followed in the next thirty years by paraldehyde, sulfonal and the barbitals. Antipyrine and acetanilide, the first of their particular group of analgesics, were introduced about 1884. For general sedative and analgesic purposes, the only drugs commonly used at this time were morphine derivatives and their disadvantages were very well known. In fact, the most attractive feature of the hemp narcotics was probably the fact that they did not exhibit certain of the notorious disadvantages of the opiates. The hemp narcotics do not constipate at all, they more often increase rather than decrease appetite, they do not particularly depress the respiratory center even in large doses, they rarely or never cause pruritis or cutaneous eruptions and, most important, the liability of developing addiction is very much less than with the opiates.

These features were responsible for the rapid rise in popularity of the drug. Several features can be recognized as contributing to the gradual decline of popularity. Cannabis does not usually produce analgesia or relax spastic conditions without producing cortical effects and, in fact, these cortical effects usually predominate. The actual degree of analgesia produced is much less than with the opiates. Most important, the effects are irregular due to marked variations in individual susceptibility and probably also to variable absorption of the gummy resin.

The reported therapeutic successes and failures of these drugs are briefly summarized below.

Among the miscellaneous conditions for which it has been used and recommended may be mentioned cough, fatigue, rheumatism, rheumatic neuralgia, asthma, and delirium tremens.

Spastic conditions. Part of the early enthusiasm for cannabis was based on its presumed value as an antagonist of spastic conditions. It was used and highly recommended in the treatment of tetanus, hydrophobia, puerperal convulsions, chorea and strychnine poisoning. In the case of strychnine poisoning, at least, its value is slight. The author, with the help of Horace Dozier, tested the influence of cannabis in so far as it affected the minimal convulsive dose of strychnine in dogs. Even large doses of cannabis did not alter the strychnine effect enough to indicate any significant antagonism. In tetanus and hydrophobia, spasticity is more cerebral in origin and the cannabis antagonism may have been more effective in such cases.

Analgesic uses. In combatting pain of various causes, cannabis preparations might be expected to be reasonably effective. See declared that it

gives relief from pain and increases the appetite in all cases, no matter on what causes the pain and loss of appetite may depend.

Hare says

> during the time that this remarkable drug is relieving
> pain, a very curious psychical condition sometimes
> manifests itself; namely, that the diminution of pain
> seems to be due to its fading away in the distance, so
> that the pain becomes less and less.

Mercer says that it does not arrest pain but has a "special
power over spasmodic pain." Wood says that

> as an analgesic, it is very much inferior to opium but
> may be tried when the latter is for any reason contra-
> indicated. In full doses, in neuralgic pains, it certainly
> often gives relief.

Audie says that

> as a remedy for the relief of supraorbital neuralgia no
> article perhaps affords better prospects than cannabis.

Headache and   Farlow considered cannabis useful in "nervous headache."
migraine.   MacKenzie says that if continued for some time it is the most
valuable remedy he has met with in the treatment of
persistent headache. Marshall does not consider that cannabis
is generally useful but says however that it appears to be
useful in headache of a dull and continuous character.
   Regarding migraine, Stevens says that *Cannabis indica* is

> sometimes very useful ... Two drops of the fluid
> extract may be given every half hour until the pain
> abates or until slight dizziness or mental confusion
> appears. Even larger doses may be used if necessary.

Osler and McCrae have said that for migraine, *Cannabis indica*
is probably the most satisfactory remedy. However, in the
latest edition of this text is is only suggested that "a
prolonged course of *Cannabis indica* may be tried." Solis-
Cohen and Githens consider that cannabis is of great service
in certain cases of migraine not dependent upon nor aggravated by eyestrain. Fantus recently recommended its use in
migraine, prescribing doses of one cc. of the fluid extract in

iso-alcoholic elixir. N. F. McConnell, Bastedo, Hare, Lewis, and Bragman have also favorably mentioned its use in migraine.

Beckman on the other hand says that whereas the drug was once considered a specific for migraine it has recently fallen into "a probably deserved disrepute."

One of the earlier experimenters with hashish declared that **Sedative and hypnotic action.**

in its hypnotic and soothing effects on the nervous system, its resemblance to morphia is very great.

Fronmueller made about one thousand observations on patients in which the soporific effects were compared with other drugs, particularly opium. He considered that the effect on the nervous system was much less dangerous than with opium. In most instances his patients are stated to have fallen asleep in about an hour without any particular side effects.

Bastedo remarks that it may promote sleep in the presence of pain. Poulsson and Dixon say that

sleep has often been seen to ensue without any, or with only slight excitement.

Miller, Berthier, McConnell, Shoemaker, Clendinning, Hiller and Florshinger have also described its usefulness in procuring sleep. Fantus and Cornbleet use it as a general sedative along with sodium bromide in the treatment of pruritis. Lees was very enthusiastic about the anodyne and soporific action of an aqueous extract, which he considered did not produce any of the excitement effects.

In current practice, the sedative effects are probably most used in veterinary work. Milks and Eichhorn say that

cannabis is a distinct depressant to the brain and cord. In man, this may be preceded by a brief period of stimulation but this action is rarely seen in a horse. It is a distinct depressant and hypnotic and probably ranks ahead of opium for this purpose in equine practice. After full doses the animals feel drowsy, sleepy, have a disinclination to move and may finally pass into a stage of narcosis which may last from twelve to twenty-four hours, and then recover.

One half ounce of the solid extract is cited as being sufficient to anesthetize a horse. This drug is relatively safe if considered simply on the basis of its effects on the circulation and respiratory center. It would seem however that a very real source of danger exists in the possible development of bronchopneumonia during the long period of semi-anesthesia.

Mental conditions. Moreau de Tours was the first to advocate using the hashish euphoria as a means of combatting mental conditions of a depressive character. He reported a number of case histories of manics and melancholics which were improved after such therapy. His conclusions were immediately criticized by Rech. There have been a few other observations agreeing in general with Moreau de Tours and there have been some who reported adversely on such treatment. Straub recently suggested that small doses of a properly standardized preparation may possibly prove useful in depressive melancholias.

Edes found it benefited patients who complained of unpleasant, tiring dreams and Birch used it in the treatment of chronic chloral and chronic opium poisoning.

Uterine dysfunction. Some have been particularly enthusiastic regarding the value of cannabis in dysmennorhea and menorrhagia. Batho says

> considerable experience of its employment in menorrhagia, more especially in India, has convinced me that it is, in that country at all events, one of the most reliable means at our disposal.

Referring to the use of Indian hemp in menorrhagia, Brown says

> there is no medicine which has given such good results; for this reason it ought to take the first place as a remedy in menorrhagia.

Effects during labor. Willis recommended its use in "tedious labor where the patient is restless." Christison used the drug during childbirth and advocated its use an an oxytocic. He believed it stimulated uterine movements more quickly than ergot. Kobylanshi, Grigor and Savignac also reported on its effects during childbirth. These observations may be taken generally as evidence that cannabis does not depress uterine movements. The drug is so lacking in peripheral actions that any special stimulation or depression would hardly be expected.

The question as to the effects of cannabis during labor was recently discussed in the *Journal of the American Medical Association.*

> The sensation of pain is distinctly lessened or entirely absent and the sense of touch is less acute than normally. Hence a woman in labor may have a more or less painless labor. If a sufficient amount of the drug is taken, the patient may fall into a tranquil sleep from which she will awaken refreshed. . . . As far as is known, a baby born of a mother intoxicated with cannabis will not be abnormal in any way.

In South Africa the native women smoke cannabis to stupefy themselves during childbirth. A requisite for the successful use of this technic would seem to be a previous familiarity with the effects of the drug. The African natives no doubt use the drug at other times and accordingly are not as likely to be distressed by the occasional terrifying phases of the episode. Also some experience is needed in order to regulate the dose when used in this way. In such obstetric use, the drug has one important advantage as contrasted with morphine, that is, the almost complete absence of any depressing effect on the respiratory mechanism.

There have been numerous suggestions that the hashish delirium may be used in psychiatric analysis as a means of removing the barriers to the subconscious. This was one of the purportedly useful features of the drug as declared in the recent legislative deliberations. Although such an application is not unreasonable, the few trials which have been made were not particularly successful. In contrast with cocaine and amytal, the patient usually becomes more absorbed and less communicative. Lindemann and Malamud observed this while

Diagnostic usefulness.

studying effects in schizophrenics and psychoneurotics. They reported that

> new experiences are created which allow new presentations or new fantasies and an increasing neglect of the outside world in favor of experiences which are in keeping with the patient's desires.

They did note that with schizophrenics there was much less change in space and time than in psychoneurotic and normal persons.

There is a fictional account of the use of the drug to obtain confessions from suspected criminals. In general, however, the usual effect of the drug is not such as to make it very useful for such purposes. Von Schrenck described some rather inconclusive experimentation involving the use of hashish in hypnotism.

Anti-epileptic Action of Marijuana-Active Substances

BY JEAN P. DAVIS, M.D., and H.H. RAMSEY, M.D.

The demonstration of anticonvulsant activity of the tetra-hydrocannabinol (THC) congeners by laboratory tests (Loewe and Goodman, *Federation Proc. 6:352, 1947*) prompted clinical trial in five institutionalized epileptic children. All of them had severe symptomatic grand mal epilepsy with mental retardation; three had cerebral palsy in addition. Electroencephalographic tracings were grossly abnormal in the entire group; three had focal seizure activity. Their attacks had been inadequately controlled on 0.13 gm. of phenobarbital daily, combined with 0.3 gm. of Dilantin per day in two of the patients, and in a third, with 0.2 gm. of Mesantoin daily.

Two isomeric 3 (1,2-dimethyl heptyl) homologs of THC were tested, Numbers 122 and 125A, with ataxia potencies fifty and eight times, respectively, that of natural marijuana principles. Number 122 was given to two patients for three weeks and to three patients for seven weeks. Three responded at least as well as to previous therapy; the fourth became almost completely and the fifth entirely seizure free. One patient, transferred to 125A after three weeks, had prompt exacerbation of seizures during the ensuing four weeks, despite dosages up to 4 mg. daily. The second patient transferred to 125A was adequately controlled on this dosage, except for a brief period of paranoid behavior three and a half weeks later; similar episodes had occurred prior to cannabinol therapy. Other psychic disturbances or toxic reactions were not manifested during the periods of treatment. Blood counts were normal. The cannabinols herein reported deserve further trial in non-institutionalized epileptics.

Reprinted from *Federation Proceedings,* Federation of American Society for Experimental Biology, vol. 8, 1949, p. 284.

Cannabis Substitution:
An Adjunctive Therapeutic Tool
in the Treatment of Alcoholism

BY TOD H. MIKURIYA, M.D.

The physical and psychosocial effects of alcoholism are varied in kind and amount, depending on each individual case. The resultant behavior is due to the complex interplay of pharmacologic effect of alcohol with the psychosocial aspects of the user. Tamarin and Mendelssohn vividly depict the destructive effects of prolonged alcohol intoxication:

> The anxiety-reduction model often utilized to explain initiation and perpetuation of episodic drinking was found inadequate to explain motivation for alcohol use by the alcoholic. Euphoria and elation were manifest only during the initial phases of intoxication. Prolonged drinking was characterized by progressive depression, guilt, and psychic pain. These unpleasant affects, however, were poorly recalled by the alcoholics following cessation of drinking.
>
> The degree of inebriation appeared to be more closely related to patterns of alcohol ingestion than to the total volume of alcohol consumed. Compulsive and constricted behavior patterns, which were present during sobriety, changed markedly during intoxication, with increased verbalization, varied expression of feelings, increased interaction, and frequent behavioral regression. During inebriation, psychic defenses appeared weakened with significant reduction of repression and reaction formation.*

Such chronic abrasive difficulties have been noted by a patient of mine, a forty-nine-year-old lady (Mrs. A.) with a

* John S. Tamert, M.D., Jack H. Mendelssohn: The Psychodynamics of Chronic Inebriation: Observation of Alcoholics during the Process of Drinking in an Experimental Group Setting. *American J. Psychiat.* 125:7 (January 1969).

Reprinted from *Medical Times*, vol. 98, no. 4, April 1970, pp. 187–191.

history of alcoholism dating back from her teens, unsuccess-fully treated by varied group and individual psychological treatments for many years. When she was referred to me, she had •been using illicitly obtained crude marijuana intermit-tently with a frequency of perhaps every weekend or so. It was noted that when she smoked marijuana she decreased her alcoholic intake. I instructed her to substitute cannabis daily —any time she felt the urge to partake in alcohol.

Just in case she should impulsively think of slipping back into her old habits, Antabuse®, (disulfiram) in the usual loading and stablizing doses was administered to afford her additional buttressing for her ego strength. As related to Cannabis, the addition of the Antabuse might be compared with providing a "stick, as well as a carrot for the donkey."

*　　*　　*

She offers me her observation in an interview after she began to substitute cannabis daily for alcohol.

A: I've been on grass every day this week. I've also been on Antabuse. I haven't had a drink since I saw you. I'm pretty proud of that. It was . . . an effort to take it, because I am depressed, and I thought, well, you know, I've got to do something now or never. So I smoked grass every day this week. And the first couple of days I was . . . I couldn't set myself a task to do anything. All I did was lay around the house and listen to music. I didn't go out of the house, I didn't do anything. But then I found that if I don't take as much, you know, just a couple of puffs is all I need, and I feel good and I can do what I have to do.

M: Such as . . . ?

A: Oh, well, this week I really did things. I finally vacuumed my apartment. I haven't unpacked all my suitcases yet, but . . . I cleaned the refrigerator, washed my hair, had company for dinner, my son and his girlfriend . . . uh . . . I was really high, though. But I got through it. They ate. I cooked it. (Laugh.)

M: Did you notice any decrement in your performance when you made up your mind you were going to do it?

A: Yeah. *But* . . . I didn't smoke as much. I'd take a couple of puffs, and then maybe an hour later, take a couple of other puffs. I had a little pipe in my kitchen.

M: How many puffs would you usually take?

A: Well, I have a little water pipe. The barrel is about that big, and I fill it up maybe three-quarters of the way, and if I smoked half of that I would be *really* stoned.

M: About how many puffs would you say that is?

A: Six or seven.

M: But taking just one or two gives you the desirable effect?

A: In alcoholic terms, you'd call it a glow.

M: Did it make you lethargic?

A: No. So I find that if I limit myself, you know, if I'm careful . . . and you know how this happened? Uh . . . I got some grass that doesn't burn, it's wet, so I can only take one or two and then I have to . . . it goes out, and then relight it, so it was easier to do it than normally, because normally I would want to . . . just get way up there real fast.

M: What do you suppose would have happened if you had set about to do the same thing with alcohol?

A: Well, I've tried that with alcohol, too. I guess you might call it playing a game, I don't know, but I've limited myself to, uh . . . well, Dr. S. said that if I could limit myself to one highball every hour, that my system would absorb the alcohol, and I would be okay, I wouldn't get drunk or intoxicated. Uh . . . sometimes I could do that, but I found that after a week or two and the more stress I had, the less able I was to wait that hour. And then I found that I just didn't give a damn, and . . . like the day before I came in here I drank almost a fifth of alcohol, which for me is a *lot*. I tend to . . . not handle it.

M: And from what I understand, grass doesn't have the same effect. It doesn't seem to call for another toke?

A: Right. There's another big difference, and that's ...
your appetite. With alcohol, you want to ... just want to get
out of it, like put yourself to sleep, and with grass, uh ...
well, I eat everything in sight.

*Her first lesson was to learn her proper dose in order to
perform routine tasks. She also discovered that she was able
to function as a hostess and cook while taking a small
amount of cannabis. Her description of the phenomenon of
tolerance to alcohol contrasts graphically with the lack of
tendency to increase the dose of cannabis.*

*Alcohol euphoria appears to cause irritability, belligerence,
and loss of control behaviorally. Cannabis euphoria in this
woman causes, if anything, a mild lethargy and mild temporal
distortion.*

M: You said you noticed that it (alcohol) somehow decreased your control?

A: Yeah. Sure. Well, for instance, I would go to a party,
expecting to have a good time, being able to mix with people,
dance, saying whatever ... was going on I would be able to
participate in it, and after every party I'd wake up the next
morning, feeling, OH, GOD, did I ever make an *ass* of myself,
because it would get away from me.

M: How would it get away from you?

A: Well, like half the time, before the party was over, I
didn't know what I said or what I did. . . . Uh, like going up
to somebody else's husband ... it was in groups where this
sort of thing just, you know ... wasn't part of the scheme of
things, you just didn't do this. . . . And another thing that
alcohol did, it gave me the courage to walk into a bar if I was
looking for a man.

M: You would pick up men in bars?

A: Yes. I was. . . . I suppose it started a long time ... a
long time ago, but, uh, the year before I came to the Center,
was really getting into messes. Really. Trying to ... just
dives. And getting drunk, and having blackouts, and waking
up not knowing where I was.

M: Does grass give you this oblivion?

A: Uh uh. No, there's a big difference. Uh . . . a real big difference. It's just not the same as drinking. With grass I . . . (laugh) I just wouldn't go into a bar . . . and pick up a man . . . it's . . . it's for one thing, I wouldn't meet the kind of man I would want to meet.

M: So these different intoxicants change your personality in most radical ways?

A: Yes. Well, I have changed a great deal in the past year. My behavior has changed, I've changed, my attitudes have changed. With alcohol, uh . . . well, there were three times in my life when I made a half-assed attempt at suicide. And . . . all three times alcohol was involved.

M: How have you changed since getting stoned on grass?

A: I just feel good, relaxed, I don't feel depressed, and I love to listen to music.

M: And in the way you feel toward others?

A: Others? Very gentle. Uh . . . I told you Sunday that my son came over. He wanted to go swimming that afternoon, and he wanted to know if he could bring a girl friend. I said, sure. And when he came over, uh, I asked them if they wanted to stay for dinner. And I had already started . . . smoking grass that day, before they came over, that was . . . Saturday. Uh . . . everything just went along fine. At least *I* thought so. I wasn't concerned about whether my table was set right, or whether I served right, or, uh . . . I mean, I just put the food on the table, and they could eat, I . . . just wasn't *bothered* about things that would normally bother me.

M: If you'd been drinking, would it have been different?

A: Uh . . . I think they would've waited until about ten o'clock at night to eat for one thing. And they probably wouldn't have waited, they would have like gone out to eat.

M: If you had been drinking?

A: Right. I probably would have gotten into a fight with Bill, said some nasty things to him, whereas I ignored him.

M: So it seems grass gives you control, and at the same time euphoria and tranquilization?

A: Yeah, except that at the dinner table, I had the feeling that . . . Bill certainly didn't know what I was talking about. And Chris didn't know what I was talking about. Leonard was laughing so he seemed to know, communicate with me . . . Uh . . . and I wasn't concerned with it, I wasn't bothered by . . . *I wasn't bothered* by little things that are unimportant, which when you are drinking are *greatly* magnified.

M: Such as?

A: Like my husband not smiling at the table. Or is eating too much, or too little, or . . . *anything.* Or not talking.

M: So you become irritable?

A: Belligerent. Hostile. . . . Nasty.

M: Makes you wonder why you'd drink at all?

A: Yeah. This week I . . . I really . . . once I took the Antabuse, it hadn't been too much of a struggle. And the only thing that I'm concerned about with marijuana is that . . . it's difficult to get, and it's uh . . . it's illegal.

M: Do you find it cheaper or more expensive than alcohol?

A: Oh, it's cheaper. Even though it's . . . gone up in price, it's still cheaper. A lot cheaper.

*   *   *

At about five months after the cannabis substitution therapy began, the patient shows an increase in insightfulness and she "revisits" the different social situations where she would drink to excess and play her compulsive games. She smokes hemp drug instead and notes that she relinquishes very little in the way of self control. At the same time, her physical health has improved, and she finds her disposition much less irritable and herself able to think and concentrate more readily.

The major difference she describes between the effects of hemp drugs as compared with alcohol is that "it made me high like alcohol, but it didn't give me that feeling in the pit of my stomach when I felt *angry.*"

She finds herself confronted with different dilemmas now, since she is afforded a new awareness and control over her life, instead of being continually sick and intoxicated and acting out in a maladaptive fashion. She finds that many of the friends that she seemed to have such warm relationships with have little in common with her anymore. She also discovers she is able to express anger more directly and in a controlled and appropriate manner as compared with her uncontrolled expression of anger under the influence of alcohol with its destructive disinhibiting characteristics.

Over two years of abstinence has afforded the opportunity in psychotherapy of working through the intricate problems of personality growth arrest facilitated by a thirty-five year history of alcoholism. I can in no way claim a total cure. At least, she has become free from repetitious cyclic frustration-rage-guilt amplified by alcohol. It is, however, quite difficult for her to give up these habits of 70 percent of her life. I am less concerned about her physical well-being for substitution of cannabis for alcohol has allowed her liver and general physical health to return to normal. Her appearance, complexion, posture and energy level have gradually improved. While all these gains make me optimistic, I realize the possibility of relapse—an unfortunate characteristic of certain cases of alcoholism.

Discussion. It would appear that for selected alcoholics the substitution of smoked cannabis for alcohol may be of marked rehabilitative value. The drug effect of cannabis, as compared with alcohol, while having a sense of euphoria and detachment in common, lacks any other similarity except the intent for which it is taken. Excessive alcohol use produces a predictable weakening and dissolution of various superego and ego functions, whereas cannabis does not seem to have this attribute, providing, if anything, any increase in ego strength. Because cannabis does not facilitate ego alien behavior as seen with alcoholic excess, a great burden of guilt is removed, thus freeing the individual for more constructive pursuits.

The fact that cannabis did not produce symptoms of irritability upon withdrawal, nor effects on the gastrointestinal tract, as compared with alcohol, also assists in the rehabilitation of the individual. Since he is not physically sick anymore, he is thus free to begin resocialization and to perceive the subtleties of the world beyond his needs for immediate gratification or succor. Certainly cannabis is not a panacea, but it warrants further clinical trial in selected cases of alcoholism.

IV

RECENT ACUTE CLINICAL STUDIES

To the detriment of readability and style, there has been a shift from the old school of "Let's try it on ourselves and the gang at the lab" to today's "controlled studies." As the plethora of instruments and laboratory tests grew, statistical evaluation methods were developed to deal with this rising flood of information. Coupled with avoidance of the use of the first person in a quasi-rationalistic anonymous stance, the writing somehow lacks the color and flavor of the old studies.

Allentuck et al. *were chiefly concerned with physiologic changes and the mental effects in inmates of a prison hospital. Individual case descriptions and acute mental symptoms observed in this setting compare unfavorably with experiences described in previous chapters for excessive morbid content.*

Ames repeats Allentuck's physiologic tests and adds a few of her own. Both report minimal physiologic effects and describe the psychological effects on subjects. Ames uses herself and eleven eager intern volunteers—very different from Allentuck's prisoners.

Weil and Crancer et al. *are interested in the more subtle but practical contemporary question of psychomotor performance impairment at low, socially used doses of smoked marijuana. Crancer compares smoked marijuana with high doses of alcohol. The Crancer driving study was rejected for publication in the* Journal of the American Medical Association, *but published in* Science, *since the findings did not support the AMA's current official stance.*

Weil uses simple machines and complicated psychological tools. Crancer uses complex machines to evaluate specifically the effects on driving performance in comparing the two social "highs."

These recent studies are rather pale by comparison with the earlier personal experiences and speculations, but are vital to the more accurate description of the low-dose marijuana states of consciousness.

Medical Aspects

BY S. ALLENTUCK, M.D.

I. SYMPTOMS AND BEHAVIOR
In Preliminary Group

The preliminary study of the five volunteer subjects had for its purpose the establishment of methods or procedures to be followed for the main group, and the obtaining of a general picture of the physical and mental effects induced by the drug. Having no knowledge of the safe limits of marijuana dosage, the dosage given to this group was restricted to from 1 to 4 cc. of the concentrate, and for smoking from one to three cigarettes.

When ingested, 1 cc. of marijuana was slightly effective, the multiples of this more so. There was noted in all subjects some increase in pulse rate and in blood pressure, dilated and sluggish pupils, dryness of the mouth and throat, ataxia, and some clumsiness and incoordination of movement. Symptoms distinctly disagreeable were dizziness in three subjects, a sense of heaviness of the extremities in two, nausea in two and faintness in two. Three showed motor restlessness. A state classed as euphoria, characterized by laughter, witticisms, loquaciousness, and lowering of inhibitions occurred in three subjects. This was not sustained but alternated with periods during which disagreeable symptoms were dominant. In one of the subjects (V.C.) there was no euphoric state, but a feeling of discomfort and depression throughout. Finally in one of the five (A.V.) with 2 cc. there was a state of depression with anxiety and with 4 cc. a psychotic episode with fear of death.

With the exception of the one individual during his psychotic episode, the subjects gave no evidence of abnormal mental content at any stage of the drug action, the only

Reprinted from *The Marijuana Problem in the City of New York* (J. Cattell, 1944), pp. 35–64. © Ronald Press Co., N.Y.

change noted being a delay in focusing attention on questions asked and difficulty in sustaining mental concentration. While there was objection at times to carrying out repetitious tests, there was no definite refusal. There was no sexual stimulation giving rise to overt expression.

With the cigarette smoking, ataxia and changes in pulse rate, blood pressure and pupils corresponded to those following oral administration. In only one of the subjects, however, was there definite euphoria. The common symptoms were dizziness and drowsiness. Two of the subjects found it difficult to concentrate.

The duration of the effects of marijuana was variable. When it was ingested, the effects usually passed off in from two to four hours, but in one instance persisted for seven hours and in another for fourteen hours. After smoking, the duration of effects was from one to three hours.

In Main Group

The evidence of the effects of marijuana was obtained by the subject's statement of symptoms and sensations, by the nurse's reports and by the examiner's observations and interpretation of changes in the subject's mental state and behavior.

The dosage of the marijuana concentrate ranged from 2 to 22 cc. and in each subject the effects of more than one dose were studied. Dosage ranging from 2 to 5 cc. was used for the largest number of subjects, and that from 14 to 21 cc. on only seven occasions. It is known that marijuana intoxication may bring about a comatose state, but no attempt was made to determine the dosage required for this. The number receiving each of the selected doses is shown in Table 1.

TABLE 1

Dosage of marijuana

Dosage	Number of Subjects	Dosage	Number of Subjects	Dosage	Number of Subjects
2 cc.	37	8 cc.	4	14 cc.	1
3 cc.	6	9 cc.	6	15 cc.	2
4 cc.	20	10 cc.	8	17 cc.	1
5 cc.	16	11 cc.	5	18 cc.	1
6 cc.	8	12 cc.	5	19 cc.	1
7 cc.	7	13 cc.	4	22 cc.	1

While the duration of action and its intensity tended to increase with dosage, this was not always the case and equal doses did not bring about uniform effects in all those receiving them. Thus, 3 cc. produced a striking effect in one individual; much less in another; in still another, 10 cc. produced less effect than 5 cc. Such variations are to be explained by differences in the mental make-up of the subject, and the particular state of his responsiveness at the time when marijuana is taken.

The number of cigarettes smoked ranged from one to eleven. The smoking of a single cigarette took about ten minutes and up to eight could be smoked in an hour. In smoking, increasing the number of cigarettes usually increased the sensation described as "high," but here also there was no uniformity in individuals or groups.

When marijuana was ingested, in dosages from 2 cc. up, its actions became evident in one half to one hour. The maximum effects were seen in two to three hours. These subsided gradually, but the time of disappearance was variable, usually three to five hours, in some instances twelve hours or more.

When marijuana cigarettes were used the effects appeared almost immediately. After one cigarette, these had usually disappeared in an hour. After several cigarettes had been smoked the effects increased progressively in intensity and reached a maximum in about an hour. In most instances they disappeared in three to four hours.

The Concentrate

Behavior Symptoms. The effects on the general behavior of the subjects taking the concentrate were variable. If left undisturbed some remained quietly sitting or lying, showing little interest in their surroundings. Others were restless and talkative. Under the heading "Euphoria" there are listed those marijuana effects which give rise to pleasurable sensations or experiences. These are a sense of well-being and contentment, cheerfulness and gaiety, talkativeness, bursts of singing and dancing, daydreaming, a pleasant drowsiness, joking, and performing amusing antics. The drowsiness, daydreaming and unawareness of surroundings were present when the subject was left alone. Other euphoric expressions required an audience and there was much contagiousness of laughing and joking where several of the subjects under marijuana were congregated. The occurrence of a euphoric state, in one or another form, was noted in most of the subjects. But, except for those who were allowed to pass the time undisturbed, the pleasurable effects were interrupted from time to time by disagreeable sensations.

Quite commonly seen, as with the preliminary group, was a difficulty in focusing and sustaining mental concentration. Thus, there would occur a delay in the subject's answers to questions and at times some confusion as to their meaning. There was, however, except in a few isolated instances, no abnormal mental content evident and the responses brought out by the examiner were not different from those in the pre-marijuana state.

Altered mental behavior which would give rise to more concern was seen in a relatively small number of subjects. In some this took the form of irritation at questioning, refusal to comply with simple requests and antagonism to certain of the examiners. There was, however, only verbal and no active opposition in any of these behaviors, caused by the subject's desire to be left undisturbed and his disinclination to carry out certain tests which in his pre-marijuana period he had considered tiresome and meaningless. With this came antipathy to those conducting the tests.

The occurrence of the disagreeable physical symptoms accompanying marijuana action would naturally lead to a feeling of disquietude and some alarm as to significance and consequences. This, however, was a prominent feature in relatively few instances. A pronounced state of anxiety reaching a panic stage, associated usually with fear of death or of insanity, was observed only in those subjects experiencing psychotic episodes and here the anxiety state led to pleas for escape and not to acts of aggression. Even in the psychotic states there were no uncontrollable outbursts of rage or acts of violence.

Some evidence of eroticism was reported in about 10 percent of the one hundred and fifty instances in which marijuana was administered to the group. The presence of nurses, attendants and other women associated with the study gave opportunity for frank expression of sexual stimulation, had this been marked. There was no such expression even during the psychotic episodes.

In some isolated instances there was evidence of marked lowering of inhibitions such as loud discharge of flatus, urinating on the floor instead of in the vessels supplied and in one instance frank exhibitionism. In the last instance the subject, who was not a regular marijuana user, had been arrested on three occasions for indecent exposure.

The frequency with which significant changes in behavior occurred is indicated in Table 2.

TABLE 2

Effects of varying doses of marijuana on behavior of users and non-users

Symptoms	2-5 c.c. Percent affected Users (41 trials)	Non-users (43 trials)	6-10 c.c. Percent affected Users (25 trials)	Non-users (12 trials)	11-22 c.c. Percent affected Users (17 trials)	Non-users (3 trials)
Euphoria	92		92		100	
Excitement	19	32	8	41	24	33
Antagonism	7	11	0	16	6	0
Anxiety	7	27	4	41	6	33
Eroticism	4	11	4	16	12	0

As used in Table 2, anxiety means the subject's expressed worry concerning what might happen to him. Excitement, shown by physical restlessness, muscular twitchings and jerky movements, loud talking, and some degree of antagonism are known to be expressions of an "alarm" or "fear" state.

It is seen from this table that, except for euphoria, the effect of marijuana was definitely more pronounced on the non-users. This might be taken as evidence of a persisting tolerance to the drug in the user group, but, on the other hand, it may have as its basis a feeling of greater apprehension in the non-users. Such a feeling would undoubtedly arise among those who have had no previous experience with marijuana and are in a state of uncertainity as to its possible harmful effects.

Physical Symptoms. Of the subjective symptoms, a feeling described as lightness, heaviness, or pressure in the head, often with dizziness, was one of the earliest and occurred in practically all subjects, irrespective of dose. Dryness of the mouth and throat were reported by over half of the subjects as was also a floating sensation. Unsteadiness in movement and a feeling of heaviness in the extremities were commonly experienced as was a feeling of hunger and a desire for sweets especially. Less commonly noted were nausea, vomiting, sensations of warmth of the head or body, burning of the eyes, and blurring of vision, tightness of the chest, cardiac palpitation, ringing or pressure in the ears and an urge to urinate or defecate.

From observation by the examiner, tremor and ataxia were present in varying degrees in practically all instances and in all dosages used, as were also dilation of the pupils and sluggish response to light. These effects were often present on the day following marijuana administration.

The frequency of the more common subjective symptoms and their relation to dosage is shown in Table 3. The figures are taken from the subjects' reports.

There is a tendency for the symptoms to be more frequent in the non-users than in the users but the differences are variable and in general not striking.

TABLE 3

Physical symptoms produced in users and non-users by varying doses of marijuana

	2–5 c.c.		6–10 c.c.		11–22 c.c.	
	Percent affected		Percent affected		Percent affected	
	Users	Non-users	Users	Non-users	Users	Non-users
Symptoms	(41 trials)	(42 trials)	(25 trials)	(12 trials)	(17 trials)	(3 trials)
Lightness in head, dizziness	83	97	80	85	100	100
Dryness of throat	69	72	48	67	76	100
Heaviness of extremities	46	51	32	41	41	67
Unsteadiness	41	39	20	33	41	33
Hunger, thirst	44	35	48	41	70	33
High floating sensation	60	63	72	66	64	33

The Cigarette

Smoking. When marijuana is smoked, there is, as has been stated, no such accuracy in dosage as is the case when it is ingested. The marijuana user acquires a technique or art in smoking "reefers." This involves special preparation of the cigarette and regulation of the frequency and depth of inhalations. In a group of smokers, a cigarette circulates from one to another, each in turn taking one or more puffs. The performance is a slow and deliberate one and the cigarette, held in a forked match stick, is smoked to its end.

When the smoke comes in contact with the respiratory mucous membrane, the absorption of the active principle is rapid and the effects are recognized promptly by the subject. He soon learns to distinguish the amount of smoking which will give pleasant effects from the amount which will give unpleasant ones and so regulates his dosages. Providing there are no disturbing factors, as is the case in gatherings of small friendly groups or parties in "tea-pads," the regulated smoking produces a euphoric state, which accounts for continued indulgence.

The effect from smoking marijuana cigarettes was studied in thirty-two subjects. Of these, twenty were classed as users, that is, prior to their arrest they had more or less extensive experience in smoking. In the study the smoking was repeated by each subject several times, the number of cigarettes smoked within an hour ranging from one to eight.

In all of the user group the smoking produced a euphoric state with its feeling of well-being, contentment, sociability, mental and physical relaxation, which usually ended in a feeling of drowsiness. Talkativeness and laughing and the sensation of floating in the air were common occurrences. These effects were of short duration, from one to three or four hours after the smoking was concluded. In none of these subjects was there an expression of antagonism or antisocial behavior.

In the non-user group the effects were similar except that in one subject a state of mental confusion occurred and in another the main effect was a feeling of dizziness, unsteadiness and muscular weakness. Finally one subject showed effects entirely different from the others. He smoked one cigarette and became restless, agitated, dizzy, fearful of his surroundings, afraid of death. He had three short attacks of unconsciousness. At one period he had visions of angels, and for a few minutes a euphoric state. The entire episode lasted a little over an hour after which he went to sleep. This subject had a similar psychotic episode after taking 120 mg. of tetrahydrocannabinol. On seven other occasions he had been given the marijuana concentrate or tetrahydrocannabinol with no unusual effects.

Of the physical symptoms occurring with smoking, dryness

of the mouth and thorat, dizziness and a sensation of hunger were the most common. None of these or other symptoms seemed to lessen materially the pleasurable effects.

The effect of smoking on the seven females, six of whom were classed as users, corresponded to that on the male group. All showed euphoric effects. One of the subjects was nauseated and another was restless, irritable and contrary. These effects were observed in both of the subjects when marijuana was taken by stomach. One of the users, euphoric after smoking six and ten cigarettes, had a psychotic episode after 8 cc. of marijuana concentrate.

*Tea-Pad Parties.** In addition to the quantitative date regularly obtained from the subject during the course of the testing program, the examiner had opportunity to make diverse observations of the subject's global reactions which threw interesting light on the general effect of the drug on the individual's personality.

When the subject became "high," his inclination was to laugh, talk, sing, listen to music, or sleep, but the requirement that he solve problems, answer questions, or remember drawings created an artificial situation, tending to bring him "down" and spoil his pleasure. In order, therefore, that the influence of the drug might be observed in less formal circumstances and in a set-up more nearly like the customary "tea-pad," two groups of men were given "parties" on the last night of their hospital sojourn. The men were consulted beforehand, and the stage was set according to their desires. They requested that nothing be done until it was really dark outside. They brought the radio into the room where the smoking took place and turned it to soft dance music. Only one shaded light burned, leaving the greater part of the room shadowy. The suggestion was made that easy chairs or floor cushions be procured but the party progressed without these.

The men were allowed as many cigarettes as they wanted. When the "reefers" were passed out they crowded around with their hands outstretched like little children begging for candy. The number of cigarettes the men smoked varied, the range being from two to twelve or thirteen. There were both users and non-users in these two groups. The users of course were highly elated at the prospect of getting much free "tea," and some of the non-users also smoked with genuine enjoyment.

* This section on "Tea-Pad Parties" was prepared by Mrs. Halpern.

In the beginning the men broke up into little groups of twos and threes to do their smoking, or in some instances went off by themselves. Smoke soon filled the atmosphere and added to the general shadowy effect. After the initial smoking there was some moving about; some men laughed and joked, some became argumentative, while some just stared out of the window. The arguments never seemed to get anywhere, although they often dealt with important problems, and the illogical reasoning used was never recognized or refuted by the person to whom it was addressed. Gradually, as though attracted by some force, all restlessness and activity ceased, and the men sat in a circle about the radio. Occasionally they whispered to one another, laughed a little, or swayed to the music, but in general they relaxed quietly in their chairs. A feeling of contentment seemed to pervade, and when one man suddenly got a "laughing jag" they were annoyed at the interruption.

In general, they gave the impression of adolescent boys doing something which was forbidden and thereby adding spice to the indulgence. Many of the adolescent personality patterns as they appear in group activities were clearly observable here. There was the eternal "wisecracker," the domineering "important" individual who tried to tell everyone what to do, the silly, giggling adolescent and the shy, withdrawn introvert. One forgot that these were actually adults with all the usual adult responsibilities. One could not help drawing the conclusion that they too had forgotten this for the time being.

Although urged to smoke more, no subject could be persuaded to take more than he knew or felt he could handle. After about an hour and a half of smoking, the men were given coffee and bread and jam, and the party broke up. They all went to bed and reported the next day that they had slept very well.

Another attempt at evaluating the effect of marijuana in less formal situations was made in the following manner. The examiner, one of the police officers and the subjects listened to Jack Benny on the Jello Program at seven o'clock Sunday evening. The police officer noted the number of times the audience laughed, and the length of time the laughter lasted. The examiner checked these items for the subjects. The first time this was done without marijuana; the following week the subjects were given several "reefers" about fifteen minutes before the radio program started. The results were as follows: Without drug, the subjects laughed forty-two times as against seventy-two laughs in the radio audience. The total time for all laughs was sixty-three seconds as compared with one hundred and thirty-nine seconds for the radio audience. With cigarettes the subjects laughed forty-three times as compared with forty-seven laughs in the audience, the total laugh time being one hundred and twenty-nine seconds as compared with one hundred and seventy-three seconds of laughter in the audience. Without the drug, the subjects laughed, roughly speaking, only half as often and as long as the audience; while under the drug they laughed almost as often and the laugh time was about 75 percent that of the audience.

It is obvious that under marijuana the subject laughs more readily and for longer time intervals. This is probably due both to the fact that things seem funnier to him and because when under the influence of the drug he is less inhibited.

Differences between Concentrate and Cigarette

When marijuana was ingested, it was in the form of the concentrate, containing all the active principles which are soluble in the menstruum used. The relative proportions of the principles present are unknown, and the effects can be assumed to give a composite picture of different actions, the dominating one being that of tetrahydrocannabinol. There is no information available concerning the principles present in marijuana smoke, and it is possible that some of those found in the concentrate have been destroyed by the heat of combustion. The effects from smoking correspond to those induced by tetrahydrocannabinol taken by stomach, so it may be assumed that this principle is present in the smoke. The rapidity with which effects occur after smoking demonstrates the quick absorption of the cannabinol from the respiratory tract and the short duration of these effects indicates its prompt excretion or detoxification. When the concentrate is taken, the absorption from the intestinal tract is slower and more prolonged. For these reasons it is not possible to make a precise comparison between the effects of the two forms of administration.

In general, the subject's consciousness of unpleasant symptoms is more marked when the concentrate is taken and this may interrupt or obscure the pleasant effects. The long duration of action and the inability of the subject to stop it serve to accentuate the physical symptoms and to cause apprehension concerning what may happen. The result of all this readily accounts for the irritability, negativism and antagonism which occurs. The lessening of inhibitions is not peculiar to marijuana. For in a few subjects who were given alcohol in intoxicating doses, the behavior corresponded to that induced by marijuana.

After smoking, the main effect was of a euphoric type. Some dizziness and dryness of the mouth were generally present, but were not pronounced enough to distract from the pleasant sensations. The conditions described as "high" came on promptly and increased with the number of cigarettes smoked, but it was not alarming or definitely disagreeable, and did not give rise to antisocial behavior. On the contrary it prompted sociability. The marijuana was under the subject's control, and once the euphoric state was present, which might come from only one cigarette, he had no inclination to increase it by more smoking. When a considerable number of cigarettes were smoked, the effect was usually one of drowsiness and fatigue.

The description of the "tea-pad parties" brings out clearly the convivial effect on the groups and the absence of any rough or antagonistic behavior.

Psychotic Episodes

What has been referred to as psychotic episodes occurred in nine subjects, seven men and two women. A description of the happenings in each instance is given.*

A.V. Male. Non-user. Given 4 cc. of marijuana concentrate. About three hours later he became restless, tremulous, agitated, fearful of harmful effects, suspicious of examiners. For short periods he was euphoric. At one time he had visual hallucinations of figures making gestures suggesting harm. He talked continuously, mainly expressing fear. His answers to questions were delayed but intelligent.

W.P. Male. Occasional user. Given 3 cc., repeated two hours later. At first there was a euphoric state; later he became resistant and negativistic. He showed antagonism to the examiner, demanding to be left alone. He vomited twice. Throughout he was highly excited and talked to himself. The effects in general resembled those seen in a maniacal state. He returned to his normal state in about three hours after the second dose.

F.D. Male. Occasional user. Given 4 cc. Five hours later he became confused, disoriented and slow in answering questions. There were periods of elation and depression with laughter and weeping. The effects passed off in six hours.

R.W. Male. Non-user. Given 5 cc. Three hours later he became disoriented with continued talkativeness and rapid shifting of thought. He had fits of laughter and weeping, grandiose ideas, some paranoid trends. He answered questions clearly but without perseveration. He returned to normal after six hours.

I.N. Female. Occasional user. Also heroin addict for many years. Given 8 cc. Three hours later she became confused and anxious with periods of laughing and weeping. There were several short episodes resembling hysterical attacks with dyspnea, pallor and rapid pulse during which she felt that she was dying and screamed for the doctor and for a priest. Throughout, her response to questioning was intelligent but delayed. There was a return to her normal state in three hours.

E.C. Male. Non-user. Given 6 cc. Two hours later he developed a marked state of anxiety accompanied by a sensation of difficulty in breathing. This began during a basal metabolism test. In the Sanborn equipment used there is a nose clip occluding nasal breathing and a rubber mouthpiece through which the air is inspired and expired. During the test the subject became confused, panicky and disoriented as to time. The anxiety over breathing continued for four hours but could be interrupted by distraction. He was then given 4 cc. more. The breathing difficulty lasted five hours more.

The condition here had features seen in claustrophobia. Before the episode the subject had taken marijuana on five occasions in 2, 4, 5, 5, and 2 cc. dosage, without any symptoms of respiratory distress. However, after the episode he took marijuana on three occasions in 2, 5, and 6 cc. dosage and each time the respiratory symptoms occurred. A certain degree of nervousness was present but there was no mental confusion. The subject realized that there was no physical obstruction to his breathing and had learned that by concentrating his thought on other lines he could keep his respiratory difficulties in abeyance and would not suffer from real anxiety. Smoking up to as many as thirteen marijuana cigarettes did not bring about the respiratory effect. It appeared then the the respiratory symptoms were precipitated by the wearing of the apparatus while under the influence of marijuana, and through suggestibility there resulted a conditioning to the marijuana concentrate which was given subsequently.

The description of these six psychotic episodes fits in with many others found in marijuana literature. They are examples of acute marijuana intoxication in susceptible individuals which comes on shortly after the drug has been taken and persists for several hours. The main features of the poisoning are the restlessness and mental excitement of a delirious nature with intermittent periods of euphoria and an overhanging state of anxiety and dread.

Three other subjects presented the features of marijuana psychosis.

R.H. Male. White. Age twenty-three. Non-user. In prison for the offense of living on prostitution. The family history was bad. His father never supported his wife or family and there was continual discord at home. When the subject was nine years old, the father deserted the family. Three brothers received court sentences, one for stealing a taxi, one for rape, and one for striking a teacher. R.H. was a problem child at school and on account of truancy and waywardness he was sent to the Flushing Parental School. He ran away from this school several times and was transferred to the House of Refuge on Randall's Island. At the age of sixteen he was discharged. Since that time he had had two jobs, one for three months in a factory, the other for four and one-half months in the W.P.A. When he was sixteen he was run over by a truck and unconscious for a time. After his return to the

Riker's Island Penitentiary from Welfare Hospital further questioning concerning his past revealed that he was subject to "fits" occurring once or twice every two months. During the attacks his body became rigid and his mouth felt stiff.

The subject was admitted to Welfare Hospital for the marijuana study on February 20th. After the usual program of examinations he was given 2 cc. of the concentrate on February 27th and February 28th. These doses brought on the symptoms of dizziness and tremor and heaviness of the head and the state called "high" which is characterized by periods of laughter and talkativeness. These effects passed off in a few hours and were followed by drowsiness and a sense of fatigue. On March 1st at 1 p.m. he smoked one marijuana cigarette. Immediately afterwards he became agitated and restless and suddenly lost consciousness. He recovered quickly and stated that he had a second short period of unconsciousness. During the afternoon he continued to be agitated and restless and had periods of laughing and weeping. After he was given phenobarbital he went to sleep. On the next day his only complaint was that he felt dizzy. Following this episode he was given 4 cc. of marijuana concentrate on March 3rd, 2 cc. on March 10th, 2 cc. of tetrahydrocannabinol on March 5th and 4 cc. on March 8th. The effects corresponded to those seen after the earlier administrations of 2 cc. doses of the concentrate.

On March 11th R.H. was given 5 cc. (75 mg.) of the tetrahydrocannabinol at 11 A.M. and 3 cc. at 2 P.M. No unusual effects were noted during the afternoon and he ate his supper with appetite at 4:30 P.M. At 6 P.M. he became restless, apprehensive and somewhat belligerent. He felt that something had happened to his mother, that everybody was acting queerly and picking on him. He continued to be agitated and fearful, refused medication and slept poorly. This condition persisted and on March 13th he was returned to Riker's Island. After four days there he became quiet and composed. The psychotic state cleared up completely. The resident psychiatrist's report was: Impression 1. Psychosis due to drugs. (Marijuana experimentally administered.) Acute delirium, recovered. 2. Convulsive disorder, idiopathic epilepsy. Petit mal on history.

H.W. Female. White. Age twenty-eight. Non-user. Drug peddler, serving a three-year indefinite sentence for unlawfully possessing a drug. Her parents died when she was about ten years old and she was raised in an orphanage. At the age of nineteen she entered a training school for nurses, but gave this up after four months and supported herself by prostitution. Her sister and her sister's husband were drug addicts and through them she began taking morphine and heroin, being, according to her account, depressed and dissatisfied at the time. She continued using these drugs up to the time of her arrest, a period of eight years. In 1938 she married a man who was also a drug addict, and engaged in the drug traffic.

On May 7th she was given 2 cc. of marijuana. Aside from a headache and a feeling of muscular weakness and incoordination, the effect was to make the subject feel gay and very good-natured. On May 8th she was given 3 cc. of the concentrate and became somewhat confused and unsteady, irritated and upset at carrying out tests, and greatly worried about the physical symptoms. Five hours after she had taken the drug the effects had largely passed off. Six hours later, however, she became restless and agitated, moving about constantly, and worried about past conduct. This state continued for a few hours. On other occasions the subject was given marijuana in doses of 2, 3, and 4 cc. Twice after the administration of 3 cc. the general effect was of a euphoric type, and after 4 cc. had been given a state of sadness set in on two occasions and one of euphoria on a third. Toward the end of her stay the subject became depressed and moody, constantly dwelling on the belief that she had committed unpardonable sins.

She was returned to the House of Detention on June 2nd, transferred to the Psychiatric Division of Bellevue Hospital on June 9th, and from there was sent to Matteawan State Hospital on July 10th. On admission to the State Hospital she appeared confused, retarded, apprehensive, and depressed. She had a marked feeling of guilt. She began to improve in September and was discharged, cured, in January. Since her return to New York she reports at frequent intervals to the parole officer. She has secured employment in a food shop and is to be promoted to the position of manager of the shop.

The diagnosis made at the State Hospital was: Psychosis, due to drugs and other exogenous poisons (morphine and heroin).

D.P. Male. Colored. Age twenty-three. Occasional user. Sentenced for unlawful possession of drugs. Since graduation from high school at the age of sixteen he had had no occupation. His criminal record dated from his graduation. He was arrested in 1934 for disorderly conduct and in the same year sentenced to Elmira Reformatory for five years for second degree assault. He was paroled in 1936, but during the same and the following year was arrested three times for assault or robbery. He was returned to Elmira where he remained until his discharge in 1940: in August 1940 he was arrested for the possession of drugs and sentenced to a three-year indefinite term. He had served eight months of this sentence when he was admitted to Welfare Hospital as a subject for the marijuana study.

During his stay at Welfare Hospital, D.P. was given marijuana in the form of a concentrate and as cigarettes on numerous occasions. His symptoms and behavior corresponded to those usually seen, lasting a few hours with no after-effects. When the time came for his return to Riker's Island he urged that he be allowed to stay at the hospital and assist in the study. Two weeks after his return to the penitentiary he developed a psychosis characteristic of schizophrenia. He was transferred to Matteawan where the diagnosis made was: Psychosis with psychopathic personality.

These three cases are of special interest from the standpoint of the relationship of marijuana to the psychosis. The first subject, R.H., had a definite history of epileptic attacks. After smoking one marijuana cigarette he experienced an acute confusional state which lasted a few hours. In the second episode which lasted six days there was a more prolonged confusional state. Epileptics are subject to such attacks, epileptic or epileptic equivalents, which may be brought on by any number of upsetting circumstances. In this case marijuana is the only known factor which precipitated the attack.

The second subject, H.W., was a heroin addict of long standing. During her stay in the hospital, in her retrospective reports on her marijuana experiences there were usually included expressions of worry and remorse at her conduct, such as her failure to answer questions or perform tests honestly, informing on the other women in her group, and denials concerning a syphilitic infection she thought she had had. Prior to this incarceration she had had no prison experience. The mental picture developed from the study at the hospital and at Matteawan and the subject's subsequent history represents a fairly typical example of what is termed a prison psychosis.

The third subject, D.P. did not develop his psychosis until two weeks after he had been returned to the Riker's Island Penitentiary. He had shown no unexpected effects from marijuana and had hoped to be allowed to stay on at the hospital instead of going back to prison to complete more than two years of an unexpired sentence. At Matteawan this subject was considered to have an underlying psychopathic personality. His case also may be taken as an example of prison psychosis. With both the second and third subjects, the exact role of marijuana in relation to the psychosis cannot be stated.

Dr. Peter F. Amoroso, Commissioner of Correction of the city of New York, has given us information concerning the prisoners sentenced to the penitentiary at Riker's Island from whom our subjects were drawn. During the year beginning July 1, 1941 and ending June 30, 1942, there were one thousand seven hundred and fifty-six inmates in this institution. They had received an indeterminate sentence, that is, from a minimum of a few months to a maximum of three years. Of this group, one hundred seventy-five were subjected to intensive study by the psychiatrist because they were considered possible psychotic cases, one hundred seventeen were sex offenders, and two hundred were miscellaneous cases referred for mental observation, making a total of four hundred ninety-two. Twenty-seven of these cases were committed to state institutions for the criminal insane, namely, twenty-five to Matteawan and two to Dannemora.

Commissioner Amoroso, after reviewing these cases, writes as follows: "This prison atmosphere may place a most severe strain on those who are physically or mentally abnormal upon commitment ... Emotionally unstable persons find themselves during incarceration denied the assertion and enjoyment of the basic human urges and impulses and it is natural to expect, therefore, that prison life may result in various types of explosions, such as psychoses, neuroses, sex perversion, and even physical and moral deterioration.

"I am indeed surprised that we had so little trouble with our volunteers upon completion of their study and sojourn at Welfare Hospital, and the few psychotic episodes that occurred are exactly what we would expect in the whole group without considering the administration and effects of excessive doses of marijuana."

Summary

In the study of the actions of marijuana in respect to subjective and objective symptoms and behavior, the marijuana was given a number of times to each of the subjects in the form of the concentrate taken by stomach. The amount given ranged from 2 to 22 cc., in most cases from 2 to 5 cc. After marijuana was taken, the systemic action became evident in one-half to one hour and the maximum effects were seen in two to three hours. They passed off gradually, usually in three to five hours, although in some instances they did not completely disappear until twelve or more hours.

Of the symptoms occurring, a feeling of lightness in the head with some dizziness, a sensation of floating in the air, dryness of the throat, hunger and thirst, unsteadiness and heaviness in the extremities were the most frequent. Tremor and ataxia, dilation of the pupils and sluggishness in responsiveness to light were observed in all subjects.

From observations on the behavior and responses of the subjects, it was found that a mixture of euphoria and apprehension was generally present. If the subjects were undisturbed there was a state of quiet and drowsiness, and unawareness of surroundings, with some difficulty in focusing and sustaining mental concentration. If they were in company, restlessness, talkativeness, laughter and joking were commonly seen. A feeling of apprehension, based on uncertainty regarding the possible effects of the drug and strengthened by any disagreeable sensations present, alternated with the euphoria. If the apprehension developed into a state of real anxiety, a spirit of antagonism was shown. However any resistance to requests made to the subjects was passive and not physical and there was no aggressive or violent behavior observed. Erotic ideas or sensations when present took no active expression.

Six of the subjects developed toxic episodes characteristic of acute marijuana intoxication. The dosage varied from 4 to 8 cc. of the concentrate, and the episodes lasted from three to six hours, in one instance ten hours. The effects were mixtures of euphoric and anxiety states, laughter, elation, excitement, disorientation and mental confusion.

The doses given were toxic to the individuals in question but not to others taking the same or larger ones. Once the drug had been taken the effects were beyond the subject's control. The actions described took unusual expression because for the particular subject at a particular time the dose was unusually effective. A corresponding toxicity did not occur from cigarettes. Here the effects came on promptly and on the appearance of any untoward effects, the smoking was stopped.

In three of the subjects a definite psychotic state occurred; in two shortly after marijuana ingestion, in one after a two-week interval. Of the first two, one was an epileptic and the other had a history of heroin addiction and a pre-psychotic personality. The third was considered a case of prison psychosis. The conclusion seems warranted that given the potential personality make-up and the right time and environment, marijuana may bring on a true psychotic state.

II. ORGANIC AND SYSTEMIC FUNCTIONS

The functions of the body organs and systems were studied in the manner common to hospital practice according to the methods and with the equipment in use at Welfare Hospital. The study was designed to show not only the effects of varying doses of marijuana but also whether subjects who had long been users of the drug gave evidence of organic damage. The tests were made before the drug was administered, during its action, and often in the after period. The heart and circulation, blood composition, kidney, liver and gastro-intestinal function, and basal metabolism received special consideration. The results of the study follow.

The Circulation

Pulse Rate

Coincident with the onset of marijuana symptoms, there usually occurred a rise in pulse rate. The peak was reached in one and one-half to three and one-half hours. The maximum increase was from thirty to forty beats per minute in most instances but in some it was from fifty to sixty beats. The decline after the peak was at times sharp, at other times gradual. The rise and its extent appeared to be dependent upon the mental state induced by the drug, that is, it was greater in states of euphoria and talkativeness, laughter, and body movement. As these symptoms subsided the pulse rate fell correspondingly.

Blood Pressure

Blood pressure changes were variable. In general, there was a rise in blood pressure coincident with the increase in pulse rate. There was no consistency in this, however. Thus, in one instance, with an increase of thirty beats per minute in pulse rate, the blood pressure rose 20 mm. Hg.; in another, with a rise in pulse rate of fifty beats per minute, the blood pressure remained unchanged. The diastolic pressure in general followed the systolic. There was no consistent relationship between the degree of change and the size of dosage.

Circulation Time

In a number of instances, ether and saccharin were injected into the antecubital vein and the time intervals required for the recognition of ether in the expired air and of the taste of saccharin were measured. The measurements made before and during marijuana action showed no differences and it was concluded that marijuana has no effect on the arm to lung and arm to tongue circulation time.

Electrocardiograms

Electrocardiographic records were made of all subjects before the administration of marijuana and during the drug action. The dose ranged from 1 cc. upwards, going as high as 17 cc. for one subject. In a number of instances a preliminary dose was given in the morning and a second, usually much larger, later, the record being taken after the second dosage. The readings and interpretations were made by Dr. Robert C. Batterman.

In eleven of the subjects abnormal electrocardiograms were noted. A description of these follows:

A.B.	Control	P split in leads 2 and 3.
	Marijuana	same
T.E.	Control	P split in leads 2 and 3. Left axis deviation.
	Marijuana	same throughout
C.H.	Control	T diphasic in leads 1 and 2.
	Marijuana	T diphasic in leads 2, 3 and 4.
J.H.	Control	Normal PR interval .19
A.B.	Control	P split in leads 2 and 3.
	Marijuana	same
T.E.	Control	P split in leads 2 and 3. Left axis deviation.
	Marijuana	same throughout
C.H.	Control	T diphasic in leads 1 and 2.
	Marijuana	T diphasic in leads 2, 3 and 4.
J.H.	Control	Normal PR interval .18
	Marijuana	P split in leads 1, 2 and 3. PR interval .22
W.J.	Control	Elevated ST segment, lead 1 and 4. P split in leads 1, 2 and 3. T diphasic in 3. P diphasic in lead 4.
	Marijuana	LA deviation. P split in leads 1, 2 and 3. T inverted in lead 3.
J.P.	Control	P split in leads 1, 2 and 3. Diphasic in lead 4. T split in 2, diphasic in 3.
	Marijuana	P split in 2.
J.R.	Control	RA deviation, P split in lead 1.
	Marijuana	RA deviation, P split in leads 1 and 2.
C.S.	Control	Deep Q in lead 3. Inverted T in lead 3. Depressed ST segment lead 2.
	Marijuana	same throughout
L.V.	Control	Ventricular rate 120. RA deviation. P split in leads 1, 2, 3, and 4. PR interval .20
	Marijuana	Ventricular rate 120. No deviation. P split in leads 1, 2, 3, and 4. PR interval .24.
B.W.	Control	Normal
	Marijuana	Sinus tachycardia. T inverted in leads 3 and 4.
H.W.	Control	T split in leads 1, 2 and 3. P inverted in lead 3. Wassermann positive.
	Marijuana	same throughout

In nine of the subjects, seven users and two non-users, abnormal electrocardiograms were noted in both the readings taken before and those taken after the administration of marijuana. In four of these the tracings resemble the pattern of those seen in patients with rheumatic heart disease, but it is impossible to state what underlying pathological conditions were present in the group as a whole. In two users the control records were normal, the marijuana ones abnormal.

In six subjects not included in the list given, a sinus tachycardia, and in two a sinus bradycardia were seen after the ingestion of marijuana.

In all the remaining subjects no abnormalities were seen before or during marijuana action.

Hematology

Blood morphology and certain chemical constituents of the blood were studied before and during marijuana action on sixty-one subjects, the dosage ranging from 2 to 21 cc. Before the administration of marijuana the hemoglobin reading was between 80 and 90 percent in thirty-six subjects and over 90 percent in twenty-two; during marijuana action it was from 80 to 90 in nineteen subjects and over 90 percent in thirty-nine. Three showed a low hemoglobin percentage before, 65, 70 and 77 percent, but a rise to 79, 90, and 95 percent during the drug action.

The blood counts showed the usual individual variations but the average counts for the sixty-one subjects were: before the administration of the drug, red blood cells 4,800,000 and white blood cells 8,900; during the drug action, 4,900,000 and 9,500 respectively.

The urea nitrogen, calcium and phosphorus blood concentration figures are given in Table 4.

TABLE 4

Blood concentrations of urea nitrogen, calcium and phosphorus
(in milligrams percent)

	Number of Subjects	Before Marijuana		After Marijuana	
		Average	Range	Average	Range
Urea nitrogen	63	12.2	6.9–24.9	12.2	8.5–20.7
Calcium	39	11.2	10.2–13.2	11.2	10.0–12.5
Phosphorus	36	3.9	2.6– 5.5	3.7	2.8– 5.0

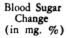

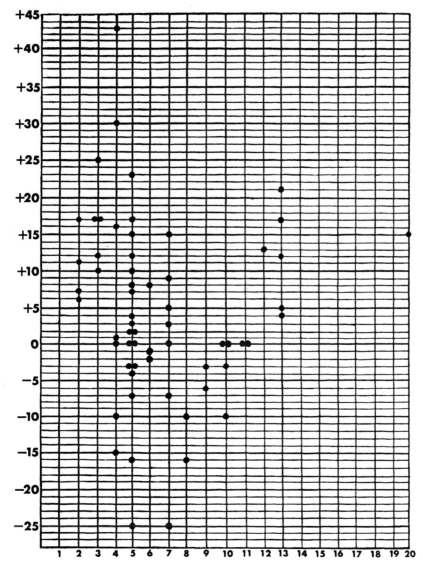

Figure 1. Increase or Decrease in Blood Sugar of Sixty-Two Subjects as a Result of Varying Doses of Marihuana.

From these blood studies it is seen that marijuana in the range of dosage stated produced no appreciable change in hemoglobin or cell count or in blood urea, calcium, and phosphorus. The blood examinations were made at varying periods during the subjects' stay at the hospital and in all instances marijuana had been given previously on a number of occasions. Thus, one subject had been given a total of 85 cc., another 143 cc., and a third 169 cc. The results show, therefore, that in addition to the lack of effect from a single dose, there was no cumulative effect from previous doses.

Blood sugar determinations were made on sixty-two subjects, forty-two users and twenty non-users. The blood samples for all tests were taken in the morning before breakfast. In the case of the tests made during marijuana action, the drug was administered two or three hours before the samples were taken.

The incidence of rise, fall, or no change in the blood sugar after the ingestion of marijuana is shown in Table 5, and the blood sugar changes in relation to dosage are shown in Figure 1.

TABLE 5

Changes in blood sugar determination of 62 subjects following the ingestion of marijuana

Blood Sugar before Marijuana (in mg. %)	Number of subjects showing		
	Rise	Fall	No change
55– 59	1	0	0
60– 69	3	0	0
70– 79	7	1	0
80– 89	19	9	5
90– 99	5	6	2
100–110	1	2	1
Total	36	18	8

For thirty-eight subjects twenty-seven users and eleven non-users, the differences between the control and marijuana figures were within plus and minus 10 mg. percent. In five, four users and one non-user, there was a rise of from 11 to 14 mg. percent, in fourteen a rise of 15 mg. percent or more, and in five a fall of 15 mg. percent or more. The blood sugar figures for subjects showing a rise or fall of 15 mg. percent or more are given in Table 6.

TABLE 6

Blood sugar changes of 15 milligrams percent or more

	15 mg. % or more rise				15 mg. % or more fall		
Dose	Before Marijuana	After Marijuana	Difference	Dose	Before Marijuana	After Marijuana	Difference
Users				*Users*			
A.R. 20 c.c.	85	100	15	J.W. 8 c.c.	90	74	-16
W.J. 13 c.c.	91	108	17	J.H. 5 c.c.	98	73	-25
J.N. 13 c.c.	91	112	21	J.B. 4 c.c.	85	70	-15
W.C. 5c.c.	55	78	23				
B.W. 5 c.c.	73	90	17				
J.T. 5 c.c.	85	100	15				
W.S. 4 c.c.	89	105	16				
W.R. 4 c.c.	60	90	30				
Non-users				*Non-users*			
E.F. 7 c.c.	90	105	15	A.T. 7 c.c.	105	80	-25
L.V. 4 c.c.	82	125	43	S.L. 5 c.c.	100	84	-16
C.C. 3 c.c.	68	85	17				
W.H. 3 c.c.	75	92	17				
P.B. 3 c.c.	75	100	25				
J.T. 2 c.c.	83	100	17				

From these tables it is seen that while there was a trend toward a rise in blood sugar levels during marijuana action, for the majority of the subjects there was no significant change from the control levels. In the instances where a rise or fall of 15 mg. percent or more occurred, a level of over 100 mg. percent was noted in only five subjects under marijuana; in the fourteen others the range kept between 70 and 100 mg. percent, which may be considered normal limits. Throughout there was no distinction between users and non-users in regard to blood sugar levels.

The Kidney

Routine examinations of twenty-four-hour urine specimens were made on all subjects for periods before and following marijuana administration. In no instance were albumin, sugar, casts, blood cells or other abnormal elements found.

Thirty-six subjects were given 1,000 cc. of water and the urine was collected for three one-hour periods. The procedure was repeated after the administration of marijuana in doses varying from 2 to 13 cc. An analysis of the figures obtained gave no evidence of a diuretic or antidiuretic effect from marijuana.

It was observed that an urge to urinate was a not infrequent occurrence during marijuana action. Since this was not accompanied by any appreciable increase in the amount of urine output, it is probable that it was a psychological reaction.

The phenolsulfonphthalein test for kidney function was carried out on forty-nine subjects before and during marijuana action. The dose ranged from 4 to 17 cc. The results are shown in Table 7.

TABLE 7

Phenolsulfonphthalein Tests. Number of subjects excreting various percentages of injected solution in two hours

Period	Number of Subjects Excreting			
	Under 40%	40–49%	50–59%	Over 60%
Before Marijuana	13	13	15	8
After Marijuana	16	13	13	7

There was a decrease of 2.5 percent in the total amount excreted by the forty-nine subjects after the administration of marijuana as compared with the amount excreted under normal conditions. This difference is well within the limits of technical error.

The results of the examinations showed therefore that the administration of marijuana brought about no structural or functional change in the kidney as determined by the techniques employed.

The Liver

No clinical evidence of liver damage was observed in any of the subjects before or after marijuana had been administered. The bromsulfalein test was given to a number of the subjects. The dye was injected in amounts of between 2 and 3 mg. for each kilogram of weight and the blood examined after thirty minutes. In twenty instances where marijuana was given in dosages ranging from 2 to 10 cc. and in one instance where 20 cc. was administered, the dye was absent from the blood after the thirty-minute interval.

The Gastro-Intestinal Tract

As has been stated, a characteristic effect of marijuana is a sensation of hunger and an increased appetite. Disagreeable effects which may occur are nausea and vomiting. The frequency with which the symptoms were noted is given in Table 8.

TABLE 8

Gastro-intestinal symptoms

Dose	Number of subjects	Number of trials	Symptoms			
			Hunger	Nausea	Vomiting	Diarrhea
Concentrate	*Men*					
1- 3 c.c.	64	184	94	5	2	occurred
4- 5 c.c.	59	186	129	7	2	in 4
6- 8 c.c.	46	106	85	6	3	of the
9-22 c.c.	33	71	50	2	1	psy-
						chotic
	Women					episodes
1- 3 c.c.	7	28	17	6	1	
4- 6 c.c.	7	35	25	1	0	
7-10 c.c.	4	5	3	0	0	
Cigarettes	*Men*					
1-8	37	54	40	3	1	
	Women					
1-8	5	7	5	2	1	
Tetrahydrocannabinol						
(natural and synthetic)	*Men*					
	34	93	61	7	5	
	Women					
	6	18	11	2	2	

As shown in the table, after the ingestion or smoking of marijuana more than half the subjects experienced hunger and increased appetites. A desire for sweets was especially strong, and users believe that the taking of candy or sweetened drinks lessens the "too high" effect which may follow marijuana smoking. The tendency toward a rise in blood sugar after the ingestion of marijuana indicates some need of the tissues for more sugar, but there is no explanation of the mechanisms involved.

While nausea and vomiting might be attributed to irritant effects of marijuana, on the other hand these symptoms occurred after smoking and in one instance after an intramuscular injection of tetrahydrocannabinol. The action here is presumably a central one.

The effects of marijuana on gastric motility and secretion were studied by Dr. Louis Gitzelter. A Miller-Abbott balloon attached to a Levine tube was passed into the stomach through one nostril and a Levine tube alone through the other nostril. The balloon was inflated with air to a pressure of approximately 10 mm. of water and connected with a tambour which registered gastric contractions on a kymograph. The other Levine tube was used to withdraw gastric contents at stated periods.

With the subjects in a fasting state, control records of gastric motility and measurements and analysis of gastric secretion were made throughout a period of an hour or more. The procedure was repeated on subsequent days following the administration of marijuana (6, 8, 6, 15, and 15 cc.) and at a time when the subjects were in a "high" state. A comparison of the two sets of findings gave no evidence that marijuana had any effect on motility or brought about any change in gastric secretion.

Roentgenograms, which were taken of the stomach of one of the subjects after a barium test meal, showed the emptying time of the stomach to be three hours both before and after the administration of marijuana. In another subject there was considerable delay in the emptying time during the marijuana action.

The Brain

Brain Metabolism

The effect of marijuana on the metabolic rate of the brain was investigated by studying the oxygen and carbon dioxide content of the arterial and venous blood drawn from the carotid artery and the internal jugular vein. The blood samples were obtained as simultaneously as possible, collected under mineral oil, and kept under anaerobic conditions until analyzed. Coagulation was prevented by the use of oxalate, and glycosis was inhibited by the addition of fluoride. The blood samples were analyzed for oxygen and carbon dioxide by the method of Van Slyke and Neil.

For analyses made when the subjects were under the influence of marijuana, the blood samples were collected two and a half or three hours after the drug was given, at a time when the subjects were in a state classed as "high."

The results presented in Table 9 show no consistent change in the metabolism of brain tissue as measured by blood oxygen and carbon dioxide concentration in four subjects showing clinical evidences of marijuana intoxication. Circumstances prevented an extension of the study.

TABLE 9

Oxygen and carbon dioxide content of arterial and venous blood of four subjects before and after the administration of marijuana

		Oxygen content			Carbon dioxide content		
		Arterial blood	Venous blood	Differ-ence	Arterial blood	Venous blood	Differ-ence
		(in volume percent)			(in volume percent)		
Before	R.S.	19.3	14.3	5.0	48.6	52.0	3.4
Marijuana	M.G.	19.4	14.9	4.5	46.7	50.8	4.1
	A.B.	20.4	16.3	4.1	45.2	50.8	5.6
	W.S.	19.4	13.7	5.7	45.4	52.9	7.5
After	R.S.	19.1	10.7	8.4	46.8	55.0	8.2
Marijuana	M.G.	20.2	14.9	5.3	44.2	48.5	4.3
	A.B.	20.2	14.9	5.3	43.3	48.4	5.1
	W.S.	18.0	12.9	5.1	47.0	49.0	2.0

Electroenchephalograms

Electroencephalographic records of fifteen subjects were made by Dr. Hans Strauss. There appeared to be a relationship between the typical euphoric reaction produced by marijuana and an associated increase in the alpha activity seen in the electroencephalogram. However, similar increase of alpha activity was observed in two subjects who received no marijuana. It is known that a high degree of alpha activity is suggestive of relaxation or perhaps the shutting off of any disturbing extraneous environmental stimuli and these findings merely suggest that marijuana is conducive to mental relaxation in some individuals.

Basal Metabolism

The basal metabolic rates of sixty-one subjects were determined before and during marijuana action. The Sanborn apparatus was used and the determinations were made in the morning before breakfast. The marijuana dosage ranged from 2 to as high as 20 cc. In the group of sixty-one subjects, forty-five were classed as users, sixteen as non-users. The accompanying table gives the data on forty-three subjects whose metabolic rates were within a range of +9 to -13 percent, both under normal conditions and while under the influence of marijuana. Of these, nineteen showed a rise in basal metabolic rate of 2 to 12 percent, twenty-three a fall of 2 to 13 percent, and in one the rate did not change.

TABLE 10

Metabolic rates (in percent) within a range of from + 9 to − 13 percent

Dose	Without Marijuana	Under Marijuana	Differ-ence	Dose	Without Marijuana	Under Marijuana	Differ-ence
Users				*Users*			
H.W. 10 c.c.	− 2	+ 5	+ 7	A.R. 20 c.c.	0	− 8	− 8
W.C. 8 c.c.	− 6	0	+ 6	E.T. 17 c.c.	− 7	− 11	− 4
C.J. 8 c.c.	+ 4	+ 5	+ 1	J.B. 13 c.c.	− 4	− 13	− 9
J.H. 8 c.c.	− 13	+ 4	+ 17	W.J. 13 c.c.	0	− 8	− 8
R.T. 7 c.c.	− 7	0	+ 7	R.S. 13 c.c.	0	− 4	− 4
L.C. 6 c.c.	− 12	− 10	+ 2	A.B. 11 c.c.	− 5	− 11	− 6
P.B. 6 c.c.	− 5	− 2	+ 3	J.W. 8 c.c.	− 3	− 5	− 2
F.W. 6 c.c.	− 11	− 7	+ 4	O.D. 7 c.c.	+ 4	− 6	− 10
M.N. 5 c.c.	− 9	− 5	+ 4	M.V. 6 c.c.	− 5	− 10	− 5
S.L. 5 c.c.	− 9	+ 2	+ 11	J.R. 5 c.c.	− 7	− 10	− 3
A.B. 4 c.c.	− 12	0	+ 12	W.B. 5 c.c.	− 6	− 13	− 7
W.S. 4 c.c.	− 5	+ 7	+ 12	H.W. 5 c.c.	− 9	− 13	− 4
R.S. 4 c.c.	− 9	− 5	+ 4	M.G. 5 c.c.	− 2	− 5	− 3
M.B. 2 c.c.	− 2	+ 5	+ 7	K.S. 4 c.c.	+ 9	− 5	− 14
C.D. 2 c.c.	− 12	0	+ 12	M.S. 2 c.c.	− 2	− 7	− 5
				A.S. 2 c.c.	+ 4	− 2	− 6
Non-users				*Non-users*			
D.L. 10 c.c.	+ 5	+ 7	+ 2	W.B. 7 c.c.	− 6	− 4	− 2
L.V. 6 c.c.	− 2	+ 6	+ 8	N.R. 6 c.c.	+ 2	− 9	− 11
E.S. 6 c.c.	− 8	− 6	+ 2	J.T. 5 c.c.	+ 2	− 2	− 4
C.S. 5 c.c.	− 11	− 5	+ 6	P.B. 4 c.c.	+ 8	− 10	− 18
H.B. 4 c.c.	− 8	0	+ 8	W.H. 3 c.c.	− 2	− 11	− 9
				S.H. 3 c.c.	0	− 5	− 5
				J.B. 4 c.c.	− 13	− 13	0

The remaining eighteen subjects had a basal metabolic rate of plus or minus 15 percent or more either before or after marijuana was administered. Of these, there was a rise in fourteen and a fall in four following the ingestion of marijuana, but in only four of these subjects was the rise significant, the rates being +30, +32, +18, and +25, after doses of 20, 2, 8, and 6 cc. respectively. The figures for this group are shown in Table 11.

TABLE 11

Metabolic rates (in percent) outside a range of from + 9 to − 13 percent

Dose	Without Marijuana	Under Marijuana	Differ- ence	Dose	Without Marijuana	Under Marijuana	Differ- ence
Users				*Users*			
J.N. 13 c.c.	− 20	− 17	+ 3	C.B. 11 c.c.	− 7	− 18	− 11
T.R. 13 c.c.	− 17	− 8	+ 9	J.B. 5 c.c.	− 2	− 15	− 13
B.W. 8 c.c.	− 22	− 14	+ 8	J.K. 5 c.c.	− 9	− 17	− 8
J.P. 8 c.c.	− 15	− 4	+ 11				
F.G. 8 c.c.	− 12	+ 18	+ 30				
H.A. 8 c.c.	− 17	− 4	+ 13				
V.L. 6 c.c.	+ 9	+ 25	+ 16				
W.R. 4 c.c.	− 17	− 13	+ 4				
R.G. 2 c.c.	+ 4	+ 32	+ 28				
E.S. 2 c.c.	− 23	− 19	+ 4				
J.T. 2 c.c.	− 15	− 12	+ 3				
Non-users				*Non-users*			
H.B. 20 c.c.	+ 2	+ 30	+ 28	C.C. 3 c.c.	− 19	− 23	− 4
J.G. 3 c.c.	− 15	− 14	+ 1				
W.D. 3 c.c.	− 16	− 14	+ 2				

The control figures are lower than those commonly reported. Of the sixty-one subjects, the rate in eleven was on the plus side, in thirty-eight on the minus side within a range of +9 and -15 percent, while for four it was 0. In eight the rate was between -16 and -23 percent. It is possible that prison life is conducive to a lowering of metabolic processes but our study is too limited to allow any generalization.

From the figures shown, it may be concluded that in the majority of subjects, marijuana caused no appreciable change in metabolic rate, although in those having an initially low rate, there was usually a rise. What changes occurred had no relationship to marijuana dosage, and there was no distinction between users and non-users.

Vital Capacity

Along with the determination of the basal metabolic rate, the measurement of vital capacity was made on sixty-six subjects before and after marijuana was administered. There was a decrease in forty-one, an increase in eleven, and no change in fourteen. Such changes as occurred were insignificant. The average vital capacity during the control period was 3.6 liters (range 2.3−5.1); after marijuana 3.5 liters (range 2.1−4.9).

Summary

The most consistent effect of marijuana observed in this division of the study was an increase in pulse rate which began shortly after the taking of the drug, reached a peak in about two hours, and gradually disappeared. In a few instances a temporary sinus tachycardia or sinus bradycardia was noted, but except for these there were no abnormalities in rhythm. The increase in pulse rate was usually accompanied by a rise in blood pressure.

There was in general an increase in the blood sugar level and in the basal metabolic rate, quite marked in some subjects, but in the majority the levels reached did not exceed the high normal limits.

An increase in the frequency of urination was often observed. There was, however, no appreciable increase in the total amount of urine passed during the drug action.

Hunger and an increase in appetite, particularly for sweets, was noted in the majority of the subjects, and the taking of candy or sweetened drinks brought down a "too high" effect of the drug. Nausea and vomiting occurred in a number of instances, diarrhea only during psychotic episodes.

On the other hand, the blood showed no changes in cell count, hemoglobin percent, or the urea nitrogen, calcium and phosphorus figures. The figures for the circulation rate and vital capacity and the results of the phenolsulfonphthalein test for kidney function and the bromsulfalein test for liver function were not different from those of the control period. The electrocardiograms showed no abnormalities which could be attributed to a direct action on the heart. In the few observation on gastric motility and secretion no evidence of marijuana action on these functions was obtained.

The positive results observed, increase in pulse rate and blood pressure, increase in blood sugar and metabolic rate, urge to urinate, increased appetite, nausea and vomiting, and diarrhea, were not intensified by an increase in dosage, for they could occur in an equal degree after the administration of any of the effective doses within the range used. All the effects described are known to be expressions of forms of cerebral excitation, the impulses from this being transmitted through the autonomic system. The alternation in the functions of the organs studied come from the effects of the drug on the central nervous system and are proportional to these effects. A direct action on the organs themselves was not seen.

A Clinical and Metabolic Study of Acute Intoxication with Cannabis Sativa and Its Role in the Model Psychosis

BY FRANCES AMES, M.D.

This paper describes an inquiry into the effects of giving oral doses of the narcotic drug variously known as hashish, marijuana and, in South Africa, dagga. The drug is a preparation from the plant *Cannabis sativa* whose narcotic effect has been known for centuries. The writer's interest in it was inspired by the work in recent years on the mental disturbances produced by the active principles of other plants, e.g. mescaline and lysergic acid. Because of the similarity of these changes to those occurring in conditions such as schizophrenia, some workers have suggested that these "model psychoses" could be used as a research tool in attempts to elucidate the mechanisms and causes of the naturally occurring psychoses. Although there has been a great deal of work on mescaline and lysergic acid, cannabis has not received much attention. This may be because its chemistry is still not fully worked out and preparations of the plant are difficult to standardize and vary in their potency.

Cannabis is widely though illegally grown in South Africa and there is no difficulty in getting supplies from the police for research purposes.

Because of possible dangers, such as addiction, in using the drug, research was confined to volunteers from the medical staff of Groote Schuur Hospital, the teaching hospital attached to the University of Cape Town. This also had the advantage that all volunteers, being medically trained, were

Reprinted from *Journal of Mental Science*, vol. 104, October 1958, pp. 972–999.

reasonably equipped to describe their experiences under the drug.

As a background to the investigation, a brief general history of the cannabis habit is given and a fuller one of the use of the plant in South Africa. The experiments and findings are described as well as the results of special investigations such as blood-sugar curves and electro-encepha-lographic changes.

Finally the implications of the findings are discussed.

The work is limited to acute intoxication. Research on the chronic effects of cannabis addiction is badly needed. There is much divergence of opinion about the chronic effects, but this question, and the interesting sociological and legal aspects of the habit are inevitably beyond the scope of this inquiry.

Although the drug is known by various names, for the sake of consistency the name cannabis has been used as far as possible.

GENERAL HISTORY

One explanation for the name cannabis is given by Lewin.[10] He says that the Assyrians used hemp as incense in the seventh or eighth century before Christ and called it "Qunubu" or "Qunnabu," a term apparently borrowed from an old East-Iranian word "Konaba," the same as the Scythian name cannabis and as the word "Kanaba" which is derived from the primitive Germanic word "Hanapaz." Lewin suggests that these words are identical with the Greek term κοναβος meaning noise, and that it would seem to originate from the noisy fashion in which the hemp-smokers expressed their feelings.

The hemp plant, *Cannabis sativa*, source of the narcotic, is a native of Central Asia and is now grown in many parts of the world. It is an herbaceous annual that grows to a height of four to eight feet or more. The leaves are long, slender and serrated and have about five to seven lobes arising from the same point, rather like the fingers of a hand spread fanwise. Male and female flowers grow on separate plants. The seed is hard and bony. The plant is covered with glandulose hairs rich in a resinous exudate. The resin contains most of the active ingredient of the hemp, though the seeds also contain a small amount. Traditionally the flowering tops of the female plant have been regarded as the richest source of resin, but this is not now generally accepted. Narcotic potency varies with the heredity of the plant and with the climate—a hot dry atmosphere tends to increase the yield of resin and some people think that this is because the resin has a protective function.

The plant is known by many names. The Chinese call it Ma; the Indians give different names to it according to how it is prepared: bhang, composed of the leaves and sometimes the fruit of the plant, ganja, made from the flowering tops of female plants and twigs covered by resinous exudate secreted by the leaves, young twigs, bark of the stem and even the young fruit of the female plant[6] ; in the Middle East it is called hashish (according to the *Shorter Oxford English Dictionary* the English word "assassin" comes from the Arabic Hashisan, meaning hashish-eaters and, later, certain Moslem fanatics who were sent out to murder the Christian leaders in the time of the Crusades); in North Africa it is called kif; in Russia, anascha; in Turkey and Persia, esrar; in Spanish-speaking America, marihuana; in Brazil, macoha; in South Africa, dagga (by Europeans and Coloured people) and mbanzhe, mbangi, matakwane, intsangu, etc. (by Africans).

As a narcotic the plant has interested men for centuries—incidentally, it is also an excellent source of fibre, hence the name hemp.

From early times religions have made use of it. The Hindus regarded it as a holy plant and had many legends about its origin, such as that it was brought out of the ocean by the god Shiva and all the gods churned it in order to extract "nectar" from it. Much of the sanctity attached to the plant was due to the belief that it "clears the head and stimulates the brain to think."

Some of the Mohammedan sects regarded the plant as an embodiment of the spirit of the prophet Khizer Elijah, the patron saint of water (Khizer means green, the colour of the drink made from bhang.[6])

The lives of some tribes in the Congo center on hemp, which is cultivated, smoked regularly and venerated. Whenever the tribe travels it takes the Riamba (huge calabash more than a yard in diameter which is used for smoking) with it. The man who commits a misdeed is condemned to smoke until he loses consciousness.[10]

Apart from its use in religions it has been widely employed

as a medicine. Its main therapeutic properties have been considered to be analgesic, sedative, anti-spasmodic and diuretic, though it has been recommended for a host of ailments both internal and external.

It was apparently introduced into Western medicine at the beginning of the nineteenth century by doctors attached to Napoleon's occupying forces in Egypt. They were sufficiently impressed by its sedative and analgesic properties to use it in the army, though the French generals were so appalled by the habit among the natives that they introduced several regulations forbidding its use.

Its use then became fairly widespread in Western Europe and it has been estimated that between 1840 and 1900 more than one hundred medical articles were written recommending it for various ailments.

Besides medical interest, it became fashionable among certain writers, artists and intellectuals to take cannabis as a "lark." Many of these people came to use it regularly and have left colourful accounts of its effects.

There were in the nineteenth century few alternatives to opium as a pain reliever, but by the beginning of the present century interest had shifted to new drugs, and sedatives such as chloral hydrate, paraldehyde and the barbiturates were being widely used. Cannabis preparations had always been difficult to standardize and if kept for long tended to deteriorate.

In addition, the chemistry of the active ingredients of cannabis had long eluded analysis.*

---

* Goodman and Gilman[7] state: "the isolation of the active principles proved most difficult. For many years it was erroneously believed that cannabinol, discovered in 1899, was the active principle of hemp. Cannabinol is a homogeneous, viscous oil obtained from purified 'red oil' derived from hemp extracts or resin. The chemical structure proved to be a dibenzopyran derivative. Cannabidiol was soon isolated from fresh hemp extracts and its structure identified. Cannabinol is the product of an inner condensation and reduction of cannabidiol. The former is virtually and the latter entirely inactive pharmacologically, but cannabidiol provides the basis for the synthesis in the laboratory of products of high potency which are probably isomers of the active principles of the red oil of hemp. Although reports of the isolation of natural active compounds and their derivatives have appeared it was not until 1942 that Wollner and his co-workers isolated and identified a

The difficulties of chemical studies of cannabis appear to have been enhanced by a series of unfortunate accidents to chemists engaged in such work. Walton[20] says that "Wood, Spivey and Easterfield, the Cambridge chemists, were not able to complete their program because of a series of tragic accidents. Wood barely escaped with his life when he took some cannabinol at the time he was preparing zinc ethyl. He lost consciousness, the zinc ethyl ignited and he was rescued from the burning room only with much difficulty. Easterfield was killed by a violent explosion while attempting to hydrogenate cannabinol. Spivey similarly perished while engaged in a synthetic study of the nitro-cannabinolactone."

The pharmacological action in animals is poorly understood. The main action is on the central nervous system and ataxia potency in animals closely parallels psychic potency in man. Samples of the crude material are such a mixture of different fractions that they vary considerably in their potency. Loewe[11] is an authority on the chemistry and pharmacology of the crude extract and the synthetic preparations. He found it poorly soluble in water and it dissolved slowly even in ideal solvents such as acetone. Consequently it is absorbed slowly. Even after intravenous injection, thirty to sixty minutes may elapse before a peak effect is attained and the effect may persist for hours or even days. The margin of safety is enormous. Despite the wide use of the drug only two cases of death in human beings have been reported. Ewens[20] reported two cases from India in which a large overdose proved fatal. Ewens said "the effect was rapid coma with vomiting of green-coloured contents of the stomach, stertorous breathing, etc. with marked congestion of the conjunctivae and coldness of the body surface. At postmortem there was a most curious congestion of all the internal organs of the body." Dogs have been killed with large doses of one of the synthetic cannabis preparations and the most striking autopsy finding was profuse intestinal

---

natural tetrahydro-cannabinol. This compound is quite active in animals and man, as is also a number of its synthetic congeners. The tetrahydro-cannabinols are the intermediate products in the conversion by the hemp plant of cannabidiol to cannabinol. Approximately eighty derivatives of tetrahydrocannabinol have been synthesized and studied pharmacologically."

haemorrhage; after intravenous injection the dogs developed fatal pulmonary oedema. (It is well known that both these findings sometimes result from acute cerebral disease in humans).

With more potent synthetic preparations of cannabis, death is associated with convulsions and appears more directly due to central nervous system damage.

Investigation into the chemistry of cannabis stimulated fresh clinical interest in the drug. In 1938 Walton wrote a comprehensive book on marihuana; in 1939 Bromberg described mental reactions seen during intoxication with the drug; in 1941–1942 Adams reported on the co-operative work of three laboratories—chemical, pharmacological and clinical; in 1942 Allentuck and Bowman described the psychiatric aspects of cannabis intoxication; in 1944 a team of workers, including doctors and police officers, issued a report on it in New York and the results of their experiments with seventy-seven subjects, and in 1957 the Narcotics Division of United Nations Publications issued a full report on cannabis in India.

Occasional reports on the therapeutic use of cannabis have appeared in recent years. In 1947 Stockings described synhexyl, one of the synthetic cannabis preparations, as a "new euphoriant." He used it in fifty cases of "neurotic depression" and claimed that thirty-six showed definite improvement: their depression lifted, they had an increased zest for work and were more accessible to psychotherapy.

Parker and Wrigley[14] tried synhexyl in sixty-two cases of melancholia and neurotic depression giving 10–20 mg. daily. They were not impressed by the drug after using the "double-blind" method, but despite this concluded their paper by saying that it is undoubtedly a euphoriant and further work should be done on it.

In 1954 Rolls and Stafford Clark described the successful use of cannabis in the treatment of a case of depersonalization. They included cannabis in the group of hallucinogens described by Osmond and Smythies and discussed its possible mode of action.

SOUTH AFRICA

Cannabis was in use for many years before Europeans settled in the country and was smoked by all the non-European races, i.e. Bushmen, Hottentots and Africans. It was probably brought to the Mozambique coast from India by Arab traders and the habit, once established, spread inland. The similarity of African names for the drug, e.g. mbangi, to the Hindi bhang, suggests this mode of entry into the country.

The term "dagga" is derived from the Hottentot "dachab"* and is applied not only to *Cannabis sativa* but also to *Leonotis leonurus* (Red or Wilde dagga) and *Leonotis leonotis* (klip-dagga). These two plants are reputed to have a mild narcotic effect (Gunn) but are not generally used for that purpose although they are apparently given to animals, e.g. racehorses, as a stimulant.

The plant has been used for many purposes in South Africa. Suto women smoke it to stupefy themselves during childbirth; they also grind up the seeds with bread or mealie pap and give it to children when they are being weaned.[21] It has often been recommended as a local application for snake-bite and some "cancer curers" use the oil from a dagga pipe as an external application. It has also been recommended for malaria, anthrax and dysentery.

* Senator Vedder, who has lived in South West Africa for many years and is an authority on the customs and language of the native inhabitants, says that the term dagga originates from the Hottentot— dachab being the singular and dachagu the plural. The term can be explained in two ways. Firstly, dacha is an Arabic word meaning "to smoke." Secondly, in the Hottentot language "da" is a verb meaning "to tread down." If "cha" is added to a verb the word receives an additional meaning that you do it with pleasure and frequently, e.g. ma means to give and macha to give gladly. Consequently, dacha might mean "to tread down gladly or frequently," i.e. the dagga smoker gladly becomes stupefied. Senator Vedder is of the opinion that both the Arabic and Hottentot languages have contributed to the name of the plant though many people might consider the Hottentot derivation given as rather too tortuous. Vedder tells a favourite story about dacha. Apparently in Karibib there was a Bergdama (one of the native people) who decided to surround his hut with a new kind of verandah. He placed barrels in a semi-circle round the hut and filled them with earth. On top of them he placed another layer of barrels so that the wall was more than the height of a man. In the top barrels he planted dacha plants. Many police passed but did not know what went on. When the plants had grown he cut them, plaited them, rolled them and fastened them with long thorns. Nobody disturbed him in this work. But a

Apart from African folklore there are four studies by Europeans on the use of cannabis in South Africa. The position before 1913 has been described by Bourhill. According to him dagga smoking was widespread among rural Africans and did not constitute a problem. Only adult males were permitted to smoke. They did so in a leisurely manner and smoking was often accompanied by the "dagga games." These games were played by blowing saliva through thin reed pipes to create intricate patterns. When the smoke was inhaled through water (the customary way of smoking) excessive salivation (it was claimed) was induced. The old men of the tribes gave their fondness for these games as one of the main reasons for continuing dagga smoking.

Bourhill states that dagga smoking was not only permitted but actually encouraged among African mine-workers because "after a smoke the natives work hard and show very little fatigue."

The usual mine practice was to allow three smokes a day. Nevertheless, the impression was growing even at that time that dagga smoking was harmful to urban Africans. Bourhill's

young Bergdama watched him and asked for an explanation. The old man said that the plant was dacha that could be smoked. The smoker would then enter into a wonderful sleep and see things that one did not normally see and he would receive a wonderful feeling of happiness and contentment. The young man asked for a pipeful of this wonderful stuff, filled his pipe and returned to his pondok to smoke it. But it did not take long before he put down his pipe, and very tired he sank into a deep sleep. When he awoke he was berserk.

In olden times the Bergdama used the plant for magic rites. They appointed one from their midst to smoke himself to sleep and his friends would watch him. If he smacked his lips they would say they could expect a year when they would find much wild honey, but if the smoker looked sad it was a foreboding of a bad year.

These people also used to dance a folk dance to an old song about dachab:

> "The water bubbles O dachab
> You little seed which grows because of the water
> The bushy tail fed by the spring
> You cover the earth—you sit in my head
> The dachab from the river has got hold of me
> Show me a kudu O dachab
> So that my hunting will be successful," etc.

discussion of this view naively reflects social attitudes to Africans at that time. He accepted uncritically the current belief that Africans were unstable and inferior in intelligence.

He paints a reasonably accurate picture of acute intoxication with cannabis, though it is doubtful whether auditory hallucinations are, as he claimed, part of the picture.

The second part of his paper dealt with "dagga insanity" among patients admitted to Pretoria Mental Asylum during the years 1908 to 1912. He claimed that 18 percent of all males admitted during this period were suffering from "dagga lunacy." In a review of one hundred three cases the average age was twenty-seven, the average period of detention in the asylum two hundred fifty-five days and relapses occurred in forty-one of the one hundred three cases.

Bourhill's labelling of his cases as "dagga insanity" is not acceptable. He himself mentions the difficulty in excluding alcohol as a factor and there is no good reason why many of his cases might not have been schizophrenics who were also cannabis smokers. His emphasis on auditory hallucinations is much more suggestive of schizophrenia than cannabis intoxication.

In 1936 Watt and Breyer-Brankwijk cleared up much confusion about the plants to which the name "dagga" applied by showing that *Cannabis sativa* was "true" dagga with undoubted narcotic properties while the other plants called dagga belonged to the Leonotis family, i.e. klip-dagga, wilde dagga, etc. Only one species, *Leonotis leonurus,* had been investigated (Gunn) and was reported to be mildly anthelmintic, feebly narcotic and probably harmless when smoked.

Watt and Breyer-Brankwijk described some of the clinical effects of smoking *Cannabis sativa* and urged a controlled investigation into the relationship of the cannabis habit to the production of acute psychosis and of permanent mental deterioration.

The third paper appeared in 1938 as the result of this suggestion by Watt and Breyer-Brankwijk. It was based on an investigation by the medical staff of Pretoria Mental Hospital on seventy-two non-European patients (twenty-two of whom had been diagnosed as "dagga psychosis"). The patients were observed while smoking cannabis and the results recorded.

The writers found that all cases showed marked mental

dulling; 35 percent of the cases showed motor excitement; 45 percent reacted with depression and 20 percent "just became silly and fatuous." The authors themselves seem to have been doubtful about the information that could be gleaned from this experiment as all the patients were psychotics and some of the effects observed might well have been due to activation of the original psychosis.

The fourth paper, 1951, is a report by a committee appointed by the Government. It is not confined to the medical aspects and is, in fact, full of valuable information and gives a balanced history and assessment of the problem as a whole. The committee felt that the picture of acute dagga intoxication was fairly well known but that there was far too little information on the effects of chronic dagga smoking. The committee pointed out that since 1928, when the cultivation of dagga had been declared illegal, there had been an unceasing prosecution of those engaged in the trade. They found it impossible to give an accurate idea of the extent of dagga smoking in the Union of South Africa, but felt that the practice was widespread among Africans (both rural and urban) and less common among the Coloured people and Europeans. Of all persons prosecuted for dagga offenses, Africans regularly constitute 75 percent although many of these are traffickers who do not themselves use the drug.

EXPERIMENTAL WORK

The investigation which is the subject of the present paper was designed to study the effect of giving a single oral dose of *Cannabis sativa* under controlled conditions. All subjects were medically trained and the writer had known them for some time before deciding to use them in the experiment so that on the whole they were articulate and fairly stable people.

The work can be divided into five sections:

1. This deals with the effect of cannabis on ten subjects (two female) in the twenty-thirty age group. Seven subjects were asked to participate and three volunteered spontaneously. They were all interns with no particular knowledge of psychiatry or chemical intoxications. During the experiment particular attention was paid to:

    (*a*) Subjective experiences and behavior.
    (*b*) Clinical changes.

(c) Certain special investigations, e.g. half-hourly blood-sugar estimations, urine output, electro-encephalographic recordings before and three hours after the cannabis had been taken.

2. The experiment was repeated on three subjects but on this occasion blood sugar estimations and electro-encephalographic recordings were not done.
3. The writer took cannabis but did not have blood-sugar estimations done.
4. One subject was inadvertently given an overdose and his reactions are described separately.
5. Four male cannabis addicts were interviewed.

TECHNIQUE

All the subjects knew that they were taking cannabis and took full responsibility for their actions.

They fasted from 10 P.M. the previous day and presented themselves in the ward at 8:30 A.M. On arrival an electro-encephalographic recording was done, blood was taken for blood-sugar estimation and the subject got into bed in pyjamas and a basal pulse rate was established. An oral dose of cannabis was taken without water. The dose varied between four to seven grains according to body weight and temperament. An observer stayed with the subject more or less continuously (in all cases the writer and one other person acted as observers, relieving each other when necessary). The observers took notes throughout the experiment and sometimes took a tape-recording or took the pulse rate if the nurse did not arrive at the correct time. In addition, blood was taken from an arm vein every half-hour and urine output was measured before the experiment began and three hours after it had started.

A second electroencephalogram was done three hours after the cannabis had been taken and three to four hours afterwards the subject was given a meal and left to sleep and drowse through the rest of the day with occasional visits.

All but two (one of whom was the writer) of the ten subjects were kept in the ward overnight. The two who returned home were driven home, one at 10 P.M. and the writer at 5:30 P.M.

All subjects submitted a report within the next few days on what they remembered of the experience.

PREPARATION

One thousand grams of powdered *Cannabis sativa* was extracted by the method given in the British P.C. (1934, p. 1229). The product yielded one hundred ten grams of concentrated resinous extract. Of this extract sufficient was taken to make one thousand pills, each containing 0.06 grams of extract, using powdered licorice root and powdered tragacanth as excipients. Each pill, therefore, contained one grain of *Cannabis sativa.*

A healthy female cat was given six grains of the extract of the *Cannabis sativa* made up into an emulsion with Pulv. Trag. Cr. Within two hours a change in its behavior was noted in that it seemed disinclined to move and remained looking apathetic on the floor of its cage. When taken out and encouraged to drink it exhibited marked ataxia and had great difficulty in lapping, continually hitting its head against the side of the saucer, splashing the milk, etc. It remained apathetic for the rest of the day and made a perfect recovery on the following day.

SUBJECTIVE EXPERIENCE AND BEHAVIOR

General.   The onset of the abnormalities of sensation was always abrupt and unmistakable. All subjects were somewhat apprehensive at the beginning of the experiment and anxious to report on every change. But once the drug really took effect there was no doubt about the reality and definiteness of the change.

A., after complaining hesitantly of various vague symptoms suddenly said, "This is it," and immediately lay down because of light-headedness and a feeling of unreality. He reported, "With me the first perceptual change was a change in the color and outline of objects. Colors became striking and vivid—the curtains were a vivid green, the room looked freshly painted and the figures in the room looked as if they had been cut out of cardboard. There was no third dimension. They were flat with bright colors and sharp outlines, and were seen through a screen of moving black dots like a newsprint photograph, with moving dots instead of still ones."

B. also experienced an abrupt onset accompanied by marked physical changes. He said, "I had been waiting for the first symptom with some curiosity. I thought I noticed a mild weariness and an aching feeling, mostly in my neck and shoulders. I was just saying perhaps this was something definite when I was 'hit' by fairly violent somatic symptoms. There was now no longer any doubt that I felt abnormal. I felt less inhibited and was no longer reluctant to talk about myself. The somatic symptoms were waves of warmth which started in the center of my abdomen and radiated up, fading out about mid-chest. This was associated with forceful, fast palpitations, dyspnea, dry mouth and waves of throbbing frontal headache." He likened these physical symptoms to adrenaline release "qualitatively the same but quantitatively more violent—it was like having the visceral effects of panic and a mental sense of panic without cause and without alarming thoughts in my head."

The onset was usually accompanied by tachycardia which was often considerable, e.g. pulse rates of one hundred thirty were not unusual.

Another striking feature about the experience was that it came in waves and several of the subjects felt compelled to communicate this fact by drawing a line rising and falling. Each dip in the curve might last only a few moments. C., after describing the onset, said a few minutes later, "Well, I'm blowed—it's gone—like a color film with the shutters coming down." Within a matter of minutes he said, "Here I go again—it's a floating away—like a balloon taking off— momentarily it's a positive exertion even to breathe, and yet it is lovely. What a silly thing to say—my emotions seem to have become dissociated from my speech but I feel I must keep on talking to keep human contact." This subject also described the wave-like alteration in consciousness as "like seeing reality in glimpses as one drives past a row of palings."

Other subjects interpreted the waves of abnormality as sleep. D., suddenly speaking after a few minutes of silence, said "I was asleep then, wasn't I?" B. would repeatedly fall silent for a moment or two then say: "I keep going off or going away from the room and the observers. I feel that if I keep banging myself I could keep in contact more easily. It reminds me a bit of driving in the early hours of the morning along a monotonous road when one is very tired."

E. said, "I had phases of losing contact with reality and at times I did not know whether I was awake or dreaming, but when I surfaced everything was quite clear."

These lapses lasted a few minutes but to the subjects they seemed an eternity. Their minds were not occupied with anything in particular at these times, except for those subjects who, on closing their eyes, saw visual images.

During these lapses the observer could always rouse the patient to give relevant replies to questions but the demeanor and intonation of the subjects suggested great languor and was in striking contrast to the briskness and alertness of the emergent phases. C. said, "Now I am in full possession of my senses—my mind is precision clear."

The mood was usually one of detachment and mild amusement. The subjects, after emerging from one of these wave-like experiences, described what had happened without apparent anxiety.

Thought Disorder.   Several subjects described their thought processes as "fragmented." One subject, F., in whom this was accompanied by extreme anguish, said, "There was no blunting of perception and no distortion, but before I could express a thought by word or action it was lost to me and displaced by another and often irrelevant thought. I thus had extreme difficulty in sorting out thought processes to a single idea goal."

Several subjects felt they were thinking more efficiently than usual. C. said with deliberate emphasis, "There is no mental or physical feat of which I do not feel capable." D. said, "I am enjoying talking because so many new associations occur to me—my talk is disconnected only because I immediately forget previous statements." G. felt that he was acquiring deeper insights into his basic personality structure, that he had a new awareness of the meaning of things; yet in the next breath he said, "My thought processes are slow and I have difficulty in expressing myself—it's like dysphasia—I've read a paragraph four to five times and it won't stick."

B. complained that he could not get the meaning of a simple cartoon he was looking at, and several subjects stared for many minutes at a book, puzzled because it had suddenly become meaningless.

One striking change was loss of recent memory or rather a difficulty in recall. Because of this, conversation became bizzarely disconnected. If a subject was asked a question about a statement he had made a few seconds earlier he was often unable to answer because he had forgotten what he had just said. When reminded of it he immediately took up the thread of conversation, saying, "How odd—I remember it now, but before it was lost to me." Direct questioning invariably elicited prompt and relevant replies and in most cases the seven from one hundred serial test was well done, but if subjects were left to themselves to pursue a train of thought this difficulty of immediate recall manifested itself.

Despite this the notes kept by the observer and the notes written by the subjects a day or so later corresponded very closely and in no instance was anything considered important forgotten.

Several subjects were struck by the dissociation between thought and action, e.g. F., when asked to sit up said, "I never thought I would be able to sit up—it is almost as though my muscles held me up without volition."

Several subjects became suspicious during the experiment. **Delusions.** H. refused on several occasions to close his eyes because he thought he was being hypnotized into seeing visual images. C. often paused before answering a question and admitted that he was examining it for hidden implications. He asked uneasily several times, "Is there someone hidden behind that screen?" I. at one time was convinced that a tape recorder had been concealed in the room and talked into the imaginary recorder when left alone for a few minutes.

A. got very suspicious when someone came in to hand the observer the electrocardiogram of a patient—he was convinced that it belonged to him (an EEG had been done on him), was abnormal and that this information was being withheld from him. He was eventually convinced by being handed the tracing with someone else's name on it.

J. became convinced that cannabis had unmasked a latent schizophrenia and when several people came in to talk to him he refused to answer any questions because he believed they had been called in to certify him. When the second EEG was done on him he was convinced that he was receiving electro-convulsive therapy in spite of the fact that three hours earlier he had been through exactly the same routine for an electro-encephalographic recording.

All subjects experienced a disorder of temporal orientation **Temporal** and it gave a remarkable quality to the experience. Events **Orientation.**

occurring immediately after each other seemed separated by an eternity of time; e.g. B. said, "The puffs between cigarette smoking seemed an eternity," and D. said that a venipuncture which had taken under a minute seemed to take about fifteen minutes. Several subjects asked uneasily when someone had just left the room, "How long is it since he left?" and were astonished at the answer because they thought it was so much longer.

Subjects could never estimate the time correctly. They invariably made an error ahead; i.e. they always thought it was much later than it was. One subject thought it was afternoon and not morning and another said he would not have been very much surprised if it had been the next day.

Because of this temporal disorientation distances seemed much longer; e.g. when subjects were wheeled down the corridor they felt that the journey was immensely long.

Disturbances of Visual Perception. Four subjects experienced disturbances of visual perception. A. said that people looked as though they were cut out of cardboard. He later described the face of one of the observers as "like an alabaster tortoise," and another as "sharply delineated through a blue haze of cellophane with acne showing up as pink excrescences and the head two or three times bigger than normal."

H., while laughing hilariously, said to the observer, "Your eyes look like large oranges—as big as a beach umbrella."

B. described one of the observers as looking like "an Egyptian pharaoh in judgment" and the ceiling as having "an iridescence like mother-of-pearl," while some wire netting formed a "rather pleasing pattern—benzene rings or stained-glass windows with two lots of colors—emerald green and grass green and red and green."

D., watching the sun's reflection on the wall, said, "It looks like a hyena or a duck-billed platypus."

After-image. Many subjects seemed to experience a greater intensity and duration of after-images, especially when objects such as windows had been looked at just before eye-closure.

Visual Hallucinations. Six subjects experienced visual hallucinations but only when their eyes were closed and usually when they were experiencing a disturbance of consciousness. H. said, "Now I see gold with blue and red stripes—flickering lights and patterns like a cartoon. Now it is changing into a technicolored cartoon with a silver ray going up into the sky." Later he said, "Whenever I shut my eyes I lose control and see my brain like a ballerina's dress going round and round in the middle of a glass cube." A. said, "I see a cross-pattern of people in old European costume—it changes so quickly—it has already changed a hundred times. Now I see a fat man in military costume running down some stairs. He is in a military uniform, has a snow-white beard and he is in a Roman tunic."

D. said, "I see church windows and mathematical shapes, mainly on the left. Now a meteor—a fiery ball that came and went."

C. said, "I see very beautiful, vivid colors like illustrated thoughts. Now there are little Chinese scenes like lace patterns—very formalized and lovely."

I. said, "I can see fixed prismatic colors racing over my head. Now intricate figures and symmetrical scenes—each half of the picture like the other as though carved out of ivory and lighted from behind. Now it has changed and I see a block of flats with a garage and stable gates and a man is leaning on the gate—it keeps changing and there are flickering bands of light going across like a forked flame."

G. had a variety of visual images. "There is a reddish glow when I close my eyes. I imagine a cat curling up—I don't like cats or scorpions—coloured lights. All based on a pattern— basic theme of glowing, with circles getting larger and larger—there seems to be a cat with long talons curled up crouching on top of me." About twenty minutes later he said, "Imagine a fellow draped like an Egyptian mummy— picture myself on a slab like a mummy—shaft of light" . . . "My teeth feel sore—feel full of holes—that damn circle keeps coming back . . . I rose out of that sarcophagus. Now there is a vague image of a ship in harbour—glowing light on the ship."

All the subjects emphasized the fleeting nature of visual images, the speed with which they changed and the inadequacy of language to describe them properly. If beautiful, they were indescribably so—the colours were of an intensity never experienced before and the patterns marvellously intricate and suffused with light. G. was the only subject who experienced unpleasant imagery, but when asked if it frightened him he said, "I did not like them, especially the cat, but then I don't like cats but they never actually frightened me."

Disturbance of Perception of Body Image. B. said, "I had a series of recurring unpleasant feelings about the shape of my own body. One was that my ribs seemed big and thick and sticking out through shrunken flesh like an anatomy body. Another was that two fairly trivial scars on my body sustained in childhood seemed so enormous that they were almost the whole of me. A third disturbance was that my penis seemed deformed. I have the idea it seemed wooden with a clubbed end but it was not erect."

C. said, "My one eye feels bigger than the other—like a Picasso picture—my face is drawing out like a Greek mask and when the corners of the mask go up I feel happy."

H. said, "In the beginning I had a pleasantly warm feeling beginning in the umbilical area and extending down both legs and genitalia—not erotic but a delightfully soothing feeling. Later I soon realized that I was having a watered-down orgasm which was constantly present—a most delightful feeling. But at the same time I seemed to have lost all sensation from my bladder and penis and had no control over the sphincter muscles or erectors and can remember being acutely disturbed as to whether I was disgracing myself by passing urine, faeces or semen into the bed. I had no idea whether I was wet or not, except by looking to see." (We had great difficulty in getting urine from this patient—he felt incapable of passing urine because his urinary apparatus seemed dissociated from him.)

F. experienced three attacks of what he described as "a sort of vertigo. I feel I am travelling a spiral course in a forward and up and down direction and the spirals are gaily coloured and all this is accompanied by acute anxiety and only occurred when his eyes were closed. This subject also complained of a "fluid-like feeling in my mouth—like a pad—it seems to make it difficult for me to articulate. Yes, it is amorphous—How amorphous can one get." (This remark accompanied by much merriment.)

I. said, "My body feels as though it is in continual motion, rocking and spinning around through space. My teeth feel strange as though they are made of plastic."

A. complained bitterly of a "horrible vibration" through his body and of difficulty in moving his tongue because it seemed "structureless." He said, "From time to time I get a feeling of descent. I could see a mental image of myself folded like a jack-knife falling through space between triangles of vivid colours set at angles and depths at variance to each other."

B., summing up, said, "The outstanding psychic experience was a loss of feeling real, an inability to know that I was really doing specific acts like talking, passing urine, etc." *Depersonalization.*

F. said he had a curious double image of himself. "It is as though I am watching myself lying in a big transparent bubble with my face pressed close to the side."

C. and I. both likened the experience to watching a film of one's own performance.

H.'s difficulty in knowing what his body was doing has already been described.

Mild euphoria was present at some time in all subjects and often one of the first abnormalities noted was a sudden unexpected burst of laughter because the whole idea of the experiment seemed suddenly very funny, or because some mildly amusing occurrence had become uproariously amusing. *Mood.*

On these occasions subjects would be unable to restrain their mirth, which was usually infectious.

One subject became extremely distressed about his "fragmentation of thought" and begged in anguish to have the experiment terminated immediately because everything had suddenly become unreal and terrifying—"this is like schizophrenia—there is a blocking between emotion and thought and it frightens me." His agony lasted only a few seconds and during this period the observer felt quite unable to make contact with him. Within a few minutes he was euphoric and with a laugh said, "In a way I can understand why people take it—if you just let your thoughts drift without worrying about them having reality or meaning it is quite relaxing."

Two subjects felt that the whole experience was extraordinarily delightful. J. said, "It is such a lovely drifting voluptuous sensation," and C. said, as the experiment was coming to an end, "I've got such a let down feeling—it is like coming out of a golden dream." These two subjects were the only ones who felt they would gladly take the drug again.

A curious detachment was common. At times the observer would become quite disturbed about some unexpected occurrence, e.g. gross muscular contractions, inability to urinate, sustained tachycardia of 140, or expiratory dyspnea, etc. But the subject, although aware of the occurrence, seemed insulated from anxiety about it. Some of the subjects mentioned headache as one of their symptoms, but when asked if it bothered them they laughed and seemed as detached as if it were someone else's headache. This detachment also extended to disorder of mental functioning, e.g., loss of recall seemed amusing more than alarming. If they had difficulty with a test they usually shrugged lazily as if to say, "What does it matter anyway?" Four subjects showed anxiety, but even then it was mild, or very transient, except in F. This was well shown by J., who became convinced that cannabis had unmasked a latent schizophrenia and that the second EEG was really electroconvulsive therapy, but this delusion was accompanied by what he called "uneasiness" even though he had thought out all the implications of being psychotic, e.g. losing his job and the distress of his parents.

Although this is the most striking example, all subjects showed inappropriateness of affect at some stage. G., while complaining bitterly of painful muscular spasms, burst out laughing.

After several hours, when the effects of the drug were wearing off, most subjects felt apathetic, disinclined to talk and vaguely depressed.

CLINICAL CHANGES

Physical Symptoms.   An invariable complaint was marked dryness of mouth. This was often one of the first symptoms noted. All subjects complained of paraesthesiae of the fingers and toes; five subjects also complained of paraesthesiae over the nose and round the mouth.

Several subjects described a "warm glowing feeling" which was experienced in the abdomen or pelvis.

Several subjects complained of intense praecordial discomfort.

Two subjects complained of expiratory dyspnea.

A most interesting and striking feature was a uniform suffusion of the conjunctiva sometimes accompanied by oedema of the eyelids. This invariably appeared about one to two hours after ingestion of the drug and persisted for many hours. It was not accompanied by any subjective discomfort and did not wax and wane. All subjects developed a sinus tachycardia—in one case the pulse rate, initially 50, rose to 80, but in all the other cases the rate rose to between 120 and 140. An ECG was done on one case and the graph showed a sinus tachycardia. In most cases the tachycardia persisted for several hours before the pulse gradually returned to its original level.

There was occasionally some rise in blood pressure in the first hour or two but this was never excessive, mainly systolic, and never exceeded 160 mm. Hg.

All subjects developed moderate coldness of the extremities and in some cases fingers and toes looked pallid.

One subject (a blonde) developed patchy flushing of the skin over the face and upper trunk which persisted for some hours.

Five subjects complained of mild frontal headache.

Nausea was common, occurring about three hours after the start of the experiment and some subjects vomited. It was the writer's impression that this symptom was related to the moving of the subject to the laboratory for the second EEG recording. The impression was that any movement at this time aggravated vasomotor imbalance. Subjects frequently became very pale and cold, but after returning to bed and being warmed, or after vomiting, they improved rapidly.

No subjects complained of hunger during the first three hours although they had not been given anything to eat or drink since 10 P.M. When given food all ate with relish—five said, "Even hospital food tastes delicious."

Reaction to venipuncture was variable. J., after the third puncture, begged to be allowed to discontinue the blood-sugar estimations because they were "agonizing." F., after the third puncture, said, "It's amazing—the drug is an analgesic—I did not feel a thing though I watched all the proceedings." Most subjects thought that the needle pricks became more and more unpleasant, but quickly added that it may well have been a cumulative effect.

Abnormal Movements.   Paucity of movement was usual and subjects ascribed this to the feeling of tranquillity and detachment. In many cases it was even an effort to speak and the observer had repeatedly to stimulate the subject by asking questions. Several subjects expressed their astonishment at the thought of anyone being impelled to violent or aggressive action by the drug.

G., however, exhibited the most astonishing muscular movements. These consisted of gross flexion-extension and abduction-adduction movements, principally of proximal muscles of the lower limbs and all muscles of the upper limbs. The movements could be stopped momentarily if he were urged to do so but immediately began again and were accompanied by much discomfort and complaint of soreness. "This is real—this is motor cortex irritation not hysterical. No, it is not a convulsion—my knee is dancing a Scottish reel." There was a certain amount of facial grimacing at the same time and a curious struggle between laughter and tears. The movements continued virtually without cessation for about three hours and the subject was left with painful, aching limbs the following day.

A. periodically gave a sort of jump with arching of the back and said it happened when he got a "vibratory feeling" passing over his whole body.

F. complained of involuntary muscular twitching involving at different times proximal limb or abdominal muscles—visible to the naked eye but not gross enough to move a limb.

Muscular Co-ordination.   Most subjects complained of slight difficulty in articulation but this was seldom objectively demonstrable. Crude tests such as the finger-nose test were usually well done, but picking up a small pin was difficult. The gait was not strikingly ataxic but subjects felt light-headed when walking and did not show any alacrity about getting out of bed for some hours after the drug had been taken, e.g., D. said, "About eight hours after the start I thought I would have a bath but felt so unsteady when I got out of bed that I decided to sleep instead."

SPECIAL INVESTIGATIONS

Electroencephalography.   Parasagittal and temporal recordings were done before cannabis was taken and repeated three hours afterwards. Of ten recordings four were reported as showing no change and in six there was some change. The reports were as follows:

E. The resting record shows a well-marked persistent 9 c.p.s. alpha rhythm in occipital and central areas.

    After cannabis the only change is a slight tendency to diminished persistence with longer and more frequent intervals of fast activity. EEG—slight change towards less persistent alpha after five grains of cannabis.

J. The resting record shows a well-marked, persistent and well-modulated 9 c.p.s. alpha rhythm which is present diffusely, except in the frontal areas where beta activity is seen.

    After cannabis the occipital alpha remains largely unchanged except that it is not quite so persistent and there is some intervening fast activity with a little random alpha over the post-central areas. EEG shows some change after cannabis—tendency to replacement of non-occipital alpha by fast activity.

G. The resting record shows a 9 c.p.s. alpha activity posteriorly, most persistent in the temporal areas and with a fair amount of fast activity in the parasagittal leads. The only change after seven grains of cannabis was one very short episode of 6 c.p.s. activity that appeared in the posterior temporal areas.

H. The initial recording shows a well-marked and almost persistent 10 c.p.s. alpha rhythm posteriorly, of rather low voltage; and low voltage beta activity anteriorly.

    Three hours after taking seven grains of cannabis the persistence of the posterior alpha activity is considerably less, it being interrupted by much irregular fast activity. The generally low amplitude remains unchanged.

K. (Clinical record of this case was not included in the series.)

    The record shows generally low voltage fast activity throughout; there is a minimal amount of posterior 11–12 c.p.s. alpha activity. After cannabis the only change is that there appears a moderate amount of bilaterally synchronous anterior temporal 6–7 c.p.s. activity.

C. The resting record shows a well-marked and persistent 10

c.p.s. alpha rhythm posteriorly with beta activity anteriorly. Three hours after the ingestion of six grains of
cannabis there is a slight quickening of the alpha rhythm
to 11 c.p.s. and it is not so persistent and uninterrupted.
The temporal leads show fast activity throughout—
probably much muscle artifact.

**Blood-sugar
Readings.**   Fasting blood-sugar estimations were done every half-
hour for two and a half hours. These did not show any
significant change. There was occasionally a tendency for the
blood sugar to show some slight elevation about one hour
after the cannabis had been taken but this was never outside
the range of normal. (See graph.)

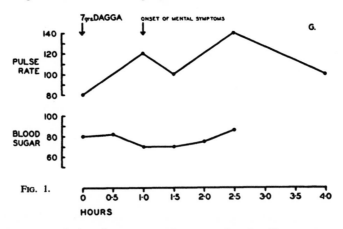

FIG. 1.

Urine Output.   Because of the frequent references in the literature to a
possible diuretic property of cannabis it was decided to
measure urine output during a fixed period before cannabis
was taken and for another fixed period after it had been
taken. The following table gives the results in seven cases:

Subject	Before Cannabis was Taken		After Cannabis was Taken	
	Period of Time	Volume of Urine	Period of Time	Volume of Urine
		ml.		ml.
A	2 hours	160	2½ hours	352
B	2 hours	224	1 hour	569
C	2½ hours	100	1½ hours	635
D	2 hours	192	50 minutes	352
I	2 hours	350	3 hours	400
J	1 hr. 45 mins.	150	3 hrs. 10 mins.	125
Writer	2 hours	250	3 hrs. 10 mins.	500

Because urine output appeared on the whole to show an increase after the ingestion of cannabis, more detailed study of two cases was done by Dr. Stewart Saunders. These showed a selective sodium and bicarbonate loss. This increase in sodium and bicarbonate is due to a tubular effect, there being no proportionate increase in the filtered load. Inhibition of carbonic anhydrase can also have this effect.

The evidence is sufficiently strong to suggest that further investigation of the diuretic properties of cannabis would be worthwhile.

The findings are tabulated below:

SUBJECT D

Excretion of Chloride Before and After Cannabis given at End of Period ONE

Period	Time (Minutes)	Urine Volume (ml.)	pH	GFR(Ccr) (ml./min.)	Filtered Load Cl. (m.eq./min.)	Urine Cl. (m.eq./min.)
1 ...	124	771	7·25	84·8	9·47	0·2395
2 ...	121	660	7·8	93·2	10·21	0·4426
3 ...	115	550	8·1	92·4	10·33	0·3139
Excretion of Sodium:						
					Na+	Na+
1 ...	124	771	7·25	84·8	11·66	0·1774
2 ...	121	660	7·80	93·2	13·51	0·7810
3 ...	115	550	8·10	92·4	9·61	0·7548
Excretion of Potassium:						
					K+	K+
1 ...	124	771	7·25	84·8	0·424	0·1581
2 ...	121	660	7·80	93·2	0·475	0·1975
3 ...	115	550	8·10	92·4	0·453	0·1148
				GFR (ml./min.)	Filtered Load m.mols./ min.	Urine Conc. m.mols./ min.
Bicarbonate:						
1 ...	124	771	7·25	84·8	2·4334	0·00435
2 ...	121	660	7·8	93·2	2·6003	0·168
3 ...	115	550	8·1	92·4	2·0882	0·1575

SUBJECT L

Excretion of Chloride Before and After Cannabis given at End of Period TWO

Period	Time (Minutes)	Urine Volume (ml.)	pH	GFR(Ccr) (ml./min.)	Filtered Load Cl. (m.eq./min.)	Urine Cl. (m.eq./min.)
1 ...	60	42	5·7	80·2	8·52	0·069
2 ...	60	46	6·0	83·7	8·89	0·113
3 ...	60	50	6·3	78·1	8·83	0·130
4 ...	60	64	6·6	89·8	10·12	0·171
5 ...	60	62		85·4	9·55	0·150

Excretion of Sodium:

					Na+	Na+
1 ...					11·15	0·076
2 ...					11·63	0·105
3 ...					11·30	0·128
4 ...					12·30	0·207
5 ...					11·61	0·212

Excretion of Potassium:

					K+	K+
1 ...					0·2887	0·035
2 ...					0·3013	0·053
3 ...					0·2812	0·036
4 ...					0·3233	0·058
5 ...					0·3577	0·080

Bicarbonate:

1 ...					2·254	0·0016
2 ...					2·351	0·0032
3 ...					2·280	0·0093
4 ...					2·028	0·0162
5 ...					2·6937	0·0274

Experiment Repeated.   The experiment was repeated on three subjects after an interval of several months. In each case the dose was reduced by one grain. It was striking that they all had the same experience the second time and one could, from their first experience, have predicted with accuracy the pattern of response on the second occasion. Several months had elapsed between the two experiments.

No blood-sugar estimations or electroencephalographic recordings were done on the second occasion and this may have accounted for the only difference observed, which was that the original tachycardia was much reduced and the main abnormality noted in heart rate was that it was more unstable than usual and accelerated rapidly on exertion.

The writer took four grains of cannabis and remained in bed in the ward until taken home by car in the late afternoon.

The Writer's Experience.

Before the cannabis was taken slight frontal headache and some apprehension was experienced. About ninety minutes after the drug had been taken some difficulty in articulation was experienced (this was not objectively demonstrable) and concurrently "I became aware of an astonishing difficulty in recall, so that I could not remember events that had just occurred. This inability of recall seemed to be associated with 'dips' in the level of consciousness when everything seemed rather unreal and hazy and in striking contrast to the periods when I emerged from the dip. It was like emerging from shadow into light. In addition, my concept of time was distorted so that it always seemed later than it really was and the journey down the corridor seemed eternally long.

"My mood change was striking. I experienced some euphoria but to me the really striking thing was detachment. This can be illustrated by the following examples: I realized that my headache (frontal and occipital) was really quite severe and yet it did not really matter and at the time I compared it to the indifference to pain apparently experienced by patients who have been leucotomized for the pain of inoperable carcinoma; when being wheeled down the corridor in full view of my patients I felt that the situation would normally have embarrassed me and I was struck by my indifference; finally, after I had been taken home and was lying in bed, I could hear my children hilariously swamping the bathroom, which normally never fails to irritate me, and I was astonished at my indifference to it. Physical symptoms were not prominent. I experienced some paraesthesiae of hands and feet, was conscious of coldness and had a bad headache. My pulse rate remained more or less normal unless I exerted myself, when it immediately rose from 80 to 120. I developed slight conjunctival suffusion and had a diuresis. The effect of the drug lasted for eleven hours."

**Report subject
who took 48
grains of Cannabis.**

About three-quarters of an hour after taking the drug the subject felt sleepy, with a heaviness of the eyes and a sense of rotation. About an hour after the drug had been taken he began to laugh uncontrollably and loudly and said that the whole idea of the experiment was killingly funny. For the next hour he laughed a great deal, spoke rapidly and excitedly and became fairly uninhibited in his behaviour, especially towards senior members of the staff whom he called by their first names. He addressed his chief, who had just been elected an F.R.C.P., by his first name and said, "You are very pleased with yourself about that F.R.C.P.—not that it was not richly deserved but really you are so self-satisfied about it." The matron of the hospital was also addressed with great familiarity and the superintendent and other members of the staff were criticized. His report on this aspect reads, "I can, of course, remember speaking a great deal, but time itself pressed on me. I was obsessed with time. There was such a lot to say and so little time and words seemed so insufficient. I remember feeling that I was behaving like a manic—with flight of ideas. I could not stick to a subject and revelled in the sheer pleasure of swinging the conversation round as it suited me. This was a time of intense activity and it all passed like a bright flash. Time and space seemed compressed into one bright minute during which all was gay talk, brilliant jokes and myself the care-free centre of it all."

At this time he experienced a "whirling of objects around a central axis which seemed placed in the middle of the ceiling," and he saw a vivid flash of colours which resembled a modern curtain set against a multi-coloured window. Objects seemed to stand out with "a lively 3-D effect" and the face of one of the observers seemed "exquisite, of very beautiful colour, and a lovely depth that made me want to sculpture his face." He was intensely hungry at this time.

After the first hour the euphoria began to wear off and he complained of various physical discomforts, e.g. intense cold in his feet which felt cold when touched and intense dryness of the mouth and nose. In addition, his hands and feet began to tingle and he complained of weakness of the extremities and several times asked anxiously whether this "peripheral neuritis" would persist. At about this time he wept when a venipuncture was done and said the needle prick was "agony."

He complained of difficulty in focusing his eyes and episodic mistiness of vision.

About three hours after the drug had been taken he became depressed and irritable, looked pale and vomited. He complained of a bitter taste in the mouth, severe abdominal cramps "like an ileus" and moaned, "What have you done to me?"

He also complained that time was passing terribly slowly.

During the "manic" phase he had a tachycardia of 120 which persisted for two and a half hours. His pulse rate then came down to 80 and eight hours later gradually settled to 70.

Five hours after the start of the experiment he looked so wretched and was in such abdominal discomfort that he was put on intravenous dextrose and given 50 mg. of Largactil* intramuscularly. Despite this he had a poor night and felt irritable and unwell and had periodic abdominal cramps for the next two days.

The report on his electroencephalograms reads: "The initial recording shows a well-marked 8 c.p.s. alpha rhythm posteriorly with irregular fast activity anteriorly and a small amount of anterior alpha. After drug ingestion there is a complete disappearance of the alpha activity and the whole record consists only of low voltage fast activity."

There was no change in blood sugar levels during the first three hours of the experiment.

(The abdominal cramps may be accounted for in part by the large amount of liquorice contained in the forty-eight pills.)

INTERVIEWS

This labourer was completely illiterate and had spent most of his life working with horses in a hawking establishment. He made a good impression, was quick-witted and had an engaging friendliness. He said that he had been smoking dagga regularly (two to three cigarettes) every night since the age of fifteen. "Once you smoke it it never lets you go. It makes your mind so that it can never fail. It makes you stronger, makes you laugh a lot and makes you like everybody. It makes me very energetic to my wife so that I even got twins. There is no crime in it—it is only with alcohol that it makes you do wrong things. It is best if you smoke it with other

Interview with coloured male aged 32 years.

---

*chlorpromazine

people but if alone you can think you hear the best band playing. Your imagination is so great that you can see someone you have not seen for a long time. But if there are other people with you you don't see or hear anything—you just enjoy yourself. If you smoke it and go to sleep immediately you feel terrible next morning. You must have a little enjoyment and exercise before you sleep and the next morning you feel fine."

He had no intention of giving up the habit and did not think it had harmed him in any way but, on the contrary, that it had enormously increased the savour of life.

This youth made a good impression. He had been in steady employment for four years, was neatly dressed, courteous and spoke intelligently. He said that he had been introduced to dagga smoking at a party eighteen months previously and although he had started the habit as a lark he had found it so pleasant that he had, since that time, regularly smoked two packets of cannabis a night. He always mixed the drug with ordinary tobacco and rolled a cigarette with the mixture. He described the effect as a "sort of light-headedness—like having a few glasses of wine and yet different because it does not make you drunk. Two cigarettes give me a very pleasant feeling for about an hour—I feel like laughing and cracking jokes and somehow one has more courage than normally. Everyone seems to be my friend and it is much more fun to smoke in company than alone. If I am alone I just fall asleep."

He was conscious of tachycardia when smoking, increased desire for food, especially ice-cream because it relieved the dryness of his mouth, and he had also noticed that he passed more urine than usual. He was not interested in alcohol and said that if he were offered alcohol or cannabis he would unhesitatingly choose cannabis. He has gone for several months without it and has not experienced any withdrawal symptoms or any cravings for the drug. The reason why he started smoking again is that he finds the habit pleasant and it does him no harm and he never has a hangover.

This youth made a poor impression. He left school at sixteen having failed to pass Standard six. He came to the interview because he thought he would be asked to volunteer to smoke some under supervision—"and then you would see how wild I get." He started smoking cannabis one year ago. It was the custom in the gang of about twenty youths of which he was a member. The gang meets about twice a week and are sometimes accompanied by girl friends. They always smoke their cannabis, mixing it with ordinary tobacco, and make a party of the meeting. They take a few bottles of wine and a vast quantity of fish, chips and bread, "because we get terribly hungry." When smoking he feels "very happy, very strong and enjoys talking a lot. I always end up by fighting someone because I feel I can't lose and if I get hurt I don't feel the pain. Once I hurt my leg but did not even know about it until the next day when I saw it was so bad a wound that it had to be stitched."

Occasionally he feels very tranquil after smoking and just wants to lie in the sun and sleep, but usually he becomes restless and either walks aimlessly for miles or picks fights. He has recently acquired a pellet gun and takes it with him when he joins the gang. After smoking several cigarettes he climbs into a tree and takes aim at the other members of the gang. The confusion and fear aroused in them pleases him very much. He said that time had no meaning for him when he was smoking and far from having a hangover he always felt very relaxed the next day and "could not worry about anything." He emphasized that the gang was not really wild—"we never do anything wrong, like breaking into houses."

This man claimed that he had smoked cannabis from the age of fourteen to thirty-two but had given up the habit because he had been rescued from this "sin" by a minister of religion. He said that after cessation of the habit he had felt a craving for the drug for six months but had not suffered any physical withdrawal effects. (Another addict said that this man was still smoking cannabis.) He gave the impression of being unstable and humourless but had a remarkable capacity for self-observation.

He started off the interview by saying "dagga means women, murder and fight." He seemed to be particularly impressed by its effect as an aphrodisiac and stated that he was obsessed with the desire for women while smoking it. He claimed that his sexual vigour was so enhanced that he had

Interview with white male aged 33 years.

on many occasions slept with four to five women in one night or had repeated intercourse with the same woman. After smoking he would follow women in the street "white or coloured—pretty or ugly—they all attracted me." If he was unable to strike up an acquaintance with the woman he would seek other women or masturbate. "A man has the energy to go on over and over and after one time my nature was still high but if I slept even for thirty minutes all desire would leave me." Recently since he began to regard the habit as sinful he would sometimes get a strange feeling while looking at a woman, that "she would seem to change into something strange and horrible, e.g., a stone mountain or a devil." One not infrequent hallucinatory experience was seeing the "devil with long claws and feet looking as though he were going to jump at me and come down on me with his long claws. Then I would cry and pray to God to deliver me from the vice. The next moment I would be laughing madly because I knew it was not really there." He described several occasions when he experienced a marked change in visual perception—"say I was looking at your face, it might change like this—the eyes might start to look Chinese and the nose to broaden until the whole face looked like a mask and then it might make me want to laugh and laugh or if it were a man's face I might go and pick a fight with him. I never felt scared and a fight only ended when I won or was knocked out."

He claimed that his thinking was better when smoking cannabis. "My thoughts get faster and continuous—it is like a verse in your brain as though the devil is talking to me." He quoted a friend of his who when taken to court "always makes a better impression of being better educated and cleverer than he really is, because if you think you are clever you seem to be cleverer." Despite the impression of accelerated thought and ideas "when one reads one sticks with one word and can't get any further." He mentioned that talking was particularly enjoyable and for this reason he always sought company when smoking. "Most smokers don't drink much with it—a man can sit the whole night with one small glass of wine in front of him as long as he has his dagga." He said that alcohol and dagga were completely different in their effect. "Dagga is 100 percent better—you walk up steady, you think a lot and you enjoy talking." An interesting observation was that he was much more reckless after drinking wine than after smoking cannabis. "Dagga makes you more scared in a way. I would never ride my bicycle or drive a car when I had been smoking because I knew the devil might mislead me and make me have an accident, but when drunk I would not mind doing these things."

He was also struck by the difficulty in estimating time. "If you walk for thirty minutes you think you have been walking for an hour and the same goes for talking."

He had also noted tachycardia and increased appetite, especially for curry and rice, and marked dryness of the mouth even after smoking through water.

He claimed that he could identify a dagga smoker at a glance by the "drooping, narrow, shining eyes."

He denied any hangover after smoking and said that the habit never interfered with his work.*

DISCUSSION

The results show quite a marked individual variation in response to cannabis. This seems to depend more on differences in the basic personality and temperament of the subjects than on difference in dosage. Apart from one subject who took forty-eight grains, the range of dosage was not wide, varying between four to seven grains. In the three subjects in whom the experiment was repeated a very similar clinical picture was obtained on the second occasion despite a reduction of the original dosage by one grain. The impression given by the addicts who were interviewed was that they always reacted in the same way to the drug.

Despite this individual variation one could discern, in all cases, a common basic pattern of response. All subjects experienced a curious disturbance of consciousness, a disorder of time perception, difficulty in immediate recall allied to thought disorder and a change in affect usually in the direction of euphoria. Accompanying these mental changes, the constant physical changes were conjunctival suffusion, paraesthesiae, dryness of the mouth, tachycardia and diuresis.

The disturbance of consciousness is difficult to define. For

* All the addicts smoked their cannabis and it is difficult to say how much of the drug was absorbed in this way.

The great advantage in smoking rather than ingesting cannabis is that the smoker can regulate the dosage so that with a little practice he can gauge with accuracy the amount that gives him the maximum satisfaction.

the first few hours there was in all cases a waxing and waning of contact with reality, or, more correctly, a constriction of the field of awareness. Despite this the capacity for self-observation appeared to be heightened and all subjects responded relevantly if stimulated. Several of them, who had no manifest disorder of perception, vigorously denied any disturbance of consciousness, maintaining that they were at all times fully aware of their surroundings and the nature and purpose of the experiment. But to the observer there was undoubtedly a definite though often subtle and elusive change in the degree or direction of awareness in all cases.

The disorder of time perception was to all subjects an incredible phenomenon and gave to the experiment a curious, slightly unearthly quality. It always took the same form, i.e. during the first few hours estimated time was always later than actual time—moments of chronological time seemed an eternity. (The only exception to this was the subject who took forty-eight grains and felt initially that time was passing incredibly quickly while later it dragged with an agonizing slowness.)

There was no clear-cut disturbance of space perception though journeys seemed eternally long. This illusion seemed to be directly related to the time that the journey took.

The change in affect usually took the form of euphoria. The subject who took forty-eight grains was in a state of sustained hilarity accompanied by great activity for about one and a half hours. All the other subjects showed a less sustained euphoria, accompanied by excited talking. Although this was to some extent infectious it was clear to the observer that it was out of all proportion to the stimulus. The idea of the experiment would suddenly seem enormously amusing, and oddly enough the subject would often remark on its inappropriateness himself; e.g., in telling some story, with much giggling, he would say that it seemed absurd that it was so funny and yet laughter was irresistible. Occasionally the laughter was bizarrely inappropriate. One subject laughed as he complained of painful muscle spasms.

Another common mood change was detachment which often alternated with euphoria. It was as though the subject was somehow insulated from everything that was happening to him. This certainly contributed to some extent to the common feeling of double consciousness, i.e., that the subject was himself an observer. Anxiety was not uncommon but seldom gross. It was usually most intense as the drug began to take effect and seemed to be greatest in those subjects who tried to resist the experience. This was well shown by one subject who asked with every indication of intense anxiety for an antidote to the drug, yet a few minutes later relaxed and said that he could understand people taking the drug for pleasure because once one "gave oneself up" to it it was pleasant.

Some degree of thought disorder was invariably present. In many cases this consisted predominantly of an inability to recall what had just happened so that the subject was often totally unable to sustain a conversation unless prompted about a recent remark by the observer. In some subjects the whole process of thinking seemed broken off abruptly, or they complained of "fragmentation" of thought and described thinking as having no beginning or end and such a tenuous reality that it was continually being shattered by other disconnected pieces of thoughts.

Mayer-Gross *et al.* (1954) stated that as long ago as the mid-nineteenth century Moreau had commented on the dissociation of ideas with cannabis. In 1932 Beringer had described three forms of thought disorder with cannabis. These were:

Fragmentation of perceptive wholes through fragmentation of thought processes. Disturbance of memory by which everything experienced is forgotten at once. Frequent and sudden interruptions of the stream of thought—the gaps only lasting a few seconds. Beringer compared these to epileptic "blanks," or the sudden disruption of the associative links in thinking of schizophrenics.

It is difficult to separate these thought disturbances from one another and they may well be closely interwoven. The sudden blockages of thought and apparent disruption of the pattern of thinking might be no more than consequences of the defect in the power of immediate recall.

The physical changes that occurred in all subjects were also of great interest.

The conjunctival suffusion, uniform and symptomless, was particularly notable. It has been mentioned by many writers and seems to appear at about the same time as the narcotic effect. It persists for many hours and disappears gradually.

Chopra and Chopra[6] state that it can persist long after the narcotic effect has disappeared. They also stated that in most addicts a permanent congestion of the transverse ciliary vessels develops. One addict interviewed showed this congestion and his addiction had been of many years standing. A marked proneness to tachycardia on exertion or a sustained sinus tachycardia was shown by all subjects. Even allowing for excitement or tension or muscular activity there appeared to be a definite autonomic imbalance. Dryness of the mouth was universal and marked, almost like an atropine effect, but dilatation of the pupils, if it existed at all, was only slight.

Paraesthesiae in the extremities and peri-oral area was a marked feature in all cases, and in the case who took forty-eight grains it was accompanied by a subjective feeling of weakness of the extremities.

The more florid symptoms were a disorder of visual perception, the appearance of formed visual images, usually intricate, when the eyes were closed, bizarre disorder of body perception and a marked feeling of dissociation not only of self, so that the subject of the experiment often said he felt as though he were the observer of the experiment, but also of the various functions of self, so that action, volition, thought and effect became chaotically disorganized.

The abnormalities of movement, which in a mild form consisted of periodic contraction of isolated muscle groups, or occasional writhing movements and in a severe form were a continuous medley of movements, are noteworthy because they are so difficult to classify. Beringer observed a great variety of motor anomalies including hyperkinetic and hypokinetic states.

Walton[20] mentions a medical man, Burr, who took cannabis and "suffered a general convulsion which lasted three minutes; he felt well; his speech was not affected. The convulsion resembled an attack of hysteria ... the convulsions appeared willful in that he willed to convulse; he knew that he was throwing his arms about, that he was writhing like a snake, acting like a clown, making silly grimaces. But he could not will to do otherwise. He could restrain a convulsion for a few minutes, but soon the will to convulse overcame the will to inhibit." This description is very like the state seen in one subject on two separate occasions, though the use of the term "convulsion" is unfortunate. One is also reminded of the peculiar contortions of the Quakers. In other works there appears to be some neural dissociation but a precise explanation for this extraordinary state eludes one.

Diuresis was suggested by the volume changes in the urine in all subjects. In two cases where the electrolytes were done there was a selective sodium and bicarbonate loss.

The electroencephalographic changes were not specific. Six out of ten showed changes but they remained within the limits of normal. Of these four showed an increase in fast activity and one showed one very short episode of 6 c.p.s. activity in the posterior temporal areas while another developed a moderate amount of bilaterally synchronous 6–7 c.p.s. anterior temporal activity. In the subject who took forty-eight grains of cannabis the alpha rhythm disappeared completely and the whole record consisted only of low voltage fast activity.

There do not seem to have been many electroencaphalographic studies done during cannabis intoxication. Wikler and Lloyd[22] reported that electroencaphalograms during marijuana smoking showed a marked increase in the number and amplitude of the fast waves but these appeared to be of muscular and not nervous origin. Williams gave *ad lib.* doses of pyrahexyl (a synthetic cannabis preparation) to six patients for twenty-six to thirty-one days and stated that during prolonged medication the dominant frequencies were markedly slowed.

The electroencephalographic tracings in this study certainly gave no indication of the site of action of cannabis and at most merely indicated a general cerebral disturbance. It is interesting that Loewe[11] has described a powerful antiepileptic effect in all the synthetic cannabinols that he tested, but at the moment the significance and practical implications of his findings are not clear.

Any attempt to explain the pathogenesis of the symptoms and signs seen in acute cannabis intoxication is purely speculative. One could envisage the process as being a diffuse neuronal change affecting not only the cerebral tissue but also peripheral nerves. The change, being temporary, suggests some subtle and reversible change in neuronal enzyme systems. Rolls and Stafford-Clark[16] have claimed that one property that all the hallucinogens have in common is their capacity to inhibit the action of amine oxidase. It is tempting to try to fit the conjunctival suffusion into the picture by suggesting that the change is primarily vascular and the suffusion a manifestation of cerebral hyperaemia. It is certainly such a striking and unusual feature that its elucidation may well yield some of the secrets of cannabis pharmacology.

Another possibility is that the principal action of cannabis is on the brainstem and thalamic structures. The chief argument in favour of this view would be the wave-like effect observed, which might suggest some disturbance of the "alerting" system between the reticular formation and the cortex. A clue to the temporal disorientation is suggested by the work of Spiegel[19] who has reported finding it in twenty-three of thirty-nine cases who underwent thalamotomy for intractable pain. The autonomic changes might also be a result of brainstem disturbance. The apparent involvement of peripheral nerves is not so easy to fit into this theory but anterior horn cells can certainly be profoundly influenced by the reticular formation and there might conceivably be an effect on the afferent nerves.

An attempt to compare the cannabis intoxication with the naturally occurring psychoses leads to immediate difficulties. The lack of any precise diagnostic criteria for schizophrenia is one difficulty and another is the nature of the experimental situation. The mental abnormality seen was not the result of a slow insidious weakening of the ties with reality but an acute disturbance produced in apparently normal well-adjusted young people. Contact with them was maintained throughout the experiment and this fact deserves special emphasis. During the experiment many subjects said that the observer seemed their one link with reality. Solitude and a cutting-off of virtually all sensory input can lead to extraordinary effects as Hebb and his co-workers have shown even without the administration of a drug that has such profound psychic effects. The fact that the observer stayed with the subjects throughout the experiment may well have profoundly modified the results so that in all cases contact with reality was never completely lost, insight in most cases was retained and florid symptoms never became overwhelming.

Despite this there are several features that deserve comment. The subject who took forty-eight grains behaved very like a manic, with much laughter, talk and flight of ideas, distractibility, lack of inhibition, etc. The other subjects showed more of a schizophrenic picture, especially as regards the apparent fragmentation of thought and the bizarre distortions of perception, notably of body image.

CONCLUSION

It is not claimed that any of the results obtained in this study are new in the sense that they have never been described before. They have all been described at one time or another, in the voluminous literature on cannabis. But each age brings some difference in attitude to an age-old problem. At the moment the quest for chemical mechanisms in the psychoses is popular and much can probably be gained from research along these lines.

It is suggested that *Cannabis sativa* may prove a valuable research tool in work of this kind. Its great advantage is its extremely low toxicity and the fact that it can be administered orally. Once its chemistry is fully understood research with it should advance rapidly.

It may well prove to have important therapeutic value as well. There has always been sporadic interest in this aspect because of the euphoria it produces, but so far the wave-like effect has been a drawback. It might be a useful adjunct to psychotherapy. Although one subject was emphatic about its value in giving him new insight into his basic personality most of the subjects did not emphasize this aspect and all of them, including the subject who took forty-eight grains, said that they had no difficulty in concealing matters that they did not wish to discuss. Obviously all subjects working together on the staff of a closed institution will have certain reservations about what they are prepared to disclose. This makes the situation different from that in a doctor-patient relationship.

Finally, an interesting sideline was the finding that cannabis is a reasonably potent oral diuretic which causes a specific sodium bicarbonate loss. With the present search for oral diuretics of this type this may well turn out to have important therapeutic implications.

Summary.

I. A clinical and metabolic study of acute intoxication with *Cannabis sativa* has been made. Special attention has been paid to its role as a research tool in the model psychoses.

II. The general history of the drug has been briefly reviewed.

III. The history of the drug habit in South Africa has been described.

IV. Experimental work comprised the

    1. Administration of a single oral dose of *Cannabis sativa* to ten medical volunteers and the observation of

       (a) Subjective experiences and behaviour;

       (b) Clinical changes;

       (c) Special investigations, e.g., blood-sugar estimations, urine output, electroencephalographic tracings.

    2. The administration of a second oral dose of *Cannabis sativa* to three of the ten subjects.

    3. The administration of the drug to the writer.

    4. The administration of an overdose to one subject.

    5. Interviews with four male cannabis addicts.

V. The implications of the experimental work have been discussed.

Acknowlegments. While deeply grateful to many people for their co-operation and encouragement I wish expressly to acknowledge my indebtedness to Dr. S. Berman, head of the Department of Neurology and Psychiatry at Groote Schuur Hospital, for not only keeping a general eye on the work and giving valuable advice and criticism but also reporting on the electroencephalographic tracings, to Professor J. M. Watt, Professor of Pharmacology of the University of the Witwatersrand, for his generosity with advice and references, Dr. Ryno J. Smit, Chief Regional Health Officer, Union Health Department for making it possible to obtain cannabis and Professor N. Sapeika, Professor of Pharmacology at the University of Cape Town and Mr. J. W. Bates of the Pharmacology Department for preparing the cannabis, Dr. I. Sakinofsky for his most generous help as an observer, Dr. S. Saunders for his enthusiastic interest in and work on the diuretic aspect, Dr. Vedder, Mrs. Glickman and her staff at the Medical Library, Sister Hoare for putting up so graciously with the disruption of her ward routine, Mr. C. C. Goosen of the Department of Surgical Research and to the Staff Research Fund for a grant. Finally my sincere thanks go to the volunteer subjects who made this investigation possible.

References

1. Adams, R., "Marihuana," The Harvey Lectures, 1942, 168.

2. Allentuck, S., and Bowman, K. M., "The psychiatric aspects of marihuana intoxication," *Amer. J. Psychiat.*, 1942, 248.

3. Beringer, K., "Clinical Symptoms of Hashish Intoxication: Psychological Disturbances," *Nervenarzt*, **5**, 346–357; cited by Mayer-Gross, Slater and Roth, *Clinical Psychiatry*, 1954, p. 357. London: Cassell & Co. Ltd.

4. Bourhill, C. J. G., "The smoking of dagga (Indian hemp) among the native races of South Africa and the resultant evils." 1913. (Thesis submitted for the degree of Doctor of Medicine, Edinburgh University.)

5. Bromberg, W., "Marihuana: A psychiatric study," *J.A.M.A.*, 1939, **113**, 4.

6. Chopra, I. C., and Chopra, N. R., "The use of cannabis drugs in India," *United Nations Bulletin on Narcotics*, 1957, **9**, 5.

Idem, ibid., 1957, **9**, 11.

Idem, ibid., 1957, **9**, 20.

7. Goodman, L. S., and Gilman, A., *The Pharmacological Basis of Therapeutics*, 1955, p. 171. New York: The Macmillan Company.

8. Gunn, J. W. C., *Arch. Internat. Pharmacodyn. Therap.*, 1929, 35, 266; cited by Watt, J. M., and Breyer-Brankwijk, M. G., *The Medicinal and Poisonous Plants of Southern Africa*, 1932, p. 35. Edinburgh: E. and S. Livingstone.

9. Hoffer, A., Osmond, H., and Smythies, J., "Schizophrenia: A New Approach. II. Result of a Year's Research," *J. Ment. Sci.*, 1954, **100**, 29.

10. Lewin, L., *Phantastica, Narcotic and Stimulating Drugs: Their Use and Abuse*, 1931, p. 109. London: Kegan Paul, Trench, Trubner and Co. Ltd. (Translated from the second German edition by P. H. A. Wirth.)

Idem, ibid., 1931, p. 114.

11. Loewe, S., "The Active Principles of Cannabis and the Pharmacology of the Cannabinols." Translated from *Archiv. für experim. Pathologie und Pharmakologie*, 1950, **211**, 175.

12. Mayor's Committee on Marihuana. *The Marihuana Problem in the City of New York: Sociological, Medical, Psychological and Pharmacological Studies*, 1944. Lancaster, Pa: The Jacques Cattel Press.

13. Moreau, J., *On Hashish and Mental Disease*, Paris 1845; cited by Mayer-Gross, Slater and Roth, *Clinical Psychiatry*, 1954, p. 357. London: Cassell & Co. Ltd.

14. Parker, C. S., and Wrigley, F., "Synthetic Cannabis Preparations in Psychiatry: (1) Synhexyl," *J. Ment. Sci.*, 1950, **96**, 276.

15. Report of the Interdepartmental Committee appointed by the Government of the Union of South Africa on the Abuse of Dagga, 1951.

16. Rolls, E. J., and Stafford-Clark, D., "Depersonalization treated by Cannabis Indica and Psychotherapy," *Guy's Hosp. Rept.*, 1954, 103, 330.

17. Russel, W., "Mental Symptoms associated with the smoking of Dagga. Report of an Investigation conducted by the Medical Staff of Pretoria Mental Hospital," *A.M.A. of S.A.*, 1938, 12, 85.

18. Stockings, G. T., "A New Euphoriant for Depressive Mental States," *Brit. med. J.*, 1947, i, 918.

19. Spiegel, E. A., Wycis, H. T., Orchinik, C. W., and Freed, H., "The Thalamus and Temporal Orientation," *Science*, 1955, 121, 771.

20. Walton R. P., *Marihuana—America's New Drug Problem*, 1938, p. 152. Philadelphia: J. B. Lippincott Co.

   Idem, ibid., 1938, p. 187.

   Idem, ibid., 1938, p. 126.

21. Watt, J. M., and Breyer-Brankwijk, M. G., *The Medicinal and Poisonous Plants of Southern Africa*, 1932, p. 35. Edinburgh: E. and S. Livingstone.

   Idem, "The Forensic and Sociological Aspects of the Dagga Problem in South Africa," *S.A.M.J.*, 1936, 10, 573.

22. Wikler, A., and Lloyd, B., "Effect of smoking Marihuana Cigarettes on Cortical Electrical Activity," *Fed. Proc.*, 1945, 4, 141.

23. Williams, E. G., Himmelsbach, C. K., Wikler, A., and Ruble, D. C., *Public Health Reports*, 1945. *Wash.*, 61, 1059–1083; cited by Parker, C. S., and Wrigley, F., "Synthetic Cannabis Preparations in Psychiatry: (1) Synhexyl," *J. Ment. Sci.*, 1950, 96, 276.

Clinical and Psychological Effects of Marijuana in Man

BY ANDREW T. WEIL, M.D.,
NORMAN E. ZINBERG, M.D.,
& JUDITH M. NELSEN, M.A.

In the spring of 1968 we conducted a series of pilot experiments on acute marijuana intoxication in human subjects. The study was not undertaken to prove or disprove popularly held convictions about marijuana as an intoxicant, to compare it with other drugs, or to introduce our own opinions. Our concern was simply to collect some long overdue pharmacological data. In this article we describe the primitive state of knowledge of the drug, the research problems encountered in designing a replicable study, and the results of our investigations.

Marijuana is a crude preparation of flowering tops, leaves, seeds, and stems of female plants of Indian hemp *Cannabis sativa* L.; it is usually smoked. The intoxicating constituents of hemp are found in the sticky resin exuded by the tops of the plants, particularly the females. Male plants produce some resin but are grown mainly for hemp fiber, not for marijuana. The resin itself, when prepared for smoking or eating, is known as "hashish." Various *Cannabis* preparations are used as intoxicants throughout the world; their potency varies directly with the amount of resin present.[1] Samples of American marijuana differ greatly in pharmacological activity, depending on their composition (tops contain most resin; stems, seeds and lower leaves least) and on the conditions

Reprinted from *Science*, vol. 162, December 13, 1968, pp. 1234–1242. © 1968 by the American Association for the Advancement of Science.

under which the plants were grown. In addition, different varieties of *Cannabis* probably produce resins with different proportions of constituents.[2] Botanists feel that only one species of hemp exists, but work on the phytochemistry of the varieties of this species is incomplete.[3] Chronic users claim that samples of marijuana differ in quality of effects as well as in potency; that some types cause a preponderance of physical symptoms, and that other types tend to cause greater distortions of perception or of thought.

Pharmacological studies of *Cannabis* indicate that the tetrahydrocannabinol fraction of the resin is the active portion. In 1965, Mechoulam and Gaoni[4] reported the first total synthesis of $(-)$-Δ^1-*trans*-tetrahydrocannabinol (THC), which they called "the psychotomimetically active constituent of hashish (marijuana)." Synthetic THC is now available for research in very limited supply.

In the United States, the use of *Cannabis* extracts as therapeutics goes back to the nineteenth century, but it was not until the 1920s that use of marijuana as an intoxicant by migrant Mexican laborers, urban Negroes, and certain Bohemian groups, caused public concern.[3] Despite increasingly severe legal penalties imposed during the 1930s, use of marijuana continued in these relatively small populations without great public uproar or apparent changes in numbers or types of users until the last few years. The fact that almost none of the studies devoted to the physiological and psychological effects of *Cannabis* in man was based on controlled laboratory experimentation escaped general notice. But with the explosion of use in the 1960s, at first on college campuses followed by a spread downward to secondary schools and upward to a portion of the established middle class, controversy over the dangers of marijuana generated a desire for more objective information about the drug.

Of the three known studies on human subjects performed by Americans, the first[5] was done in the Canal Zone with thirty-four soldiers; the consequences reported were hunger and hyperphagia, loss of inhibitions, increased pulse rate with unchanged blood pressure, a tendency to sleep, and unchanged performance of psychological and neurological tests. Doses and type of marijuana were not specified.

The second study, known as the 1944 La Guardia Report,[6] noted that seventy-two prisoners, forty-eight of whom were previous *Cannabis* users, showed minimum physiological responses, but suffered impaired intellectual functioning and decreased body steadiness, especially well demonstrated by non-users after high doses. Basic personality structures remained unchanged as subjects reported feelings of relaxation, disinhibition, and self-confidence. In that study, the drug was administered orally as an extract. No controls were described, and doses and quality of marijuana were unspecified.

Williams *et al.* in 1946[7] studied a small number of prisoners who were chronic users; they were chiefly interested in effects of long-term smoking on psychological functioning. They found an initial exhilaration and euphoria which gave way after a few days of smoking to indifference and lassitude that somewhat impaired performance requiring concentration and manual dexterity. Again, no controls were provided.

Predictably, these studies, each deficient in design for obtaining reliable physiological and psychological data, contributed no dramatic or conclusive results. The 1967 President's Commission on Law Enforcement and the Administration of Justice described the present state of knowledge by concluding:[3] ". . . no careful and detailed analysis of the American experience [with marijuana] seems to have been attempted. Basic research has been almost nonexistent. . . ." Since then, no other studies with marijuana itself have been reported, but in 1967 Isbell[8] administered synthetic THC to chronic users. At doses of 120 μg/kg orally or 50 μg/kg by smoking, subjects reported this drug to be similar to marijuana. At higher doses (300 to 400 μg/kg orally or 200 to 250 μg/kg by smoking), psychotomimetic effects occurred in most subjects. This synthetic has not yet been compared with marijuana in non-users or given to any subjects along with marijuana in double-blind fashion.

Investigations outside the United States have been scientifically deficient, and for the most part have been limited to anecdotal and sociological approaches.[9-12] So far as we know, our study is the first attempt to investigate marijuana in a formal double-blind experiment with the appropriate controls. It is also the first attempt to collect basic clinical and psychological information on the drug by observing its effects on marijuana-naive human subjects in a neutral laboratory setting.

Research Problems.   That valid basic research on marijuana is almost nonexistent is not entirely accounted for by legislation which
restricts even legitimate laboratory investigations or by public
reaction sometimes verging on hysteria. A number of
obstacles are intrinsic to the study of this drug. We now
present a detailed description of our specific experimental
approach, but must comment separately on six general
problems confronting the investigator who contemplates
marijuana research.

1. Concerning the route of administration, many pharmacologists dismiss the possibility of giving marijuana by smoking because, they say, the dose cannot be standardized.[13] We
consider it not only possible, but important to administer the
drug to humans by smoking rather than by the oral route for
the following reasons. (i) Smoking is the way nearly all
Americans use marijuana. (ii) It is possible to have subjects
smoke marijuana cigarettes in such a way that drug dosage is
reasonably uniform for all subjects. (iii) Standardization of
dose is not assured by giving the drug orally because little is
known about gastrointestinal absorption of the highly water-
insoluble cannabinoids in man. (iv) There is considerable
indirect evidence from users that the quality of intoxication
is different when marijuana or preparations of it are ingested
rather than smoked. In particular, ingestion seems to cause
more powerful effects, more "LSD-like" effects, longer-
lasting effects, and more hangovers.[12,14] Further, marijuana
smokers are accustomed to a very rapid onset of action due
to efficient absorption through the lungs, whereas the latency
for onset of effects may be forty-five or sixty minutes after
ingestion. (v) There is reported evidence from experiments
with rats and mice that the pharmacological activities of
natural hashish (not subjected to combustion) and hashish
sublimate (the combustion products) are different.[14]

2. Until quite recently, it was extremely difficult to
estimate the relative potencies of different samples of marijuana by the techniques of analytical chemistry. For this
study, we were able to have the marijuana samples assayed
spectrophotometrically[15] for THC content. However, since
THC has not been established as the sole determinant of
marijuana's activity, we still feel it is important to have
chronic users sample and rate marijuana used in research.
Therefore, we assayed our material by this method as well.

3. One of the major deficiencies in previous studies has been the absence of negative control or placebo treatments, which we consider essential to the design of this kind of investigation. Because marijuana smoke has a distinctive odor and taste, it is difficult to find an effective placebo for use with chronic users. The problem is much less difficult with non-users. Our solution to this dilemma was the use of portions of male hemp stalks,[16] devoid of THC, in the placebo cigarettes.

4. In view of the primitive state of knowledge about marijuana, it is difficult to predict which psychological tests will be sensitive to the effects of the drug. The tests we chose were selected because, in addition to being likely to demonstrate effects, they have been used to evaluate many other psychoactive drugs. Of the various physiological parameters available, we chose to measure (i) heart rate, because previous studies have consistently reported increases in heart rate after administration of marijuana;[5] (ii) respiratory rate, because it is an easily measured vital sign, and depression has been reported;[11, 17] (iii) pupil size, because folklore on effects of marijuana consistently includes reports of pupillary dilatation, although objective experimental evidence of an effect of the drug on pupils has not been sought; (iv) conjunctival appearance, because both marijuana smokers and eaters are said to develop red eyes;[11] and (v) blood sugar, because hypoglycemia has been invoked as a cause of the hunger and hyperphagia commonly reported by marijuana users, but animal and human evidence of this effect is contradictory.[6,10,11] [The La Guardia Report, quoted by Jaffe in Goodman and Gilman,[18] described hyperglycemia as an effect of acute intoxication.] We did not measure blood pressure because previous studies have failed to demonstrate any consistent effect on blood pressure in man, and we were unwilling to subject our volunteers to a nonessential annoyance.

5. It is necessary to control set and setting. "Set" refers to the subject's psychological expectations of what a drug will do to him in relation to his general personality structure. The total environment in which the drug is taken is the setting. All indications are that the form of marijuana intoxication is particularly dependent on the interaction of drug, set, and setting. Because of recent increases in the extent of use and

in attention given this use by the mass media, it is difficult to find subjects with a neutral set toward marijuana. Our method of selecting subjects (described below), at the least, enabled us to identify the subjects' attitudes. Unfortunately, too many researchers have succumbed to the temptation to have subjects take drugs in "psychedelic" environments or have influenced the response to the drug by asking questions that disturb the setting. Even a question as simple as, "How do you feel?" contains an element of suggestion that alters the drug-set-setting interaction. We took great pains to keep our laboratory setting neutral by strict adherence to an experimental timetable and to a prearranged set of conventions governing interactions between subjects and experimenters.

6. Medical, social, ethical, and legal concerns about the welfare of subjects are a major problem in a project of this kind. Is it ethical to introduce people to marijuana? When can subjects safely be sent home from the laboratory? What kind of follow-up care, if any, should be given? These are only a few specific questions with which the investigator must wrestle. Examples of some of the precautions we took are as follows. (i) All subjects were volunteers. All were given psychiatric screening interviews and were clearly informed that they might be asked to smoke marijuana. All non-users tested were persons who had reported that they had been planning to try marijuana. (ii) All subjects were driven home by an experimenter; they agreed not to engage in unusual activity or operate machinery until the next morning and to report any unusual, delayed effects. (iii) All subjects agreed to report for follow-up interviews six months after the experiment. Among other things, the check at six months should answer the question whether participation in the experiment encouraged further drug use. (iv) All subjects were protected from possible legal repercussions of their participation in these experiments by specific agreements with the Federal Bureau of Narcotics, the Office of the Attorney General of Massachusetts, and the Massachusetts Bureau of Drug Abuse and Drug Control.[19]

Subjects.   The central group of subjects consisted of nine healthy, male volunteers, twenty-one to twenty-six years of age, all of whom smoked tobacco cigarettes regularly but had never tried marijuana previously. Eight chronic users of marijuana also participated, both to "assay" the quality of marijuana received from the Federal Bureau of Narcotics and to enable the experimenters to standardize the protocol, using subjects familiar with their responses to the drug. The age range for users was also twenty-one to twenty-six years. They all smoked marijuana regularly, most of them every day or every other day.

The nine "naive" subjects were selected after a careful screening process. An initial pool of prospective subjects was obtained by placing advertisements in the student newspapers of a number of universities in the Boston area. These advertisements sought "male volunteers, at least twenty-one years old, for psychological experiments." After nonsmokers were eliminated from this pool, the remaining volunteers were interviewed individually by a psychiatrist who determined their histories of use of alcohol and other intoxicants as well as their general personality types. In addition to serving as a potential screening technique to eliminate volunteers with evidence of psychosis, or of serious mental or personality disorder, these interviews served as the basis for the psychiatrist's prediction of the type of response an individual subject might have after smoking marijuana. (It should be noted that no marijuana-naive volunteer had to be disqualified on psychiatric grounds.) Only after a prospective subject passed the interview was he informed that the "psychological experiment" for which he had volunteered was a marijuana study. If he consented to participate, he was asked to sign a release, informing him that he would be "expected to smoke cigarettes containing marijuana or an inert substance." He was also required to agree to a number of conditions, among them that he would "during the course of the experiment take no psychoactive drugs, including alcohol, other than those drugs administered in the course of the experiment."

It proved extremely difficult to find marijuana-naive persons in the student population of Boston, and nearly two months of interviewing were required to obtain nine men. All those interviewed who had already tried marijuana volunteered this information quite freely and were delighted to discuss their use of drugs with the psychiatrist. Nearly all persons encountered who had not tried marijuana admitted this somewhat apologetically. Several said they had been meaning to try the drug but had not got around to it. A few said they had no access to it. Only one person cited the current laws as his reason for not having experimented with marijuana. It seemed clear in the interviews that many of these persons were actually afraid of how they might react to marijuana; they therefore welcomed a chance to smoke it under medical supervision. Only one person (an Indian exchange student) who passed the screening interview refused to participate after learning the nature of the experiment.

The eight heavy users of marijuana were obtained with much less difficulty. They were interviewed in the same manner as the other subjects and were instructed not to smoke any marijuana on the day of their appointment in the laboratory.

Subjects were questioned during screening interviews and at the conclusion of the experiments to determine their knowledge of marijuana effects. None of the nine naive subjects had ever watched anyone smoke marijuana or observed anyone high on marijuana. Most of them knew of the effects of the drug only through reports in the popular press. Two subjects had friends who used marijuana frequently; one of these (No. 4) announced his intention to "prove" in the experiments that marijuana really did not do anything; the other (No. 3) was extremely eager to get high because "everyone I know is always talking about it very positively."

Setting.   Greatest effort was made to create a neutral setting. That is, subjects were made comfortable and secure in a pleasant suite of laboratories and offices, but the experimental staff carefully avoided encouraging any person to have an enjoyable experience. Subjects were never asked how they felt, and no subject was permitted to discuss the experiment with the staff until he had completed all four sessions. Verbal interactions between staff and subjects were minimum and formal. At the end of each session, subjects were asked to complete a brief form asking whether they thought they had smoked marijuana that night; if so, whether a high dose or a low dose; and how confident they were of their answers. The experimenters completed similar forms on each subject.

Marijuana used in these experiments was of Mexican origin, supplied by the Federal Bureau of Narcotics.[20] It consisted of finely chopped leaves of *Cannabis*, largely free of seeds and stems. An initial batch, which was judged to be of low potency by the experimenters on the basis of the doses needed to produce symptoms of intoxication in the chronic users, was subsequently found to contain only 0.3 percent of THC by weight. A second batch, assayed at 0.9 percent THC, was rated by the chronic users to be "good, average" marijuana, neither exceptionally strong nor exceptionally weak compared to their usual supplies. Users consistently reported symptoms of intoxication after smoking about 0.5 gram of the material with a variation of only a few puffs from subject to subject. This second batch of marijuana was used in the experiments described below; the low dose was 0.5 gram, and the high dose was 2.0 grams.

All marijuana was administered in the form of cigarettes of standard size made with a hand-operated rolling machine. In any given experimental session, each person was required to smoke two cigarettes in succession (Table 1).

TABLE 1

Composition of the dose. The placebo cigarette consisted of placebo material, tobacco filter, and mint leaves for masking flavor. The low dose was made up of marijuana, tobacco filler, and mint leaves. The high dose consisted of marijuana and mint leaves.

Dose	Marijuana in each cigarette (g)	Total dose marijuana (2 cigarettes) (g)	Approximate dose THC
Placebo	–	–	–
Low	0.25	0.5	4.5 mg
High	1.0	2.0	18 mg

Placebo material consisted of the chopped outer covering of mature stalks of male hemp plants; it contained no THC. All cigarettes had a tiny plug of tobacco at one end and a plug of paper at the other end so that the contents were not visible. The length to which each cigarette was to be smoked was indicated by an ink line. Marijuana and placebos were administered to the naive subjects in double-blind fashion. Scented aerosols were sprayed in the laboratory before smoking, to mask the odor of marijuana. The protocol during an experimental session was as follows. The sessions began at approximately 5:30 P.M.

Time	Procedure
0:00	Physiological measurements; blood sample drawn
0:05	Psychological test battery No. 1 (base line)
0:35	Verbal sample No. 1
0:40	Cigarette smoking
1:00	Rest period
1:15	Physiological measurements; blood sample drawn
1:20	Psychological test battery No. 2
1:50	Verbal sample No. 2
1:55	Rest period (supper)
2:30	Physiological measurements
2:35	Psychological test battery No. 3
3:05	End of testing

Experimental Sessions. Chronic users were tested only on high doses of marijuana with no practice sessions. Each naive subject was required to come to four sessions, spaced about a week apart. The first was always a practice session, in which the subject learned the proper smoking technique and during which he became thoroughly acquainted with the tests and the protocol. In the practice session, each subject completed the entire protocol, smoking two hand-rolled tobacco cigarettes. He was instructed to take a long puff, to inhale deeply, and to maintain inspiration for 20 seconds, as timed by an experimenter with a stopwatch. Subjects were allowed 8 to 12 minutes to smoke each of the two cigarettes. One purpose of this practice smoking was to identify and eliminate individuals who were not tolerant to high doses of nicotine, thus reducing the effect of nicotine on the variables measured during subsequent drug sessions.[21] A surprising number (five) of the volunteers who had described themselves in screening interviews as heavy cigarette smokers, "inhaling" up to two packs of cigarettes a day, developed acute nicotine reactions when they smoked two tobacco cigarettes by the required method. Occurrence of such a reaction disqualified a subject from participation in the experiments.

In subsequent sessions, when cigarettes contained either drug or placebo, all smoking was similarly supervised by an experimenter with a stopwatch. Subjects were not permitted to smoke tobacco cigarettes while the experiment was in progress. They were assigned to one of three treatment groups listed in Table 2.

TABLE 2

Order of treatment.

	Drug Session		
Group	1	2	3
I	High	Placebo	Low
II	Low	High	Placebo
III	Placebo	Low	High

The physiological parameters measured were heart rate, respiratory rate, pupil size, blood glucose level, and conjunctival vascular state. Pupil size was measured with a millimeter rule under constant illumination with eyes focused on an object at constant distance. Conjunctival appearance was rated by an experienced experimenter for dilation of blood vessels on a 0 to 4 scale with ratings of 3 and 4 indicating "significant" vasodilatation. Blood samples were collected for immediate determinations of serum glucose and for the serum to be frozen and stored for possible future biochemical studies. Subjects were asked not to eat and not to imbibe a beverage containing sugar or caffeine during the 4 hours preceding a session. They were given supper after the second blood sample was drawn.

Physiological and Psychological Measures.

The psychological test battery consisted of (i) the Continuous Performance Test (CPT)—5 minutes; (ii) the Digit Symbol Substitution Test (DSST)—90 seconds; (iii) CPT with strobe light distraction—5 minutes; (iv) self-rating bipolar mood scale—3 minutes; and (v) pursuit rotor—10 minutes.

The Continuous Performance Test was designed to measure a subject's capacity for sustained attention.[22] The subject was placed in a darkened room and directed to watch a small screen upon which six letters of the alphabet were flashed rapidly and in random order. The subject was instructed to press a button whenever a specified critical letter appeared. The number of letters presented, correct responses, and errors of commission and omission were counted over the 5-minute period. The test was also done with a strobe light flickering at 50 cycles per second. Normal subjects make no or nearly no errors on this test either with or without strobe distraction; but sleep deprivation, organic brain disease, and certain drugs like chlorpromazine adversely affect performance. Presence or absence of previous exposure to the task has no effect on performance.

The Digit Symbol Substitution Test is a simple test of cognitive function (see Fig. 1). A subject's score was the

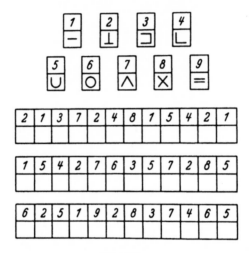

FIGURE 1

This is a sample of the Digit Symbol Substitution Test as used in these studies. On a signal from the examiner the subject was required to fill as many of the empty spaces as possible with the appropriate symbols. The code was always available to the subject during the ninety-second administration of the test. [The figure appeared originally in *Psychopharmacologia* 5, 164 (1964)]

number of correct answers in a 90-second period. As in the case of the CPT, practice should have little or no effect on performance.

The self-rating bipolar mood scale used in these experiments was one developed by Smith and Beechner[23] to evaluate subjective effects of morphine. By allowing subjects to rate themselves within a given category of moods, on an arbitrary scale from +3 to -3, it minimizes suggestion and is thus more neutral than the checklists often employed in drug testing.

The pursuit rotor measures muscular coordination and attention. The subject's task was to keep a stylus in contact with a small spot on a moving turntable. In these experiments, subjects were given ten 30-second trials in each battery. The score for each trial was total time in contact with the spot. There is a marked practice effect on this test, but naive subjects were brought to high levels of performance during their practice session, so that the changes due to practice were reduced during the actual drug sessions. In addition, since there was a different order of treatments for each of the three groups of naive subjects, any session-to-session practice effects were minimized in the statistical analysis of the pooled data.

At the end of the psychological test battery, a verbal sample was collected from each subject. The subject was left alone in a room with a tape recorder and instructions to describe "an interesting or dramatic experience" in his life until he was stopped. After exactly 5 minutes he was interrupted and asked how long he had been in the recording room. In this way, an estimate of the subject's ability to judge time was also obtained.

Results. *1. Safety of marijuana in human volunteers.* In view of the apprehension expressed by many persons over the safety of administering marijuana to research subjects, we wish to emphasize that no adverse marijuana reactions occurred in any of our subjects. In fact, the five acute nicotine reactions mentioned earlier were far more spectacular than any effects produced by marijuana.

In these experiments, observable effects of marijuana were maximum at 15 minutes after smoking. They were diminished between 30 minutes and 2 hour, and they were largely dissipated 3 hours after the end of smoking. No delayed or persistent effects beyond 3 hours were observed or reported.

2. Intoxicating properties of marijuana in a neutral setting. With the high dose of marijuana (2.0 grams), all chronic users became "high"[24] by their own accounts and in the judgment of experimenters who had observed many persons under the influence of marijuana. The effect was consistent even though prior to the session some of these subjects expressed anxiety about smoking marijuana and submitting to tests in a laboratory.

On the other hand, only one of the nine naive subjects (No. 3) had a definite "marijuana reaction" on the same high dose. He became markedly euphoric and laughed continuously during his first battery of tests after taking the drug. Interestingly, he was the one subject who had expressed his desire to get high.

3. Comparison of naive and chronic user subjects. Throughout the experiments it was apparent that the two groups of subjects reacted differently to identical doses of marijuana. We must caution, however, that our study was designed to allow rigorous statistical analysis of data from the naive group—it was not designed to permit formal comparison between chronic users and naive subjects. The conditions of the experiment were not the same for both groups: the chronic users were tested with the drug on their first visit to the laboratory with no practice and were informed that they were to receive high doses of marijuana. Therefore, differences between the chronic and naive groups reported below—although statistically valid—must be regarded as trends to be confirmed or rejected by additional experiments.

4. Recognition of marijuana versus placebo. All nine naive subjects reported that they had not been able to identify the taste or smell of marijuana in the experimental cigarettes. A few subjects remarked that they noticed differences in the taste of the three sets of cigarettes but could not interpret the differences. Most subjects found the pure marijuana cigarettes (high dose) more mild than the low dose or placebo cigarettes, both of which contained tobacco.

The subjects' guesses of the contents of cigarettes for their three sessions are presented in Table 3. It is noteworthy that

TABLE 3

Subjects' appraisal of the dose

Actual dose	Guessed dose			Fraction correct
	Placebo	Low	High	
Placebo	8	1		8/9
Low	3	6		6/9
High	2	6	1	1/9

one of the two subjects who called the high dose a placebo was the subject (No. 4) who had told us he wanted to prove that marijuana really did nothing. There were three outstanding findings: (i) most subjects receiving marijuana in either high or low doses recognized that they were getting a drug; (ii) most subjects receiving placebos recognized that they were receiving placebos; (iii) most subjects called their high dose a low dose, but none called his low dose a high dose, emphasizing the unimpressiveness of their subjective reactions.

5. *Effect of marijuana on heart rate.* The mean changes in heart rate from base-line rates before smoking the drug to rates at 15 and 90 minutes after smoking marijuana and placebo (Table 4) were tested for significance at the .05 level

TABLE 4

Change in heart rate (beat/min) after smoking the best material. Results are recorded as a change from the base line 15 minutes and 90 minutes after the smoking session.

	15 minutes			90 minutes		
Subject	Placebo	Low	High	Placebo	Low	High
			Naive subjects			
1	+ 16	+ 20	+ 16	+ 20	− 6	− 4
2	+ 12	+ 24	+ 12	− 6	+ 4	− 8
3	+ 8	+ 8	+ 26	− 4	+ 4	+ 8
4	+ 20	+ 8			+ 20	− 4
5	+ 8	+ 4	− 8		+ 22	− 8
6	+ 10	+ 20	+ 28	− 20	− 4	− 4
7	+ 4	+ 28	+ 24	+ 12	+ 8	+ 18
8	− 4	+ 20	+ 24	− 3	+ 8	− 24
9		+ 20	+ 24	+ 8	+ 12	
Mean	+ 7.8	+ 16.9	+ 16.2	+ 0.8	+ 7.6	− 2.9
S.E.	2.8	2.7	4.2	3.8	3.2	3.8
			Chronic subjects			
10		+ 32			+ 4	
11		+ 36			+ 36	
12		+ 20			+ 12	
13		+ 8			+ 4	
14		+ 32			+ 12	
15		+ 54			+ 22	
16		+ 24				
17		+ 60				
Mean		+ 33.2			+ 15.0	
S.E.		6.0			5.0	

by an analysis of variance; Tukey's method was applied for all possible comparisons (Table 5). In the naive subjects, marijuana in low dose or high dose was followed by increased heart rate 15 minutes after smoking, but the effect was not demonstrated to be dose-dependent. The high dose caused a statistically greater increase in the heart rates of chronic users than in those of the naive subjects 15 minutes after smoking.

Two of the chronic users had unusually low resting pulse rates (56 and 42), but deletion of these two subjects (No. 11 and No. 15) still gave a significant difference in mean pulse

TABLE 5

Significance of differences (at the .05 level) in heart rate. Results of Tukey's test for all possible comparisons.

Comparison	15 Minutes	90 Minutes
Low dose versus placebo	Significant	Significant
High dose versus placebo	Significant	Not significant
Low dose versus high dose	Not significant	Significant
Chronic users versus high dose	Significant	Significant

rise of chronic users compared to naives. Because the conditions of the sessions and experimental design were not identical for the two groups, we prefer to report this difference as a trend that must be confirmed by further studies.

6. *Effect of marijuana on respiratory rate.* In the naive group, there was no change in respiratory rate before and after smoking marijuana. Chronic users showed a small but statistically significant increase in respiratory rate after smoking, but we do not regard the change as clinically significant.

7. *Effect of marijuana on pupil size.* There was no change in pupil size before and after smoking marijuana in either group.

8. *Effect of marijuana on conjunctival appearance.* Significant reddening of conjunctivae due to dilatation of blood vessels occurred in one of nine subjects receiving placebo, three of nine receiving the low dose of marijuana, and eight of nine receiving the high dose. It occurred in all eight of the chronic users receiving the high dose and was rated as more prominent in them. The effect was more pronounced 15 minutes after the smoking period than 90 minutes after it.

9. *Effect of marijuana on blood sugar.* There was no significant change in blood sugar levels after smoking marijuana in either group.

10. *Effect of marijuana on the Continuous Performance Test.* Performance on the CPT and on the CPT with strobe distraction was unaffected by marijuana for both groups of subjects.

11. *Effect of marijuana on the Digit Symbol Substitution Test.* The significance of the differences in mean changes of scores at the .05 level was determined by an analysis of variance by means of Tukey's method for all possible com-

parisons. Results of these tests are summarized in Tables 6 and 7.

TABLE 6

Significance of differences (at the .05 level) for the Digit Symbol Substitution Test. Results of Tukey's test for all possible comparisons.

Comparison	15 minutes	90 Minutes
Low dose versus placebo	Significant	Significant
High dose versus placebo	Significant	Significant
Low dose versus high dose	Significant	Not significant
Chronic users versus high dose	Significant	Significant

TABLE 7

Digit Symbol Substitution Test. Change in scores from base line (number correct) 15 and 90 minutes after the smoking session.

	15 Minutes			90 Minutes		
	Placebo	Low	High	Placebo	Low	High
			Naive subjects			
1	− 3	−	+ 5	− 7	+ 4	+ 8
2	+ 10	− 8	− 17	− 1	− 15	− 5
3	− 3	+ 6	− 7	− 10	+ 2	− 1
4	+ 3	− 4	− 3		− 7	
5	+ 4	+ 1	− 7	+ 6		− 8
6	−	− 1	− 9	− 3	− 5	− 12
7	+ 2	− 4	− 6	+ 3	− 5	− 4
8	− 1	+ 3	+ 1	+ 4	+ 4	− 3
9	− 1	− 4	− 3	+ 6	− 1	− 10
Mean	+ 0.9	− 1.2	− 5.1	+ 0.4	− 2.6	− 3.9
S.E.	1.4	1.4	2.1	1.9	2.0	2.0

The results indicate that: (i) Decrements in performance of naive subjects following low and high doses of marijuana were significant at 15 and 90 minutes after smoking. (ii) The decrement following marijuana was greater after high dose than after low dose at 15 minutes after taking the drug, giving preliminary evidence of a dose-response relationship. (iii) Chronic users started with good base-line performance and improved slightly on the DSST after smoking 2.0 grams of marijuana, whereas performance of the naive subjects was grossly impaired. Experience with the DSST suggests that absence of impairment in chronic users cannot be accounted for solely by a practice effect. Still, because of the different procedures employed, we prefer to report this difference as a trend.

12. Effect of marijuana on pursuit rotor performance. This result is presented in Table 8. Again applying Tukey's

TABLE 8

Pursuit rotor (naive subjects). Changes in scores (averages of ten trials) from base line (seconds).

Subject	15 Minutes			90 Minutes		
	Placebo	Low	High	Placebo	Low	High
1	+ 1.20	− 1.04	− 4.01	+ 1.87	− 1.54	− 6.54
2	+ 0.89	− 1.43	− 0.12	+ 0.52	+ 0.44	− 0.68
3	+ 0.50	− 0.60	− 6.56	+ 0.84	− 0.96	− 4.34
4	+ 0.18	− 0.11	+ 0.11	+ 0.06	+ 1.95	− 1.37
5	+ 3.20	+ 0.39	+ 0.13	+ 2.64	+ 3.33	+ 0.34
6	+ 3.45	− 0.32	− 3.46	+ 2.93	+ 0.22	− 2.26
7	+ 0.81	+ 0.48	− 0.79	+ 0.63	+ 0.16	− 0.52
8	+ 1.75	− 0.39	− 0.92	+ 2.13	+ 0.40	+ 1.02
9	+ 3.90	− 1.94	− 2.60	+ 3.11	− 0.97	− 3.09
Mean	+ 1.8	− 0.6	− 2.0	+ 1.6	+ 0.3	− 1.9
S.E.	0.5	0.3	0.8	0.4	0.5	0.8

TABLE 9

Significance of differences (at the .05 level) for the pursuit rotor. Results of Tukey's test for all possible comparisons, 15 and 90 minutes after the smoking session.

Comparison	15 Minutes	90 Minutes
Low dose versus placebo	Significant	Significant
High dose versus placebo	Significant	Significant
Low dose versus high dose	Significant	Significant

method in an analysis of variance, we tested differences in mean changes in scores (Table 9). Decrements in performance of naive subjects after both low and high doses of marijuana were significant at 15 and 90 minutes. This effect on performance followed a dose-response relation on testing batteries conducted at both 15 minutes and 90 minutes after the drug was smoked.

All chronic users started from good baselines and improved on the pursuit rotor after smoking marijuana. These data are not presented, however, because it is probable that the improvement was largely a practice effect.

13. Effect of marijuana on time estimation. Before smoking, all nine naive subjects estimated the 5-minute verbal sample to be 5 ± 2 minutes. After placebo, no subject changed his guess. After the low dose, three subjects raised their estimates to 10 ± 2 minutes, and after the high dose, four raised their estimates.

14. Subjective effects of marijuana. When questioned at the end of their participation in the experiment, persons who had never taken marijuana previously reported minimum subjective effects after smoking the drug, or, more precisely, few effects like those commonly reported by chronic users. Non-users reported little euphoria, no distortion of visual or auditory perception, and no confusion. However, several subjects mentioned that "things seemed to take longer." Below are examples of comments by naive subjects after high doses.

Subject 2: "It was stronger than the previous time (low dose) but I really didn't think it could be marijuana. Things seemed to go slower."

Subject 2: "I think I realize why they took our watches. There was a sense of the past disappearing as happens when you're driving too long without sleeping. With a start you wake up to realize you were asleep for an instant; you discover yourself driving along the road. It was the same tonight with eating a sandwich. I'd look down to discover I'd just swallowed a bite but I hadn't noticed it at the time."

Subject 6: "I felt a combination of being almost drunk and tired, with occasional fits of silliness—not my normal reaction to smoking tobacco."

Subject 8: "I felt faint briefly, but the dizziness went away, and I felt normal or slightly tired. I can't believe I had a high dose of marijuana."

Subject 9: "Time seemed very drawn out. I would keep forgetting what I was doing, especially on the continuous performance test, but somehow every time an 'X' (the critical letter) came up, I found myself pushing the button."

After smoking their high dose, chronic users were asked to rate themselves on a scale of 1 to 10, 10 representing "the highest you've ever been." All subjects placed themselves between 7 and 10, most at 8 or 9. Many of these subjects expressed anxiety at the start of their first battery of tests after smoking the drug when they were feeling very high.

Then they expressed surprise during and after the tests when they judged (correctly) that their performance was as good as or better than it had been before taking the drug.

15. The effect of marijuana on the self-rating mood scale, the effect of marijuana on a 5-minute verbal sample, and the correlation of personality type with subjective effects of marijuana will be reported separately.

Discussion.   Several results from this study raise important questions about the action of marijuana and suggest directions for future research. Our finding that subjects who were naive to marijuana did not become subjectively "high" after a high dose of marijuana in a neutral setting is interesting when contrasted with the response of regular users who consistently reported and exhibited highs. It agrees with the reports of chronic users that many, if not most, people do not become high on their first exposure to marijuana even if they smoke it correctly. This puzzling phenomenon can be discussed from either a physiological or psychosocial point of view. Neither interpretation is entirely satisfactory. The physiological hypothesis suggests that getting high on marijuana occurs only after some sort of pharmacological sensitization takes place. The psychosocial interpretation is that repeated exposure to marijuana reduces psychological inhibition, as part of, or as the result of a learning process.

Indirect evidence makes the psychological hypothesis attractive. Anxiety about drug use in this country is sufficiently great to make worthy of careful consideration the possibility of an unconscious psychological inhibition or block on the part of naive drug takers. The subjective responses of our subjects indicate that they had imagined a marijuana effect to be much more profoundly disorganizing than what they experienced. For example, subject No. 4, who started with a bias against the possibility of becoming high on marijuana, was able to control subjectively the effect of the drug and report that he had received a placebo when he had actually gotten a high dose. As anxiety about the drug is lessened with experience, the block may decrease, and the subject may permit himself to notice the drug's effects.

It is well known that marijuana users, in introducing friends to the drug, do actually "teach" them to notice subtle effects of the drug on consciousness.[25] The apparently enormous influence of set and setting on the form of the marijuana response is consistent with this hypothesis, as is the testimony of users that, as use becomes more frequent, the amount of drug required to produce intoxication decreases—a unique example of "reverse tolerance." (Regular use of many intoxicants is accompanied by the need for increasing doses to achieve the same effects.)

On the other hand, the suggestion arising from this study that users and non-users react differently to the drug, not only subjectively but also physiologically, increases the plausibility of the pharmacological-sensitization hypothesis. Of course, reverse tolerance could equally well be a manifestation of this sensitization.

It would be useful to confirm the suggested differences between users and non-users and then to test in a systematic manner the hypothetical explanations of the phenomenon. One possible approach would be to continue to administer high doses of marijuana to the naive subjects according to the protocol described. If subjects begin reporting high responses to the drug only after several exposures, in the absence of psychedelic settings, suggestions, or manipulations of mood, then the likelihood that marijuana induces a true physiological sensitization or that experience reduces psychological inhibitions, permitting real drug effects to appear, would be increased. If subjects fail to become high, we could conclude that learning to respond to marijuana requires some sort of teaching or suggestion.

An investigation of the literature of countries where anxieties over drug use are less prominent would be useful. If this difference between responses of users and non-users is a uniquely American phenomenon, a psychological explanation would be indicated, although it would not account for greater effects with smaller doses after the initial, anxiety-reducing stage.

One impetus for reporting the finding of differences between chronic and naive subjects on some of the tests, despite the fact that the experimental designs were not the same, is that this finding agrees with the statements of many users. They say that the effects of marijuana are easily suppressed—much more so than those of alcohol. Our observation, that the chronic users after smoking marijuana performed on some tests as well as or better than they did before taking the drug, reinforced the argument advanced by chronic users that maintaining effective levels of performance for many tasks—driving, for example—is much easier under the influence of marijuana than under that of other psycho-active drugs. Certainly the surprise that the chronic users expressed when they found they were performing more effectively on the CPT, DSST, and pursuit rotor tests than they thought they would is remarkable. It is quite the opposite of the false sense of improvement subjects have under some psychoactive drugs that actually impair per-formance.

What might be the basis of this suppressibility? Possibly, the actions of marijuana are confined to higher cortical functions without any general stimulatory or depressive effect on lower brain centers. The relative absence of neuro-logical—as opposed to psychiatric—symptoms in marijuana intoxication suggests this possibility.

Our failure to detect any changes in blood sugar levels of subjects after they had smoked marijuana forces us to look elsewhere for an explanation of the hunger and hyperphagia commonly reported by users. A first step would be careful interviewing of users to determine whether they really be-come hungry after smoking marijuana or whether they simply find eating more pleasurable. Possibly, the basis of this effect is also central rather than due to some peripheral physiological change.

Lack of any change in pupil size of subjects after they had smoked marijuana is an enlightening finding especially be-cause so many users and law enforcement agents firmly believe that marijuana dilates pupils. (Since users generally observe each other in dim surroundings, it is not surprising that they see large pupils.) This negative finding emphasizes the need for data from carefully controlled investigations rather than from casual observation or anecdotal reports in the evaluation of marijuana. It also agrees with the findings of others that synthetic THC does not alter pupil size.[27]

Finally, we would like to comment on the fact that marijuana appears to be a relatively mild intoxicant in our studies. If these results seem to differ from those of earlier experiments, it must be remembered that other experi-menters have given marijuana orally, have given doses much higher than those commonly smoked by users, have administered potent synthetics, and have not strictly controlled the laboratory setting. As noted in our introduction, more powerful effects are often reported by users who ingest preparations of marijuana. This may mean that some active constituents which enter the body when the drug is ingested are destroyed by combustion, a suggestion that must be investigated in man. Another priority consideration is the extent to which synthetic THC reproduces marijuana intoxication—a problem that must be resolved before marijuana research proceeds with THC instead of the natural resin of the whole plant.

The set, both of subjects and experimenters, and the setting must be recognized as critical variables in studies of marijuana. Drug, set, and setting interact to shape the form of a marijuana reaction. The researcher who sets out with prior conviction that hemp is psychotomimetic or a "mild hallucinogen" is likely to confirm his conviction experimentally,[10] but he would probably confirm the opposite hypothesis if his bias were in the opposite direction. Precautions to insure neutrality of set and setting, including use of a double-blind procedure as an absolute minimum, are vitally important if the object of investigation is to measure real marijuana-induced responses.

1. It is feasible and safe to study the effects of marijuana on human volunteers who smoke it in a laboratory.   **Conclusions.**

2. In a neutral setting persons who are naive to marijuana do not have strong subjective experiences after smoking low or high doses of the drug, and the effects they do report are not the same as those described by regular users of marijuana who take the drug in the same neutral setting.

3. Regular users of marijuana do get high after smoking marijuana in a neutral setting but do not show the same degree of impairment of performance on the tests as do naive subjects. In some cases, their performance even appears to improve slightly after smoking marijuana.

5. Marijuana increases heart rate moderately.

6. No change in respiratory rate follows administration of marijuana by inhalation.

7. No change in pupil size occurs in short term exposure to marijuana.

8. Marijuana administration causes dilation of conjunctival blood vessels.

9. Marijuana treatment produces no change in blood sugar levels.

10. In a neutral setting the physiological and psychological effects of a single, inhaled dose of marijuana appear to reach maximum intensity within one-half hour of inhalation, to be diminished after 1 hour, and to be completely dissipated by 3 hours.

REFERENCES AND NOTES

1. R. J. Bouquet, *Bull. Narcotics* 2, 14 (1950).

2. F. Korte and H. Sieper, in *Hashish: Its Chemistry and Pharmacology*, G. E. W. Wolstenholme and J. Knight, Eds. (Little, Brown, Boston, 1965), pp. 15-30.

3. Task Force on Narcotics and Drug Abuse, the President's Commission on Law Enforcement and the Administration of Justice, *Task Force Report: Narcotics and Drug Abuse* (1967), p. 14.

4. R. Mechoulam, and Y. Gaoni, *J. Amer. Chem. Soc.* 67, 3273 (1965).

5. J. F. Siler, W. L. Sheep, L. B. Bates, G. F. Clark, G. W. Cook, W. A. Smith, *Mil. Surg.* (November 1933), pp. 269-280.

6. Mayor's Committee on Marihuana, *The Marihuana Problem in the City of New York*, 1944.

7. E. G. Williams, C. K. Himmelsbach, A. Winkler, D. C. Ruble, B. J. Lloyd, *Public Health Rep.* 61, 1059 (1946).

8. H. Isbell, *Psychopharmacologia* 11, 184 (1967).

9. I. C. Chopra and R. N. Chopra, *Bull. Narcotics* 9, 4 (1957).

10. F. Ames, *J. Ment. Sci.* 104, 972 (1958).

11. C. J. Miras, in *Hashish: Its Chemistry and Pharmacology*, G. E. W. Wolstenholme and J. Knight, Eds. (Little, Brown, Boston, 1965), pp. 37-47.

12. J. M. Watt, in *Hashish: Its Chemistry and Pharmacology*, G. E. W. Wolstenholme and J. Knight, Eds. (Little, Brown, Boston, 1965), pp. 54-66.

13. AMA Council on Mental Health, *J. Amer. Med. Ass.* 204, 1181 (1968).

14. G. Joachimoglu, in *Hashish: Its Chemistry and Pharmacology*, G. E. W. Wolstenholme and J. Knight, Eds. (Little, Brown, Boston, 1965), pp. 2–10.

15. We thank M. Lerner and A. Bober of the U.S. Customs Laboratory, Baltimore, for performing this assay.

16. We thank R. H. Pace and E. H. Hall of the Peter J. Schweitzer Division of the Kimberly-Clark Corp. for supplying placebo material.

17. S. Garattini, in *Hashish: Its Chemistry and Pharmacology*, G. E. W. Wolstenholme and J. Knight, Eds. (Little, Brown, Boston, 1965), pp. 70–78.

18. J. H. Jaffee, in *The Pharmacological Basis of Therapeutics*, L. S. Goodman and A. Gilman, Eds. (Macmillan, New York, ed. 3, 1965), pp. 299–301.

19. We thank E. L. Richardson, Attorney General of the Commonwealth of Massachusetts, for permitting these experiments to proceed and N. L. Chayet for legal assistance. We do not consider it appropriate to describe here the opposition we encountered from the governmental agents and agencies and from university bureaucracies.

20. We thank D. Miller and M. Seifer of the Federal Bureau of Narcotics (now part of the Bureau of Narcotics and Dangerous Drugs, under the Department of Justice) for help in obtaining marijuana for this research.

21. The doses of tobacco in placebo and low-dose cigarettes were too small to cause physiological changes in subjects who qualified in the practice session.

22. K. E. Rosvold, A. F. Mirsky, I. Samson, E. D. Bransome, L. H. Beck, *J. Consult. Psychol.* 20, 343 (1956); A. F. Mirsky and P. V. Cardon, *Electroencephalogr. Clin. Neurophysiol.* 14, 1 (1962); C. Kornetsky and G. Bain, *Psychopharmacologia* 8, 277 (1965).

23. G. M. Smith and H. K. Beecher, *J. Pharmacol.* 126, 50 (1959).

24. We will attempt to define the complex nature of a marijuana high in a subsequent paper discussing the speech samples and interviews.

25. H. S. Becker, *Outsiders: Studies in the Sociology of Deviance* (Macmillan, New York, 1963), chap. 3.

26. Although the motor skills measured by the pursuit rotor are represented in driving ability, they are only components of that ability. The influence of marijuana on driving skill remains an open question of high medico-legal priority.

27. L. E. Hollister, R. K. Richards, H. K. Gillespie, in preparation.

28. Sponsored and supported by Boston University's division of psychiatry, in part through PHS grants MH12568, MH06795-06, MH7753-06, and MH33319, and the Boston University Medical Center. The authors thank Dr. P. H. Knapp and Dr. C. Kornetsky of the Boston University School of Medicine, Department of Psychiatry and Pharmacology, for consistent support and excellent advice, and J. Finkelstein of 650 Madison Avenue, New York City, for his support at a crucial time.

Comparison of the Effects of Marijuana and Alcohol on Simulated Driving Performance

BY ALFRED CRANCER, JR., Ph.D.,
JAMES M. DILLE, M.D.,
JACK C. DELAY, M.D.,
JEAN E. WALLACE, M.D.,
& MARTIN D. HAYKIN, M.D.

We have determined the effect of a "normal social marijuana high" on simulated driving performance among experienced marijuana smokers. We compared the degree of driving impairment due to smoking marijuana to the effect on driving of a recognized standard—that is, legally defined intoxication at the presumptive limit of 0.10 percent alcohol concentration in the blood. This study focused attention on the effect of smoking marijuana rather than on the effect of ingesting $\triangle^9$-tetrahydrocannabinol ($\triangle^9$-THC), the principal active component.

Weil et al.[1] have studied the clinical and psychological effects of smoking marijuana on both experienced and inexperienced subjects. They suggest, as do others,[2] that experienced smokers when "high" show no significant impairment as judged by performance on selected tests; they also establish the existence of physiological changes that are useful in determining whether a subject smoking marijuana is "high." A review of the relation of alcohol to fatal accidents[3] showed that nearly half of the drivers fatally injured in an accident had an alcohol concentration in the blood of 0.05 or more.

Crancer[4] found a driving simulator test to be a valid indicator for distinguishing driving performance; this result was

Reprinted from *Science*, vol. 164, May 16, 1969, pp. 851–854.

based on a five-year driving record. Further studies[5] indicated that a behind-the-wheel road test is not significantly correlated to driving performance. We therefore chose the simulator test, which presents a programmed series of emergency situations that are impractical and dangerous in actual road tests.

Subjects were required to be (i) experienced marijuana smokers who had been smoking marijuana at least twice a month for the past six months, (ii) licensed as a motor vehicle operator, (iii) engaged in a generally accepted educational or vocational pursuit, and (iv) familiar with the effects of alcohol. The subjects were given (i) a physical examination to exclude persons currently in poor health or under medication, and (ii) a written personality inventory (Minnesota Multi-phasic Personality Inventory) to exclude persons showing a combination of psychological stress and inflexible defense patterns. Seven of the subjects were females and twenty-nine were males (mean age, 22.9).

We compared the effects of a marijuana "high," alcohol intoxication, and no treatment on simulated driving performance over a four and a half hour period. We used a Latin-square analysis of variance design[6] to account for the effects of treatments, subjects, day, and the order in which the treatments were given. To measure the time response effects of each treatment, simulator scores were obtained at three constant points in the course of each experimental period. A sample of thirty-six subjects was determined to be sufficient in size to meet the demands of this experimental design.

Three treatments were given to each subject. In treatment M (normal social marijuana "high"), the experimental subject stated that he experienced the physical and psychological effects of smoking marijuana in a social environment comparable to his previous experiences. This subjective evaluation of "high" was confirmed by requiring a minimum consumption of marijuana established with a separate test group, and by identifying an increase in pulse rate.[1]

In treatment M, the subjects smoked two marijuana[7] cigarettes of approximately equal weight and totaling 1.7 g. They completed smoking in about thirty minutes and were given their first simulator test thirty minutes later.

Some confirmation that the amount of marijuana smoked was sufficient to produce a "high" is found in Weil's[1] study.

His subjects smoked about 0.5 g of marijuana of 0.9 percent Δ^9-THC.

In treatment A, subjects consumed two drinks containing equal amounts of 95 percent alcohol mixed in orange or tomato juice. Dosage was regulated according to subject's weight with the intended result of 0.10 blood alcohol concentration as determined by a Breathalyzer reading.[8] Thus, a subject weighing 120 pounds received 84 ml of 95 percent laboratory alcohol equally divided between two drinks. This was equivalent to about six ounces of 86 proof liquor. The dosage was increased 14 ml or one-half ounce for each additional fifteen pounds of body weight. A Breathalyzer reading was obtained for each subject about one hour after drinking began; most subjects completed drinking in thirty minutes.

Treatment C consisted of waiting in the lounge with no treatment for the same period of time required for treatments M and A. The experimental subject stated that his physiological and psychological condition were normal. Subjects were requested to refrain from all drug or alcohol use during the time they were participating in the experiment.

A driver-training simulator was specially modified to obtain data on the effect of the treatments. The car unit was a console mockup of a recent model containing all the control and instrument equipment relevant to the driving task. The car unit faced a six by eighteen foot screen upon which the test film was projected. The test film gave the subject a driver's eye view of the road as it led him through normal and emergency driving situations on freeways and urban and suburban streets. From the logic unit, located to the rear of the driver, the examiner started the automated test, observed the subject driving, and recorded the final scores.

A series of checks was placed on the twenty-three-minute driving film which monitored driver reactions to a programmed series of driving stimuli. The test variables monitored were: accelerator (164 checks), brake (106 checks), turn signals (59 checks), steering (53 checks), and speedometer (23 checks). There was a total of 405 checks, allowing driver scores to range from zero to 405 errors per test. Errors were accumulated as follows:

1. Speedometer errors. Speedometer readings outside the range of 15 to 35 mile/hour for city portion of film and 45 to 65 mile/hour for freeways. The speed of the filmed presentation is not under the control of the driver. Therefore, speedometer errors are not an indication of speeding errors, but of the amount of time spent monitoring the speedometer.

2. Steering errors. Steering wheel in other than the appropriate position.

3. Brake errors. Not braking when the appropriate response is to brake, or braking at an inappropriate time.

4. Accelerator errors. Acceleration when the appropriate response is to declerate, or deceleration when it is appropriate to accelerate.

5. Signal errors. Use of turn signal at an inappropriate time or position.

6. Total errors. An accumulation of the total number of errors on the five test variables.

Two rooms were used for the experiment. The lounge, designed to provide a familiar and comfortable environment for the subjects, was approximately twelve feet square and contained six casual chairs, a refrigerator, a desk, and several small movable tables. The room was lighted by a red lava lamp and one indirect red light, and contemporary rock music was played. Snacks, soft drinks, ashtrays, wastebaskets, and a supply of cigarettes were readily available. Subjects remained in this room except during simulator tests.

The driving simulator was located in a larger room about fifty feet from the lounge. The simulator room was approximately twenty by thirty feet and was kept in almost total darkness.

Each subject took three preliminary tests on the driving simulator to familiarize himself with the equipment and to minimize the effect of learning through practice during the experiment. Subjects whose error scores varied by more than 10 percent between the second and third tests were given subsequent tests until the stability criterion was met.

The experiment was conducted over a six-week period. Six subjects were tested each week. On day 1, six subjects took a final test on the driving simulator to assure recent familiarity with the equipment. A "normal" pulse rate was recorded, and each was given two marijuana cigarettes of approximately 0.9 g each. Subjects smoked the marijuana in the lounge to become acquainted with the surroundings and other test subjects, and with the potency of the marijuana. A second pulse reading was recorded for each subject when he reported that he was "high" in order to obtain an indication of the expected rate increase during the experiment proper. They remained in the lounge for approximately four hours after they had started smoking.

Three of the subjects were scheduled for testing in the early evening of days 2, 4, and 6; the remaining three subjects for days 3, 5, and 7. A single treatment was given each evening. Within a given week, all subjects received treatments in the same order. Treatment order was changed from week to week to meet the requirement of a Latin-square design. Procedure for each evening was identical except for the specific treatment.

Subject 1 arrived at the laboratory and took the usual simulator warm-up test. Treatment A, M, or C was begun at zero hour and finished about a half hour later. One hour after treatment began, subject 1 took simulator test 1, returning to the lounge when he was finished. He took simulator test 2 two and a half hours after treatment began, and test 3 four hours after treatment began. Pulse or Breathalyzer readings, depending on the treatment, were taken immediately before each simulator test.

Subject 2 followed the same schedule, beginning a half hour after subject 1. Time used in testing one subject each evening was four and a half hour, with a total elapsed time of five and a half hours to test three subjects.

The three simulator tests taken after each treatment establish a time response effect for the treatment. For each treatment the total error scores for each time period were subjected to an analysis of variance. Table 1 presents the analysis

TABLE 1

Analysis of variance of total driving simulator error scores for three treatments; marijuana (M), control (C), and alcohol (A).

Source of variation	Sum of squares	Degrees of freedom	Mean square	Mean square ratios
Treatments	2,595.1	2	1,297.5	6.7*
M versus C	(11.7)	(1)	11.7	0.1
A versus M and C	(2,583.4)	(1)	2,583.4	13.3†
Days	738.5	2	369.3	1.9
Subjects	40,872.5	24	1,703.0	9.7†
Squares	13,708.5	11	1,247.2	6.4†
Pooled error	13,253.8	68	194.9	
Total	71,168.4	107		

* $P < .05$.   † $P < .01$.

of variance for period 1 scores; results comparable to these were obtained for scores in periods 2 and 3.

The simulated driving scores for subjects experiencing a normal social marijuana "high" and the same subjects under control conditions are not significantly different (Table 1). However, there are significantly more errors ($P < .01$) for intoxicated than for control subjects (difference of 15.4 percent). This finding is consistent with the mean error scores of the three treatments: control, 84.46 errors; marijuana, 84.49 errors; and alcohol, 97.44 errors.

The time response curves for "high" and control treatments are comparable (Figure 1). In contrast, the curve for

FIGURE 1

Display of the effect of each treatment on simulator error scores over a four-hour period. Alcohol (A), marijuana (M), and control (C).

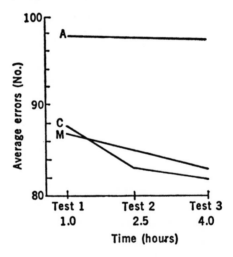

alcohol shows more total errors ($P < .01$). These higher error scores for alcohol persist across all three time periods with little evidence of the improvement shown under the other two treatments.

A separate Latin-square analysis of variance was completed for each test variable to supplement the analysis of total errors (Table 2). In comparison of intoxicated and control subjects, significant differences ($P < .05$) were found for accelerator errors in periods 1 and 2, for signal errors in periods 1, 2, and 3, for braking errors in periods 2 and 3, and for speedometer errors in period 1. In the comparison of mari-

TABLE 2

Significant treatment differences from Latin-square analysis of variance ($P < .05$). Accelerator, signal, and total errors are significantly correlated with driving performance for normal drivers. No correlation was found for brake, speedometer, and steering errors; A $>$ C, M $>$ C indicate that error scores for alcohol (A) or marijuana (M) treatment are greater than control (C).

Simulator test	Test variable errors					
	Accelerator	Signal	Total	Brake	Speedometer	Steering
Period 1	A $>$ C	A $>$ C	A $>$ C	None	A $>$ C M $>$ C	None
Period 2	A $>$ C	A $>$ C	A $>$ C	A $>$ C	None	None
Period 3	None	A $>$ C	A $>$ C	A $>$ C	None	None

juana smokers and controls, a significant difference ($P<.05$) was found for speedometer errors in period 1. In all of these cases, the number of errors for the drug treatments exceeded the errors for the control treatment.

Other sources of variation are Latin squares, subjects, and days. In all of the analyses, the effect of subjects and Latin squares (representing groups of subjects) were significant ($P<.05$). In contrast, the effect of days was not significant, thus indicating that no significant amount of learning was associated with repeated exposure to the test material.

For normal drivers, Crancer[4] found a significant correlation ($P<.05$) between the three simulator test variables (signals, accelerator, and total errors) and driving performance. An increase in error scores was associated with an increase in number of accidents and violations on a driving record. In the same study, error scores for brake, speedometer, and steering were not correlated with driving performance.

It may not be valid to assume the same relationship for persons under the influence of alcohol or marijuana. However, we feel that, because the simulator task is a less complex but related task, deterioration in simulator performance implies deterioration in actual driving performance. We are less willing to assume that nondeterioration in simulator performance implies nondeterioration in actual driving. We therefore conclude that finding significantly more accelerator, signal, and total errors by intoxicated subjects implies a deterioration in actual driving performance.

Relating speedometer errors to actual driving performance

is highly speculative because Crancer[4] found no correlation for normal drivers. This may be due in part to the fact that the speed of the filmed presentation is not under the control of the driver. However, speedometer errors are related to the amount of time spent monitoring the speedometer. The increase of speedometer errors by intoxicated or "high" subjects probably indicates that the subjects spent less time monitoring the speedometer than under control conditions.

This study could not determine if the drugs would alter the speed at which subjects normally drive. However, comments by marijuana users may be pertinent. They often report alteration of time and space perceptions, leading to a different sense of speed which generally results in driving more slowly.

Weil *et al.*[1] emphasize the importance and influence of both subject bias (set) and the experimental environment (setting). For this study, the environmental setting was conducive to good performance under all treatments.

Traditional methods for controlling potential subject bias by using placebos to disguise the form or effect of the marijuana treatment were not applicable. This is confirmed by Weil *et al.*[1]; they showed that inexperienced subjects correctly appraised the presence or absence of a placebo in twenty-one of twenty-seven trials.

The nature of selection probably resulted in subjects who preferred marijuana to alcohol and, therefore, had a set to perform better with marijuana. The main safeguard against bias was that subjects were not told how well they did on any of their driving tests, nor were they acquainted with the specific methods used to determine errors. Thus, it would have been very difficult intentionally and effectively to manipulate error scores on a given test or sequence of tests.

A further check on subject bias was made by comparing error scores on the warm-up tests given before each treatment. We found no significant difference in the mean error scores preceding the treatments of marijuana, alcohol, and control. This suggests that subjects were not "set" to perform better or worse on the day of a particular treatment.

In addition, an inspection of chance variation of individual error scores for treatment M shows about half the subjects doing worse and half better than under control conditions. This variability in direction is consistent with findings reviewed earlier, and we feel reasonably certain that a bias in favor of marijuana did not influence the results of this experiment.

A cursory investigation of dose response was made by retesting four subjects after they had smoked approximately three times the amount of marijuana used in the main experiment. None of the subjects showed a significant change in performance.

Four additional subjects who had never smoked marijuana before were pretested to obtain control scores, then given marijuana to smoke until they were subjectively "high" with an associated increase in pulse rate. All subjects smoked at least the minimum quantity established for the experiment. All subjects showed either no change or negligible improvement in their scores. These results suggest that impairment in simulated driving performance is not a function of increased marijuana dosage or inexperience with the drug.

A significant difference ($P<.01$) was found between the pulse rates before and after the marijuana treatment. Similar results were reported[1] for both experienced and inexperienced marijuana subjects. We found no significant difference in pulse rates before and after drinking.

Thus, when subjects experienced a social marijuana "high," they accumulated significantly more speedometer errors on the simulator than under control conditions, but there were no significant differences in accelerator, brake, signal, steering, and total errors. The same subjects intoxicated from alcohol accumulated significantly more accelerator, brake, signal, speedometer, and total errors. Furthermore, impairment in simulated driving performance apparently is not a function of increased marijuana dosage or inexperience with the drug.

REFERENCES AND NOTES

1. A. T. Weil, N. E. Zinberg, J. M. Nelsen, *Science* **162**, 1234 (1968).

2. Mayor's Committee on Marihuana, *The Marihuana Problem in the City of New York* (1944).

3. W. J. Haddon and V. A. Braddess, *J. Amer. Med. Ass.* **169**, No.

14, 127 (1959); J. R. McCarroll and W. J. Haddon, *J. Chronic Dis.* 15, 811 (1962); J. H. W. Birrell, *Med. J. Aust.* 2, 949 (1965); R. A. Neilson, *Alcohol Involvement in Fatal Motor Vehicle Accidents in Twenty-Seven California Counties in 1964,* (California Traffic Safety Foundation, San Francisco, 1965).

4. A. Crancer, *Predicting Driving Performance with a Driver Simulator Test* (Washington Department of Motor Vehicles, Olympia, 1968).

5. J. E. Wallace and A. Crancer, *Licensing Examinations and Their Relation to Subsequent Driving Record* (Washington Department of Motor Vehicles, Olympia, 1968).

6. A. E. Edwards, *Experimental Design in Psychological Research* (Holt, Rinehart & Winston, New York, 1968), pp. 173–174.

7. The marijuana was an assayed batch (1.312 percent Δ^9-THC) from NIH through the cooperation of Dr. J. A. Scigliano.

8. L. A. Greenberg, *Quart. J. Studies Alcohol* 29, 252 (1968).

V

CHEMICAL
AND PHARMACOLOGICAL
STUDIES

The strength and quality of cannabis products was always a problem to the pharmaceutical industry. Before the 1900s, the drug industry was dependent on shipments from India. The shipments varied in strength. To make up for a lack of chemical assay techniques, the industry developed highly sophisticated animal assay criteria for purposes of standardization.

In the early twentieth century, the industry began marijuana cultivation for medicinal purposes in suburban Philadelphia and at Rochester, Michigan. Parke Davis and Eli Lilly collaborated in the development of standardized domestic strains of marijuana to U.S. Pharmacopoeia standards. This laboratory came into being in 1918 and was closed in 1938, a year after the new drug laws called for the proof of safety of marijuana preparations.

1887: Hare provides a summary of current therapeutic applications, his clinical observations and speculation as to the mechanism of cannabis analgesia, before describing his animal studies.

1898: Marshall describes a method for refining Red oil and other more potent active components from charas. He studies the effects on animals, noting it to be non-toxic. While recommending it therapeutically as a sedative hypnotic, he cautioned against its habitual use—after making and personally using various cannabis derivatives at high oral dosage thirty-three times over a period of two and a half years.

The 1918 twentieth edition of The Dispensatory of the U.S.A. *described the state of the art of pharmaceutical treatment of crude U.S. and imported cannabis products.*

Little significant pharmacochemical research was done until the work by Walton, Loewe, and Adams in the late thirties.

Adams in 1942 reported his chemical studies, describing chemical structures of the active principles of cannabis and of his and his friends' personal experiences on tetrahydrocannabinol synthesized in his laboratory. He also summarizes findings of medical and psychiatric studies on prisoner patients.

Loewe is concerned with chemical Structure and Activity Relationships (SAR). He reviews psychological and physiological responses with regard to possible therapeutic applications of different THC homologs. In a highly detailed fashion he describes evaluation of anticonvulsant, hypnotic and analgesic properties of marijuana homologs in his animal experiments.

Shulgin ends the section with a complicated discussion of the chemistry of cannabis congeners and their derivatives.

Clinical and Physiological Notes on the Action of Cannabis Indica

BY HOBART AMORY HARE, M.D.

Cannabis Indica has been before the profession for many years as a remedy to be used in combating almost all forms of pain, yet, owing to the variations found to exist as to its activity, it has not received the confidence which I think it now deserves. At present certain improvements made in the method of obtaining the extract from the crude drug have very materially increased its reliability, so that by selecting an article made by a responsible firm we may be fairly sure of receiving a preparation in which we can place confidence. Within a few years this drug has become particularly prominent in connection with its use in migraine, particularly when used in conjunction with gelsemium, although of the two remedies the hemp is by far the most active agent in subduing the pain and preventing other attacks.

Heretofore the profession has used the remedy in such cases purely from an empirical stand-point, but I shall in a moment explain more fully its true physiological action. Aside from this, however, I have certainly seen very severe and intractable cases of migraine successfully treated by this remedy, not only in regard to the attack itself, but by acting as a prophylactic. The best use of the remedy under such circumstances is as follows, in case the drug obtained be fairly active.

If the attacks are frequent then the remedy should be used constantly in small doses, in such a way that the patient is not conscious of any influence of the drug, and about

Reprinted from *The Therapeutic Gazette*, vol. II, 1887, pp. 225-228.

one-eighth of a grain of the solid extract may be taken night and morning, or, if this produces any tendency to sleep, the whole amount may be taken at night. At the beginning and during the attack it should be freely administered, until either the pain is diminished or very marked symptoms of its physiological action assert themselves; and that this line of treatment is not one calculated to produce serious results is proved by my own experiments, and by the fact that so far no case of fatal poisoning from its ingestion has been recorded as occurring in the human being.

I myself have taken as much as one grain of the solid extract of a very active preparation without producing any disagreeable symptoms other than that of a deep sleep, which lasted for nearly eighteen hours, preceded by a period of great hilarity, which did not pass into any sensation of dread, such as has been described by some persons.

When gelsemium is used in addition to the hemp, its usefulness is limited only to its action in warding off an immediately impending attack, and I do not believe it possesses much power for good unless it be given when the first symptoms of the malady appear. Its exceedingly poisonous properties necessarily prohibit any repetition of a dose, and for this and the reasons above stated the drug should be administered in one single dose of fifteen to twenty drops of the tincture at the first sign of an attack.

Cases of migraine treated in this way, when the disease does not depend on any distinct organic lesion, are in a large proportion of instances either entirely cured or greatly benefited, the attacks even when they recur being considerably farther apart.

In neuralgias depending on a condition of debility in nursing women and in overworked men cannabis indica alone acts very favorably; not by acting in any way as a stimulant to the system, but rather by allaying any irritability of the nerve-trunks. Again, in many cases of irritative cough, depending either upon some nervous irritability or upon some actual irritated condition of the air-passages, cannabis indica will be of service in allaying the troublesome symptom, and is often found useful in the chronic winter cough of old people, provided no great outpouring of mucus or liquid is in the lungs.

In certain stages of phthisis it is a very valuable remedy,

not on account of any influence possessed by it on the pathological processes, but by quieting restlessness and anxiety, and by turning the mind of the patient to other channels. Indeed, in cases of advanced phthisis I believe it would be justifiable to push the drug almost to the condition known as euthanasia, and this has been done quite frequently by many practitioners. Under these circumstances, the patient, whose most painful symptom has been mental trepidation, may become more happy or even hilarious.

The advantages in its use over that of opium consist chiefly in the absence of prostration and nausea after its ingestion, and in the partial lack of soporific power which it possesses as compared to the opiate, for in certain cases sleep is not always desirable when pain is to be removed. That cannabis indica has, however, marked powers as a soporific is not to be denied. Added to these advantages is the fact of its failure to produce serious symptoms even if very large doses be taken, although I have found the efficient dose of a pure extract of hemp to be as powerful in relieving pain as the corresponding dose of the same preparation of opium.

That it is capable of producing a habit there can be no doubt, although whether its devotees are as devoted as are those of opium I cannot say. In my own practice I have seen a case of a young man who took his first dose as an experiment, and who afterwards had such a constant desire for its repeated use that he was forced to abstain from it entirely. He also said he could readily understand how the drug might have devotees, and that the pleasurable sensations excited were far preferable to those of alcohol.

During the time that this remarkable drug is relieving pain a very curious psychical condition sometimes manifests itself; namely, that the diminution of the pain seems to be due to its fading away in the distance, so that the pain in a delicate ear would grow less and less as a beaten drum was carried farther and farther out of the range of hearing.

This condition is probably associated with the other well-known symptom produced by the drug, namely, the prolongation of time.

Turning from the clinical stand-point of the drug to its physiological effects, we find that its clinical uses rest on a scientific basis, and I shall, therefore, detail one or two experiments showing in what manner the drug acts.

If a considerable quantity (10 minims)* of the fluid extract be given to a twenty-pound dog, by the jugular vein, in the course of two or three minutes he becomes very playful and happy, and gambols over the floor. In the course of about five minutes more there appears a slight stagger in the walk, which gradually increases, and is most marked in the forelegs, the condition of mental exhilaration continuing. Soon after this equilibration is partly lost, for the animal, sitting on its haunches, places its forefeet wide apart; nevertheless, in the course of ten minutes more he seems to partially recover his balancing powers, and to be as happy and frolicsome as ever, barking and running. In the course of twenty or twenty-five minutes more he vomits, and the swaying and staggering reassert themselves, now affecting both hind and front legs. This condition rapidly passes into a drowsy state, which, in turn, deepens into a profound sleep, from which it is difficult to arouse the animal to consciousness, although the reflexes are markedly accentuated, particularly to sounds. This sleep lasts for many hours, and finally the dog wakes up himself again. In some instances a lack of co-ordination, due evidently to failure of sensation, appears, so that the animal places his feet on the floor as if it were uneven, or higher or lower than it is.

That the drug may be given in enormous amounts by the jugular vein in the dog without producing death is proved by the fact that I have injected as much as 10 c.c. of the fluid extract without producing serious symptoms. Thus, at 1:20 P.M. the injection was given. At 1:25 the dog was sound asleep and groaning, as if having bad dreams. At this time pinching the ear called out no sign of discomfort, and the respirations were eight per minute.

At 5 P.M. the animal was as sound asleep as before, but was unfortunately killed by the laboratory assistant, owing to a misunderstanding of my orders. Just before death the respirations had risen to ten per minute, and several movements had been made by the dog.

Again, I have given by the jugular vein 22 c.c. of a fluid extract, which I knew to be active, without producing death or any marked change in either arterial pressure or pulse-rate, as may be seen from the following condensed table:

* A minim is a sixtieth part of a dram, which is in turn an eighth of a fluid ounce. It is thus a small drop.

DOG; ETHERIZED; WEIGHT, 40 POUNDS; FULL GROWN

Time	Drug	Pressure	Pulse	Remarks
3.01.10	.....	114-144	186	
3.01.20	.....	114-142	180	
3.01.30	.....	116-142	192	
3.01.40	2 c.c.	144-100	192	Injection begun.
3.01.56	.....	86-136	198	Injection ended.
3.02.06	.....	118-154	168	
3.02.16	.....	134-154	150	
3.02.26	.....	132-150	162	
3.07	.....	126-138	156	
3.09	.....	126-142	144	
3.09.10	.....	126-140	146	
3.09.20	.....	126-142	144	
3.09.38	.....	128-148	150	Vagi cut in order to determine if the slowing was due to pneumogastric stimulation.
3.09.48	.....	136-164	168	
3.11	.....	134-166	180	
3.12	.....	168-194	162	
3.12.23	5 c.c.	168-190	150	Injection begun.
3.12.35	.....	110-190	162	Injection ended.
3.12.45	.....	78-112	162	
3.13.05	.....	164-178	180	
3.13.25	.....	176-184	162	
3.25	.....	154-172	186	
3.35	.....	148-170	162	
3.37	.....	148-168	180	
3.37.12	8 c.c.	162-174	144	Injection begun.
3.37.22	.....	166-88	132	Injection ended.
3.37.32	.....	56-84	156	
3.39.00	.....	88-136	180	
3.41.10	.....	126-156	174	
3.41.20	.....	126-150	174	
3.41.37	7 c.c.	138-150	144	Injection begun.
3.41.42	.....	136-154	138	Injection ended.
3.41.52	.....	148-118	168	
3.42.02	.....	90-140	150	
3.42.12	.....	104-70	168	
3.42.22	.....	98-68	156	
3.42.5	.....	88-116	96	
3.44	.....	118-92	102	
3.44.16	10 c.c.	98-124	105	Injection begun.
3.44.20	.....	74-146	88	
3.44.40	.....	54-34	96	
3.45	.....	28-24	66	
3.45.10	.....	26-22		Pulse imperceptible; heart stopped; respiration continued for ninety seconds after heart.

The only influence exercised on the circulation by the drug consists, as is seen by the above table, in a slight slowing of the pulse and fall of arterial pressure. That the slowing is due to direct cardiac depression and not to stimulation of the vagal centres is proved by the failure of the pulse to return to its normal rate when the vagi were cut. The fall in arterial pressure seems to depend entirely on the failure of cardiac power.

The 22 c.c. were given between 3:01 and 3:41, in four doses, ranging from 2 to 8 c.c. At 3:44, 10 c.c. more of the extract was given rapidly into the jugular, producing death in about sixty seconds. In other words, it required 32 c.c. of the strong fluid extract, by the jugular vein, to produce death in a dog weighing forty pounds.

When we consider that this extract was active in doses of 8 minims to man, it must be conceded that this drug has but slight lethal power.

Respiration continues after the heart ceases to beat in those cases in which the drug is sent into the cardiac apparatus *en masse* through the jugular vein; but when death is not due to this cause, there seems to be a simultaneous failure of heart-power and respiration.

The action of the drug on the nervous system is, of course, the most interesting part of the investigation, and we find that in the frog, as in the dog, the greater portion of its action is on the brain.

When a very large dose of the fluid extract (5–20 minims) is given hypodermically to the frog, it immediately becomes quiet, and in a moment or two will lie flat on its back, apparently in a deep sleep, with slow and full respirations. That the condition of relaxation is due to sleep or cerebral depression was proved by oft-repeated experiment, reflex action being increased very markedly, proving that the motor and sensory nerve-trunks were unaffected, as well as the motor and receptive centres in the cord. Reflex action, however, rapidly diminishes after remaining for five or ten minutes, and total relaxation comes on. That this is not due to motor-nerve or spinal palsy is proved by electric stimulation of the cord and nerve-trunks, which is always followed by contractions of the tributary muscles.

The loss of reflex power, therefore, must depend on depression of the sensory apparatus, and further experiment confirms this reasoning, for, as was again and again proven, the drug, when applied locally to the exposed sciatic, invariably prevented the passage of the most powerful impulses from the foot to the cord. The poisoned foot could be burnt off without any response, while if the opposite leg was burned the batrachian instantly leaped away, using both the poisoned and unpoisoned leg, showing again that cannabis indica does not have much effect on the motor nerve-filaments even when directly applied to them.

Under these latter circumstances, however, the poisoned leg is not moved quite as rapidly as its fellow, showing that the motor nerve has not escaped absolutely the direct application of the drug. That the sensory tract of the cord is affected was proved by tying the common iliac in order to protect the nerve-trunks of the posterior extremities, and then injecting the poison into the body. Under these circumstances there is, as usual, the first stage of heightened reflex action, followed by corresponding depression of the same, and irritation of the protected sensory nerve fails to call forth any response from the spinal cord.

To summarize these conclusions, we find that cannabis indica produces in the lower animals a period of happiness followed by more or less deep sleep, according to the amount of the drug. That in both the dog and frog we have a stage of heightened reflex action following the dose.

That this increased reflex action is replaced by reflex palsy which is not due to motor-nerve or motor-spinal-tract palsy, but to failure of the sensory side of the cord and nerve-trunks.

That the chief action of the drug is upon the centres in the cerebrum, that the action on the sensory tract of the spinal cord and nerve-trunks is secondary to its cerebral action.

Before closing this paper I desire to call the attention of practitioners to the local anaesthetic action of this curious substance. As already detailed, when applied directly to the nerve-trunks it paralyzes them, and I have found that when applied to the mucous membrane of the tongue in considerable quantity it diminished sensibility to a considerable degree. Dentists, I am told, constantly use it for sensitive dentine. The drug is too irritating to be used on delicate membranes such as the eye, for I have proved in the dog that it is apt to bring on severe inflammation.

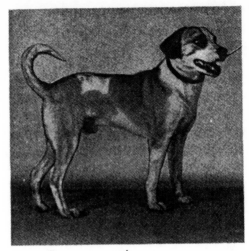

A

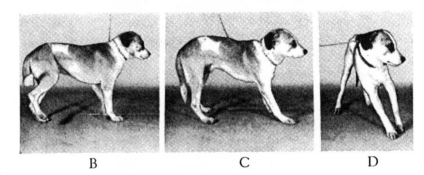

B   C   D

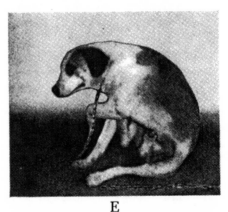

E

Various effects: A. Normal dog. B–E. Same dog in various stages following intravenous injection of "Cannabinol." B. Swaying to side. C. Swaying backward. D. Pitching backward. E. Prolonged scratching movements. From Robert P. Walton, Marihuana: America's New Drug Problem, *Philadelphia, 1938.*

A Contribution
to the Pharmacology
of Cannabis Indica

BY C.R. MARSHALL, M.D.

Notwithstanding the large amount of labor which has been expended on Indian hemp, we know comparatively little of its pharmacology. The active principle, it is true, has been isolated, in a more or less impure form, by O'Shaughnessy, Robertson, the brothers Smith, and more recent investigators, but the more important question of the changes this undergoes has not, as far as I am aware, until recently, been attempted. To me this is the most interesting part of the inquiry. Apart from the great financial loss entailed by the growing inertness with age of the drug, the variability in the strength, its preparation has led to numerous misfortunes in medical practice, and a distrust in its use as a therapeutic agent. The isolation of the active principle of the drug would not matter if we could only insure our preparations being of constant strength. But, without knowing the cause of the increasing inertness, this it is impossible to do. With this cause, among other questions, I intend to deal in this paper.

As I have dealt elsewhere[1] with the history of the active principles of Indian hemp, I shall confine myself in this communication to the work of the most recent observers. Two ·and a half years ago three Cambridge chemists—Wood, Spivey and Easterfield—commenced a re-investigation of the chemistry of Indian hemp. They worked with charas, as being the most active preparation of the plant, and by extraction with organic solvents (alcohol, ether, petroleum ether, etc.)

Reprinted from *American Medical Journal,* vol. 31, 1898, pp. 882–891.

302

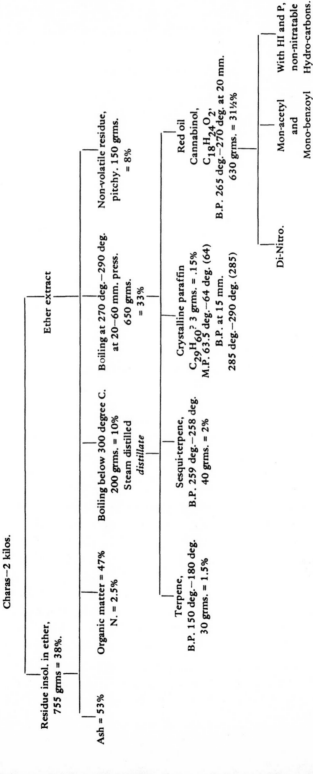

and subsequent fractional distillation, they isolated a mono- and sesqui-terpene, a crystalline paraffin and a resinous body (cannabinol); an indistillable pitch and an insoluble sandy residue were left behind.[2] The proportions of these substances are shown in the subjoined table, taken from a communication by Easterfield and Wood to the Cambridge Philosophical Society.[3]

Other samples more recently examined have not been found to be so good as this. A second lot contained only 15 per cent. cannabinol; and a third only 10 per cent. Furthermore, the cannabinol from these samples was not so pure as that obtained from the first sample and from the cannabinol obtained from the last the acetyl derivative of a higher homologue of the pure substance has been prepared. This homologue was present to the amount of 10–20 per cent.

The products (with the exception of the paraffin) and certain impure intermediate substances were passed on to me for pharmacologic examination. I naturally turned my attention first to the resin. The terpenes were present in too small an amount, and their chemic constitution and physical character were not such as to suggest a cannabis-like action. Personne,[4] it is true, attributed the activity of the drug to an oily liquid, *cannabene* ($C_{18} H_{20}$), which Valenti,[5] and more recently Vignola,[6] have shown to be an impure sesqui-terpene; but Roux[7] has proved physiologically that cannabene is not the active principle. On the other hand, numerous investigators had shown that the active principle is of a resinous nature. The paraffin was only present in very small amounts, and from its constitution and properties it is easy to infer that it possesses no marked physiologic properties.

The resin was found to be active. It possessed, as far as I could see, all the peculiar effects of the hemp plant. The question to be settled was its purity. As it boils at 265 to 270 degrees C, under 20 m.m. Hg pressure, and possesses a constant composition, the presence of an impurity seemed improbable. At least it could only be due to a stereo-chemical isomer or a substance with closely allied composition and properties. The possible presence of an alkaloid was avoided by treating the crude drug with dilute sulphuric acid before commencing the investigation. But no alkaloid has been found in charas.

In a more or less impure form cannabinol has been isolated

from various commercial preparations, viz.: Merck's cannabinon, extractum cannabis Indicae ethereum, resina cannabis Indicae, and T. & H. Smith's cannabin.

Physiologic   Experiments have been carried out on cats, dogs, rabbits
investigations. and myself, and the investigations have been mainly confined
to the administration of the various substances by the
mouth—a condition necessitated by the comparative insolubility of the drugs. With the experiments in detail I do not
intend to deal—admirable descriptions have been given by
various observers, both in this and other countries—but in
appendix I will be found types of experiments and in
appendix II a synopsis of the experiments made. By combining these and referring to the text, little difficulty will be
experienced in forming mental pictures of the condition in
each individual experiment.

Most of my experiments were made upon two dogs. One
was a mongrel puppy something like an Airedale terrier in
breed; the other was a young adult fox-terrier. Later a third
dog, an English terrier, was added. The first two dogs were of
very different temperament; the one (Airedale terrier) was
self-reliant and intelligent; the other was affectionate, but
nervous to an extreme degree. The English terrier, although
timid, possessed much more character than the last one. This
question of temperament, I believe, is of considerable importance in dealing with the finer effects of cannabis indica. The
cats were adults; the rabbits young, usually three to four
months old.

The *terpene* in the comparatively small doses in which I
was able to give them, produced no noteworthy symptoms
beyond slight diuresis. In rabbits there seemed to be slight
transient excitement, but the compound given to these
animals was impure. On myself 0.5 c.c. produced no effect; 2
c.c. (sesqui-terpene) slight and transient listlessness and heaviness of the head.

The *resin*, cannabinol, in dogs constantly produced the
same qualitative effect, although it varied slightly in the
different animals and in the same animal from time to time.
The first noticeable symptom (one-half to two hours) was
slight lassitude and an appearance of heaviness about the
eyes. Gradually the depression increased and sleepiness and
usually sleep followed; yawning and sighing were not infre-

quent; the body when standing swayed from side to side and this gradually increased until the animal fell over or suddenly pulled himself up with an effort. Usually, after falling, he remained in the position and went to sleep. Sometimes the rocking motion occurred in an antero-posterior direction, especially in the fox-terrier. In this animal, too, the standing position was more characteristic, the hind legs being half bent. In this position and markedly unsteady he usually stood gazing into the fire. Distinct ataxia during walking was present or absent according to the dose. After large doses the attention was blunted, but after small ones no effect in this direction was noticed. After three to six hours the animals began to improve. At this period the larger sometimes became extremely frolicsome and if played with would run about barking in a high-pitched voice. Usually both animals slept or lay before the fire until taken to the kennel for the night.

When under the influence of the drug, the pupils were sometimes slightly dilated, sometimes unaffected., occasionally contracted; the pulse and respiration were slowed, but whether more than could be accounted for by the condition of rest it was often difficult to decide. My general impression is that the pulse was slower than during ordinary sleep. The temperature, with one exception, invariably fell; at the most not more than 3 degrees C., usually not more than 1 or 2 degrees C. The fall naturally varied with the temperature of the room. It was most marked in the fox-terrier, and in this dog trembling was not an infrequent symptom. The reflexes were always present and the sense of pain was doubtfully blunted; the olfactory sense, however, seemed depressed. Vomiting was a frequent symptom; salivation, independent of any emesis, a rare one. In the fox-terrier, increased micturition was occasionally obtained. The influence of dose was not marked. Generally speaking, the symptoms were fairly constant; but owing to the insolubility of the material complete absorption was difficult to insure. Consequently, in dogs at least, a strictly quantitative comparison could not be made. Occasionally a small dose produced more marked symptoms than a larger one, but this was rare, and in the fox-terrier the onset of the symptoms as a rule was later and they lasted longer than in the other dogs. On the whole, however, the symptoms were fairly proportioned to the amount given. After small doses (0.02 g. per kg.) quietude, heaviness about the eyes, sleepiness and usually slight un-steadiness occurred; attention was not appreciably affected, and the symptoms almost passed away in five or six hours. In the English terrier this dose produced a very marked effect, the ataxia being as severe as after much larger doses to other dogs. After large doses (0.1 g. per. kg.) there were marked depression, ataxia, vomiting and sleepiness, although sleep was not an invariable symptom. In the evening food was refused, but the following morning they seemed quite well.

In cats effects similar to those occurring in dogs were obtained, but the action was more severe and prolonged. After a dose of 0.058 g. per. kg. improvement did not commence until after twenty-five hours. The depression and muscular weakness were more marked than in dogs, and salivation was a more constant symptom. Total anorexia and consequent loss of weight occurred after large doses. A detailed description of an experiment will be found in appendix I.

On rabbits preparations of cannabis indica exert compara-tively little effect. This was observed by O'Shaughnessy, and it has been noted by more recent investigators. The same effect was obtained in my own experiments with cannabinol. But I am inclined to believe that the immunity is more apparent than real. After large doses, slight depression and quietude are the only observable symptoms, but on further examination a fall in the number of heart-beats and respira-tion and the temperature was found to occur; the animal refuses to eat and death usually ensues. The low cerebral development of these animals prevents them showing unmis-takable signs of cannabis poisoning, and these are only found in observations on the vegetative functions. The lethal dose, however, is much larger than for dogs or cats.

The effect on myself was very similar to that described by other observers as peculiar to Indian hemp. After large doses (0.1 g.) there was a sensation of dryness of the lips, and of increased viscidity of the buccal mucus, a pleasurable tingling throughout the body, muscular weakness, slight ataxia, risi-bility and loss of time sensation. My pulse was said to be increased in frequency, sensation was somewhat blunted, and the pupils were not often forthcoming.

After intermediate doses (0.05 g.) the ability to work was lost altogether. I usually sat before the fire doing nothing,

almost thinking of nothing. There was a marked unwilling-
ness to move. Pleasurable tingling in the limbs, very slight
ataxia and other symptoms similar to those obtained after a
larger dose were present. Time passed quickly. Sleepiness was
sometimes, but not always, present. As an early symptom a
peculiar indistinctness of the periphery of the visual field
occurred, and later it was found that the point of regard was
made to travel with greater difficulty, as along the line of a
page. Depression usually continued throughout the following
day.

The residual *pitch*, when dissolved in oil, was active, but
much less so than cannabinol. The symptoms were the same.
Given in the solid form it exerted little effect. In all
probability the activity was due to unchanged cannabinol
present. Certain intermediate impure products were tried, but
none of these was as active as cannabinol. The insoluble
residue was inactive.

Thus, by a process of elimination, cannabinol was found to
be the most active ingredient of the charas products. But in
order to determine its comparative activity, control experiments were made with the crude material and extracts
obtained from it. The natural product exerted much the same
action as cannabinol, but both spirituous and oily extracts
were somewhat more active; a similar result was obtained
with Merck's cannabinon. This raised the question as to
whether cannabinol is the sole active ingredient of the plant.
I think we must assume that it is, at least, the active
principle. The symptoms produced by the natural product
and the resin are practically the same, and this is an
important point. It suggests that we must look for changes
occurring in the resin either during its manufacture or
subsequently; or to a diminished absorbability as compared
with extracts of the crude product. That faulty manufacture,
etc., will produce a more or less inert substance, will be seen
from evidence given later; but I am inclined to attribute to
the lessened absorption the more important role. The terpenes probably increase the rapidity of absorption of crude
extracts, but this I have not yet been able to put to the test.
That cannabinol does not possess all the activity of the hemp
plant I am prepared to admit; but this is the case with most
other crude drugs and their so-called active principles. In the

The active principle.

case of charas the terpenes probably aid in its physiologic action, as the crude drug seemed to produce more excitement than pure cannabinol; and when the drug is smoked it is possible that pyrodene and other bases, which are produced by the destructive distillation of the substance, may aid in its intoxicating effects. If any other substance aids in its action, we have at present no indication of it. Moreover, that cannabinol is the chief active ingredient is supported by the fact that the activity of different products is roughly proportionate to the amount of cannabinol they contain, and that the growing inertness of Indian hemp can be explained by changes occurring in this resin.

The question of the purity of cannabinol can only be settled by further research, and this, I may add, is being undertaken. The only demonstration of its purity in the present state of our knowledge, viz: the reconversion of the crystalline acetylized derivative into cannabinol, failed. The acetyl derivative was not crystalline, and the reconverted cannabinol was much less active, physiologically, than the parent substance. This might be explained in many ways, but at present it is idle to speculate.

The last and worst sample of charas yielded a substance which contained a higher homologue of pure cannabinol. This homologue regenerated from its acetyl compound was physiologically inactive. Whether it is active previous to acetylizing is at present impossible to say.

The cause of the inactivity of Indian hemp. The different samples of the same preparation of Indian hemp possess varying physiologic effects, and that good samples darken and deteriorate in keeping has long been known; but until recently no satisfactory explanation of this has been offered. In 1894 Leib Lapin,[8] by means of fractional precipitation prepared a substance which he termed *cannabindon*. This presented the appearance of "a beautiful dark cherry-red mass of thick consistency, which took the form of the vessel in which it stood, and showed a smooth horizontal surface." Its formula he gives as $C_8H_{12}O$. It possessed distinct reducing properties, and rubbed up with chocolate and left a week, its physiologic action was in great part lost. The latter he explains as being due to an oxidation of the preparation resulting from its finely divided state and its contact with fat and air; and he strengthens his position by a reference to the similar behavior of ergot, which undergoes oxidation less readily than cannabindon. The oxidation product he states "is inactive or very slightly active."

Although I was aware of Leib Lapin's views, my own researches were carried out independently. What first drew my attention to the matter was the gradual darkening which cannabinol underwent when left exposed to the air in a test-tube; the darkening commenced on the surface and gradually extended downward; the superficial layers being affected rapidly, the deeper layers very slowly. In order to determine whether this was due to oxidation, and whether in consequence the activity was affected, oxygen was slowly passed through cannabinol kept fluid by immersion in a sulphuric acid bath at 150 to 160 degrees C. The material rapidly darkened and the consistency increased. After passing the oxygen through for six hours the activity was found to be decidedly less. It was then bubbled through for thirteen hours more, the temperature toward the end of the experiment being raised to 185 degrees C. in order to keep the substance fluid. On cooling, the substance set to a hard, brittle mass, exactly resembling pitch in appearance. No loss or gain of weight, within the limits of experimental error occurred. This pitchy material given in the solid form possessed scarcely any action, but this in part is due to the lessened solubility and higher melting-point, for if previously discolored in oil, a distinct, though comparatively slight, effect is obtained. Dr. Easterfield, who has made all the analyses in connection with the charas research kindly undertook one of the oxidized cannabinol. The percentages obtained, compared with those of cannabinol, were:

Calculated for $C_{18}H_{24}O_2$ (cannabinol)	Found	Calculated for $C_{18}H_{22}O_3$
C = 79.4	C = 77.7	C = 75.0
H = 8.8	H = 7.5	H = 8.3

The product obtained was therefore not completely oxidized, and the activity it retained was in all probability due to unchanged cannabinol. As a control experiment carbon dioxide was passed through a similar sample of cannabinol similarly treated. Very slight darkening, probably owing to slight admixture with air occurred, but there was no increase in consistency. Only a slight diminution in activity was observed.

The influence of temperature was tried. Cannabinol distilled at 400 degrees C. under atmospheric pressure was found to be slightly less active than cannabinol distilled at 265 degrees C. under 20 M.m. Hg. pressure, but when the substance was heated in sealed tubes at 220 to 260 degrees C. for twenty-four hours, no very great loss of activity occurred, although this was distinct. As slight oxidation may have resulted during the process, the influence of temperature *per se* may be disregarded. The action of aqueous vapor has not been determined.

It would therefore seem as if the loss of activity of Indian hemp was due to oxidation of the active ingredient. The terpenes, like other members of this class, readily hydrolyze, and this, doubtless, exerts some effect in the deterioration of the crude drug. The obvious remedy is to keep cannabis preparations in air-tight vessels until they can be used. For practical purposes a well-corked bottle seems to be sufficiently protective but hermetically sealed packages, especially for transport purposes, are to be prepared. In sealed tubes we have kept cannabinol for seventeen months without the slightest change.

The limitation of the oxidation to the superficial layers probably explains many of the accidents occurring in practice. If the preparation has been long in stock and imperfectly protected, these may have become comparatively inert, and scarcely any effect may be produced, while a renewal of the prescription from deeper parts—or the substitution of a more recent preparation—may produce very marked effects. I am certain that the accidental administration of superficial and deep layers of cannabinol will explain some discrepancies in my own results, which previously were inexplicable.

As regards a chemical test for the physiologic activity of cannabis compounds, none exists; and the only indication at present is in the direction of their reducing power. This will probably give us some information, and I hope to deal with the question later. As far as cannabinol is concerned, the transparency is the best ready indication of its purity. When placed in an ordinary test-tube print ought to be read through it with ease; any blackening is due to admixture with oxidized material. If not carefully prepared impure products are readily obtained, and such gives no more constant results than the ordinary preparations on the market. The transparency, however, is not an absolute indication of its purity, for the higher homologue of cannabinol, which, when derived from its acetyl compound is inactive, is almost as transparent as cannabinol itself. What the physiologic effect of this compound is in the natural state, it has not been possible to determine.

But the variation in activity of the preparations of Indian hemp will not account for all the differences in effect produced. A difference in individual susceptibility also exists. What this is due to we do not know. It is probable that certain types of men are more susceptible than others, and that certain habits, such as the alcoholic, have an inhibiting influence on this direction. The subject is a difficult one to treat from a purely experimental point of view. In the dogs the greatest effect seemed to be connected with greatest mental stability, but how much of this was due to variability of absorption and how much to individual differences it is difficult to say.

Susceptibility.

The following case which recently came under my notice is of interest in this connection, as it enabled me to compare the effect of the same dose on myself. A gentleman suffering from neuralgia took ¼ grain extractum cannabis indicae (B. P.) in the form of a pill. The pills were made up by a well-known London druggist. The following account was written by the patient himself: "At about 4:30 on Sunday, feeling neuralgic pain in the right eye, I took one of the pills. I then had tea and read aloud for some time, feeling nothing unusual. But about 7:30, when dressing for dinner, I began to suffer from very curious feelings. I felt giddy and seemed to lose command of my actions; thoughts seemed to pass rapidly through my brain and I hardly felt responsible for myself. I went to my wife's room and described my feelings. She was alarmed at my appearance and said I was very white. I felt a sort of burning uncomfortable feeling inside and I tried to make myself vomit by drinking several tumblerfuls of hot mustard and water. This was partially successful, but I felt very ill and a doctor was called in. When he came I was unable to speak coherently; sentences were disjointed, and my memory partially failed me. I was ordered to bed and undressed with difficulty. I then shook violently all over, and my hands were cold and tended to contract. I was given some brandy and water and gradually I became more natural. Afterward I took some soup and fish. During my sleep I felt inclined to laugh, but I do not think I actually did so. The next morning I was comparatively well, but throughout this day and the next I did not feel quite well; there was a numbness and coldness in my legs and I feared I was in for an attack of influenza, but my temperature was normal." The neuralgia was cured, but afterward he told me he would rather bear the pain than the effects of the remedy. The ramainder of the pills were given to me and on two occasions I tried them on myself. On both occasions the usual effects of Indian hemp were produced, viz., paresthesia in the extremities, inability to do mental work, and sleepiness, but not the giddiness and other symptoms produced in the case cited. The less effect may in part be due to my previous experience, and the absence of fear in consequence, but this is insufficient to account for all the difference. The prescription was dispensed by a first-class pharmacist and there was no reason to believe that the extract was unequally shared.

The absorption of cannabinol. For all practical purposes, cannabis preparations may be regarded as being quite insoluble in water. They are soluble in fats and organic solvents generally, but with the exception of fats these are not common constituents of the contents of the alimentary canal. It is even doubtful what part fats play in the absorption of the drug. If Moore and Rockwood's[9] view of fat absorption be accepted, the only influence they could have would be a physical one—the substance would be brought into a state of finer division and thereby rendered more susceptible to other agencies. When given dissolved in oil, the onset of the symptoms is not distinctly earlier than in other cases, but as absorption probably only occurs from the intestine this observation is of little consequence. The more important question is the solubility of the active principle in dilute acids and alkalies respectively. According to Kionka[10] the resin of Indian hemp is insoluble in alkalies. From the therapeutic point of view Germain Sée[11] states that cannabis is the peculiar sedative of the stomach. Both these statements suggest that the active principle is soluble in an acid medium, and this is supported by the fact that cannabinol is actually soluble in strong sulphuric acid and glacial acetic acid. But my results for dilute acids are opposed to this view, and contrary to the statement of Kionka, I find it soluble in dilute alkalies. The following experiment proves this: Two Erlenmeyer's flasks were taken; into one (A) was put 2.127 grammes cannabinol; into the other (B) put 2.335 grammes. Both were left over sulphuric acid until they attained a constant weight; 100 c.c., 1 per cent. caustic soda solution was then added to A and 100 c.c., 1 per cent. hydrochloric acid (gas) to B. Both were shaken occasionally and left twenty-four hours. The alkaline solution soon became of a purplish color, which deepened; the acid solution remained perfectly clear. After standing twenty-four hours, both solutions were poured off and the remaining cannabinol was rapidly washed with distilled water until the washings were free from acid and alkali respectively. The flasks were again put over sulphuric acid and left until the weight became constant. The alkali-containing flask (A) had lost 0.03 gramme cannabinol; the acid-containing flask (B) 0.005 gramme, the latter being within experimental error.

It is therefore probable that the cannabis resin is absorbed under the influence of the alkaline juices of the upper part of the intestine. In the mouth, solution occurs to a slight extent, as is evidenced by the peculiar unpleasant taste, but this can not be of practical importance. The influence of other alimentary conditions has not been determined.

The condition of the stomach, however, plays an important part in the time of appearance of the symptoms, probably by hastening or retarding the course of the drug to the intestines. Thus in one case, when the drug was taken on an almost empty stomach, four hours passed before the onset of the symptoms, whereas if taken just before a meal, the first symptoms invariably occurred within one and a half hours. Taken after meals the appearance of the first symptoms is variable. In atony and dilatation of the stomach cannabis is said to be inactive (as a gastric sedative). The small solubility of the drug, even in alkalies, probably accounts for the insidious onset of the symptoms and its prolonged effect.

Habituation.   In order to determine roughly the influence of continued dosage on the activity of cannabinol, the two dogs were given very large doses every day for a week. A small dose, similar to one given just before the experiment, was then adminisered and its effects watched. The influence was certainly less than on the previous occasion, but the diminution was not marked. Whether habituation to this remedy occurs less readily than with other hypnotics can only be determined by practical experience. I know of no reliable observations on the subject, although it must be well known. In any case the tolerance is not likely to be so great as in the case of opium.

During my experiments with the two dogs, this question of tolerance often presented itself, and it was on this account that a third dog was obtained. Of the greater susceptibility of this there could be no doubt; but to a certain extent it was only apparent. The experience was new to him; he walked about and stumbled when the other dogs would have laid down. The same thing happened in the earlier experiments with these dogs; the ataxia was marked; later, they learned wisdom by experience, and laid down soon after the drug was given. It was often difficult to get them to stand sufficiently long for any indications to develop.

Although my experiments did not show any great amount of tolerance, they seemed to me to show some mental depression; the normal physical life of the animals seemed to run on a lower level, although this was difficult of proof. That cannabis indica exerts a powerful depressing influence, on some individuals at least, there can be no doubt, and from experiments on myself I have little hesitation in joining the ranks of those clinicists who regard Indian hemp as a causal factor of insanity. But this point, and others, I hope to develop in a later communication.

Effects on special organs.   Owing to the insolubility of cannabis preparations and the pressure of other work, exact experiments on the different organs have not been carried out. A solution of cannabinol was made by heating an excess of the substance in a 1 per cent. solution of sodium bicarbonate on a water bath, but the resulting product, which was of a brownish color and probably contained about 1 in 1000 cannabinol, had no distinct influence on blood-pressure. A solution of cannabinol phosphate (8 per cent.) in one experiment caused a slight fall and subsequent rise of blood-pressure, but from other points of view this substance was but slightly active.

Cannabinol is, however, somewhat depressant to the heart. A fall in the number of beats was constant, and in many cases this seemed greater than could be accounted for by the rest and sleep. Thus, in the largest dog, a pulse of 108 fell to one of 48, and a slight irregularity, also noticed in rabbits, occasionally occurred. That the blood-vessels were not dilated was inferred from a comparison with the action of chloral. After this drug, there was not the same marked fall in the number of the heart-beats, and the character of the beat was slightly different. After a large dose of cannabinol my own pulse increased in frequency; after a small dose no effect was noticed; after intermediate doses I invariably forgot to take it. No distinct effect on the respiration was observed. It was slower and deeper, as in ordinary sleep.

In the fox-terrier increased micturition was not infrequent; but this was not observed in the other dogs. Constipation was not an obvious symptom. After continued dosage some evidence of it existed, but this was not seen after single doses. In myself it was rarely present. Salivation was an occasional symptom, but as this occurs in dogs and cats after the exhibition of drugs possessing no specific properties in this direction, it is not probable that cannabinol exerts any specific action in this way. In my own case dryness of the mouth was a more constant feature.

The main action of cannabinol, however, is on the nervous system, and probably on the cerebral cells. From introspective analysis it is difficult to avoid the conclusion that some peripheral action exists, but as all the symptoms can be explained by a central influence, it is simpler, in absence of proof, to accept this.

One of the most prominent physical symptoms is the loss of time-sensation. This is mentioned by most writers. But it is not peculiar to Indian hemp, as it occurs after mescal button and other drugs of a similar nature. Its explanation, to my mind, is simple. The estimation of time is a complex act and dependent upon our calling to consciousness a series of events. When the physical state is depressed by Indian hemp a succession of ideas cannot be maintained; time ceases to exist, and it can not therefore be estimated. Even the apparently slowly travelling second hands of a watch, which is observed when under the influence of Indian hemp, may be explained in a similar way. The power of conception is more or less lost; current events are rapidly forgotten, while those fixed in the memory by older associations may still be recalled. Under the full influence of the drug, even those too are forgotten, and one's whole previous existence seems to be blotted out.

A most interesting condition, after large doses, is the occurrence, alternately, of loss of control and lucid intervals. During the latter, all the elements of complete sanity are present, but the physical state is below the normal level. In it the processes on which consciousness depends are readily exhausted, and the condition of irresponsibleness develops. Slight mental strain during the lucid periods seems to hasten the occurrence of a state of irresponsibility. A more complete rest from thought brings back the rational intervals. The over-estimation of distance was never distinctly observed by me, except to a slight degree on one occasion. The effect is probably connected with the increased effort made to accommodate the ocular muscles to the required distance, and is dependent on deficient will-power. Hallucinations, too, of a very slight character, were only present in one instance—a result probably attributable to my lack of imagination. In dogs, after large doses, the attention was blunted, and they became less obedient. As far as I can see, there seems to be no selective influence on any psychical phenomenon. All such processes are depressed, but whether to an equal degree I am not prepared to state. With this question, however, I hope to deal at some future time.

Ill effects.   The most common ill effect, or rather after effect, I have experienced, has been depression, lasting the whole or greater part of the following day, after a large dose (0.1g.) This, and the accompanying mental exhaustion, were decidedly painful, and the effect was markedly prolonged by attempts to do an ordinary day's work.

In dogs, vomiting was not an uncommon symptom but this was much less marked than with morphine. A slight, occasional irregularity of the heart in these animals and rabbits, has been mentioned; and a similar condition, viz: an increase in the cardiac irregularity of heart disease has been observed by Prior[12] after cannabis preparations, in men.

These have been investigated in connection with experiments on the constitution of this body. Oxycannabin $(C_{12}H_{11}NO_4)$ is inactive, at least in moderate doses. Acetylcannabinol and the cannabinol regenerated from it were but slightly active. The acetyl compound of the higher homologue of cannabinol, as well as the substance (regenerated from the acetyl compound) itself, was inactive.

Tri-brom-cannabinol, a brownish powder, was found to possess hypnotic properties. In dogs the action was very slight, but on myself (after 0.1g) sleep and depression were marked, and three days of mental exhaustion followed.

Attempts were made to obtain a more soluble preparation of cannabinol, and this was best accomplished by making a phosphoric ester. Cannabinol was heated to 100 degrees C. with phosphoric anhydride. The melt was boiled out with alkalies, which dissolved nearly the whole of it, and this was then neutralized by hydrochloric acid. An amorphous substance was obtained, which, on analysis, gave results agreeing with the supposition that is was cannabinol phosphate. Physiologically, however, the substance was not very active and injected subcutaneously into a dog produced an abscess.

Therapeutically, cannabinol is likely to be a valuable hypnotic. It is purer and more reliable than the cannabis preparations on the market, but it does not appear to possess any other advantages over them. It is not a powerful cerebral depressant (except in relation to its dose), and belongs rather to the substances termed "sleep producers" than "sleep forcers." Owing to its comparative insolubility its action is prolonged, and this in my own case leads to depression. Its advantages are, that its lethal dose is considerable; it does not inhibit secretory activity; and it does not readily induce habituation. Its disadvantages are, the excitement produced by early doses and the depression which follows its use. It appears to be a slight analgesic, but how far its activity goes in this direction it is impossible, in the absence of experiments in which pain is present, to say. This can only be proved by clinical observation. Purely pharmacologic investigations do not support any other actions of this drug, but so far as they have been carried they do not deny their existence.

In conclusion, I express my thanks to Messrs. Wood,

Spivey and Easterfield, for the material supplied me, and especially to Dr. Easterfield for the help he has given me during the progress of the work.

Appendix I.

Descriptions of personal experiments will be found in the *Lancet.* P = heartbeat; R = respiration; T = respiration; T = rectal temperature.

Dog (English terrier); wt. 7180 grams; P., 102; R., 16; T., 38.2 degrees C.; (room temperature 20 to 22 degrees C.); 12:10 o'clock, 0.14 gram cannabinol; 12:40, slight depression, distinct unsteadiness; 12:45, ataxia more marked, head unsteady, eyes heavy; 12:55, very unsteady, will not lie down, pricked up ears when cart passed window, no dilatation of pupils; 1:10, extremely unsteady, continually falling over; will not touch milk, P. 96, T. 37.7 C.; 1:40, ataxia rather worse, still walking about; 1:50, vomited small quantity, mainly yellowish fluid; 1:54, vomited again; 2:10, condition same, constantly falling over, P. 108, T. 38.6 C.; 2:20, vomited again; 2:30, circus movements, then sat down, got up and repeated several times; 2:40, vomited; 2:50, vomited; 3:10, slightly better; but still falling over, P. 108, T. 38.9 C.; 3:40, been laid down last twenty minutes, slept partly, just got up, ataxia very much better at first but soon developed again; 4:10, sleepy, P. 96, T. 38.5 C.; 4:40 still marked ataxia but much better; 5:15, further improvement, still unsteady and depressed, P. 96, T. 38.9 C; following morning, apparently well. This was the only case in which a rise of temperature was noted.

Dog (Airedale puppy), wt. 6500 grams. 10:30 o'clock, 0.5 gram cannabinol given in bread, P. 192; 11:30, lively, no obvious effect; 11:45, sleepy, lay down; 12:30, still in same position, yawning, came when called but seems rather stupid; 1:00, walking about, when played with commenced to run about and bark in a higher pitched voice; 2:00, been asleep for last half hour, does not answer to name so readily, weak on legs, can not stand steadily; 3:00, condition same, asleep, P. 96; 4:00, still asleep, occasionally wakes up, yawns and stretches, will not answer to name; 5:30, condition much the same, still weak on legs and tired, sent to kennel, would not eat; following morning, apparently normal.

Cat, wt. 3600 grams. 1:30 o'clock, 0.15 gram cannabinol given in meat; 2:30, no apparent effect; 3:00, sleeping; 3:45, awakened, rather weak on legs, gait slightly unsteady; 5:00, much worse, distinct inco-ordinate gait but does not move about much, has been laid down mostly, with chin on ground, passed a loose motion, would not drink milk although seemed eager for it and only ate two small pieces of meat.

Second day, 9:30 o'clock, no apparent alteration, still stupid, would not come when called, distinct muscular weakness, gait still unsteady, pupils somewhat dilated, would not drink milk although a little had been drunk during the night; 2:30, slightly better, gait less unsteady; 5:30, still better, looks up when called, ataxia still present; following morning, seemed quite normal.

Rabbit, wt. 620 grams; P., 300; R., 76; T., 38.4 C.

First day, 2:25 o'clock; 2.4 grams cannabinol given in mucilage; 5:25, has been quiet since drug was given, eyelids partially closed, slightly depressed, doubtful muscular weakness; P. 216, R. 30, T. 34.1 C.

Second day, 10:00 o'clock, somewhat worse, head trembles slightly, sensation blunted but kicks on being handled, has not eaten any food, P. 204, R. 54, T. 31.4 C., placed before fire; 5:45, seems slightly better, P. 150, R 30, T. 32.7 C.

Third day, 12:15 o'clock, condition much the same, trembling of head present, eyes half closed, P. 168, R. 60, T. 29.1 C.; 5:30, slightly increased muscular weakness, pupils more dilated, been laid before the fire all day. P. 204, R. 36, T. 31.8 C.

Fourth day, 11:00 o'clock, no noticeable change. P. 138, R. 39, T. 30.6 C.; 6:00 much worse, trembling very marked.

Fifth day, 9:00 o'clock, found dead, rigor mortis, cold; afternoon, few small petechia in stomach, otherwise normal, stomach and cecum full of food.

Appendix II.

This appendix contains a summary of the experiments made on which the foregoing account is based. Only the briefest description is given, but some attempt has been made to indicate the comparative value of the experiments. The experiments are given in the order they were made. The time in parentheses indicates the period after administration of the drug at which the preceding symptom was noted; m., minute; h., hour.

Three dogs were used; at first only two. All were fed at 9 o'clock P.M. Unless otherwise indicated the individual substances were given in gelatine capsules by the mouth. **Experiments on dogs.**

1. May 5, 1897; Airedale terrier; weight 3100 gms.; 0.4 g. cannabinol phosphate; slight depression and sleepiness.

2. June 4, 1897; Airedale terrier, 4400 gms.; 0.4 g. cannabinol phosphate hypodermically; slight depression and sleepiness, fall in pulse

rate; longer effect than in last case.

3. June 16, 1897; Airedale terrier, 5400 gms.; 1.1 g. acetyl-cannabinol; sleepiness and depression (30 m.), unsteadiness, occasional slight excitement, vomiting·(3 h.), dilatation of pupils. Quite well next morning.

4. July 1, 1897; Airedale terrier; 0.5 g. cannabinol; slight sleepiness (75 m.), stupidity, muscular weakness and unsteadiness; slept most of day; normal next morning; effect more marked than 3.

5. July 15, 1897; Airedale terrier; 7520 gms.; 1 g. charas; tired, yawning (30 m.), sleepy, ataxia, etc., pupils somewhat dilated, very much excited (6 h.); seemed normal next day; effect somewhat greater than 4.

6. July 22, 1897; Airedale terrier; 0.3 c.c. 1/6 alcoholic extract charas; depression (60 m.), temporary excitement (100 m.), weakness and unsteadiness (most marked 5 to 6 h.), shivering, involuntary micturition; slightly excited next morning; very marked effect.

7. July 28, 1897; Airedale terrier; 1 c.c. 1/6 alcoholic extract charas; lay down (75 m.), but excited if played with; sleepiness, unsteadiness, etc., as in 6, but symptoms less severe; normal next morning.

8. July 30, 1897; Airedale terrier; 0.9 c.c. mono-terpene from charas; no effect.

9. Aug. 2, 1897; Airedale terrier; 1.1 c.c. sesqui-terpene from charas; no effect.

10. Aug. 3, 1897; Airedale terrier; 0.5 g. cannabinol distilled at 406 degrees C. (atmospheric pressure); lay down (30 m.), vomited (55 m.), depressed, head falling to one side (75 m.), afterward sleepiness, unsteadiness, etc., vomited twice (6 h.); effect almost as marked as 4.

11. Aug. 11, 1897; Airedale terrier; 1 c.c. greenish oil, intermediate between sesqui-terpene and cannabinol, unpleasant smell, vomited (45 m.); no effect beyond slight depression.

12. Oct. 19, 1897; Airedale terrier, 9650 gms,; 9.97 ·g. intermediate product between sesqui-terpene and cannabinol (distils below 300 degrees C.); slight depression, increased micturition; no other effect.

13. Fox-terrier, 7550 gms.; 0.75 g. intermediate product between sesqui-terpene and cannabinol (distills below 300 degrees C.); vomited four times (70 to 100 m.), increased micturition; no other effect.

14. Oct. 27, 1897; Airedale terrier, 10,700 gms.; 1.15 g. cannabinol, from Merck's cannabinon; depression (40 m.), sleepiness, muscular weakness and unsteadiness, dilated pupils, vomiting (140 m., 240·m., 255 m.); somewhat better, but still severely affected (5½ h.): would not touch food; apparently well next morning. Most marked effect yet.

15. Fox-terrier, 7950 gms.; 1.04 g. cannabinol, from T. and H. Smith's cannabin. Unsteadiness (35 m.), which increased; became tired and sleepy but walked about much, vomited (4¼ h.); more unsteady but less depressed than other dog; would not touch food; well next morning.

16. Nov. 11, 1897; Airedale terrier, 11,250 gms.; 0.99 g. Merck's cannabinon. No effect (30 m.), usual symptoms marked (60 m.), continued to 180 m., afterward gradual improvement, very much better (6½ h.), salivation (2 h. continued 1 h.), vomiting (2 h.); depression and unsteadiness more marked than 14 but more transient.

17. Fox-terrier, 8100 gms.; 1.04 g. ext. cannab. indic. ether (Merck). Slight effect (60 m.), unsteadiness (75 m.), vomited (3½ h.), ataxia main symptom; not much better (6½ h.); very little sleep, apparently well next morning; effect about the same as 15.

18. Nov. 18, 1897; Airedale terrier; 0.19 g. ext. cannab. indic. ether (Merck). Depression (45 m.), marked unsteadiness (60 m.), slight salivation (90 m.), sleepy, excited, vomited (3 h.), ataxia not much better when left (4 h.).

19. Nov. 22, 1897; Airedale terrier; 1.95 g. cannabinol. Slight effect (30 m.): unsteadiness, sleepiness, etc., developed, but symptoms not more severe than 18.

20. Fox-terrier; 1 g. ext. cannab. indic. (Merck). Commencing weakness (45 m.), more marked (60 m.), afterward became very severe; incontinence of urine, vomited (130 m., 135 m.), trembling from cold; slight improvement (3½ h.).

21. Nov. 26, 1897; Airedale terrier; 0.19 g. cannabinon (Merck) given in a piece of meat. Slight effect (2 h.); distinct unsteadiness (2½ h.), subsequently worse, depressed but not sleepy.

22. Fox-terrier; 0.55 g. extract cannab. indic. Sicc. (Merck). No distinct effect.

23. Dec. 1, 1897; Airedale terrier, 12,400 gms.; 0.15 g. alcohol ether extract charas [previously heated three times with dil. H_2SO_4]. Sleep main symptom, depression (60 m.), unsteadiness (90 m.), vomiting (2½ h. 3½ h.); distinct improvement (5 h.).

24. Fox-terrier; 8800 gms.; 0.15 g. alcohol ether extract charas [previously heated three times with dil. H_2SO_4]. Slight depression (35 m.), slight unsteadiness (75 m.), afterward very distinct; slept, salivation (3 h.), vomited (4 h.), not much improvement (6 h.); well next morning.

25. Dec. 3, 1897; Airedale terrier; 0.15 g. alcohol-ether extract charas [previously heated 14 hours at 260 degrees C.]. Effects similar to 23, but somewhat less marked and delayed—no obvious action except slight depression and sleepiness for three and one-half hours.

26. Fox-terrier; 0.21 g. alcohol-ether extract charas [previously heated 14 hours at 260 degrees C.]. Slight depression (60 m.), slight unsteadiness (3 h.), much more marked (3½ h.); improvement (4½ h.).

27. Dec. 6, 1897; Airedale terrier; 0.15 g. cannabinol rapidly distilled from alcohol-ether extract. No apparent effect (70 m.), later, usual symptoms developed, very distinct unsteadiness.

28. Fox-terrier; 0.54 g. pitch from extract, contains a little cannabinol. Slight depression; no other distinctive action.

29. Dec. 9, 1897; Airedale terrier; 0.15 g. distillation fraction previous to cannabinol than latter. Depression (30 m.), sleepiness, unsteadiness (85 m.), but not marked; attention good, excited (5½ h.).

30. Fox-terrier; 0.21 g. distillation fraction previous to cannabinol than latter. Mostly laid down at first; slight unsteadiness (2 h.), worse (3½ h.), slight sleepiness; symptoms not marked.

31. Airedale terrier; 0.21 g. charas extract, further heated for 60 hours at 220 to 260 degrees C. (c. 25). Depression (60 m.), unsteadiness (105 m.), slept fairly well, much better (5½ h.); symptoms more marked than 25 but less than 23.

32. Fox-terrier; 0.39 g. charas extract, further heated for 60 hours at 220 degrees C. (c. 25). Slight depression and unsteadiness (90 m.), much more marked (2 h.), still severe (5½ h.), sleepy, symptoms about equal to 24.

33. Dec. 28, 1897; Airedale terrier; 1.07 g. cannabinol (oldest). Laid down at first, could not be induced to stand long; very slight unsteadiness (3 h.) and depression, more severe (5 h.) but still fairly well; normal next morning.

34. Fox-terrier; 1.03 g. cannabinol (oldest); Slight depression (60 m.), unsteadiness (90 m.), still distinct (5 h.); depressed following morning.

35. Dec. 29, 1897; Airedale terrier; 0.92 g. cannabinol, distilled from another sample of charas. Asleep (55 m.), very unsteady (90 m.), continued as long as observed (6 h.); slept mostly.

36. Fox-terrier; 0.96 g. cannabinol, distilled from another sample of charas. Unsteadiness (55 m.), became very marked afterward, vomited (65 m. and 5 h.); slight improvement (6 h.).

37. Dec. 31, 1897; Airedale terrier; 1.1 g. cannabinol (oldest). Slight depression and unsteadiness (70 m.), increased later, slept mostly; more marked effect than 33.

38. Fox-terrier; 0.97 g. cannabinol (oldest). Unsteadiness (70 m.), which increased, still marked (5½ h.); effect greater than 34.

39. Jan. 3, 1898; Airedale terrier; 0.97 g. cannabinol, distilled from another sample of charas. No effect (60 m.), afterward slept, very slight unsteadiness, (2 h.), did not increase, lay down occasionally; slept remainder of day, playful when aroused.

40. Fox-terrier; 0.95 g. cannabinol, distilled from another sample of charas. No effect (60 m.), very slight unsteadiness (2 h.), soon became more marked, continued as long as observed, slept somewhat; slightly depressed next morning.

41. Jan. 4, 1898; Airedale terrier; 1.1 g. cannabinol, distilled from another sample of charas. Slight depression; no marked symptoms.

42. Fox-terrier; 0.99 g. cannabinol, distilled from another sample of charas. Depression and unsteadiness (2 h.) not very marked; slight depression next morning.

43. Jan. 5, 1898; Airedale terrier, 12,110 gms.; 1.03 g. cannabinol, distilled from another sample of charas. Slight depression (60 m.), slight unsteadiness, slept mostly; unsteadiness increased, vomited (125 m.), awakened to be taken to kennel, very unsteady.

44. Fox-terrier, 8210 gms.; 0.97 g. cannabinol, distilled from another sample charas. Slight depression and unsteadiness (60 m.), became more marked and continued as long as under observation (6½ h.), vomited a little (5¼ h.), slept partly; apparently normal next morning.

45. Jan. 6, 1898; Airedale terrier; 1.01 g. cannabinol, distilled from another sample of charas. Slight depression (60 m.), slept mostly, unsteadiness less marked than 43; apparently well the following morning.

46. Fox-terrier; 0.97 g. cannabinol, distilled from another sample of charas. Slight depression (60 m.), unsteadiness (70 m.), effects similar but ataxia less marked than 44.

47. Jan. 7, 1898; Airedale terrier; 0.98 g. cannibinol, distilled from another sample of charas. Depression (30 m.), unsteadiness (60 m.), became very distinct, laid down mostly, slept partly; very slight depression next morning.

48. Fox-terrier; 0.97 g. cannabinol, distilled from another sample. of charas. Depression (30 m.), unsteadiness (60 m.), became very distinct, laid down mostly, slept partly; very slight depression next morning.

49. Jan. 8, 1898; Airedale terrier; 1.04 g. cannabinol, distilled from another sample of charas. Depression (60 m.), unsteadiness (90 m.), not further observed.

50. Fox-terrier; 0.97 g. cannabinol, distilled from another sample of charas. No apparent effect (90 m.); not further observed; apparently normal next morning.

51. Jan. 9, 1898; Airedale terrier; 1.02 g. cannabinol, distilled from another sample of charas. Not observed.

52. Fox-terrier; 1 g. cannabinol, distilled from another sample of charas. Not observed.

53. Jan. 10, 1898; Airedale terrier; 1.02 g. cannibinol, distilled from another sample of charas. Depression, distinct ataxia, but not marked; slept most of the time.

54. Fox-terrier; 1 g. cannabinol, distilled from another sample of charas. Sleepiness, depression and slight unsteadiness, symptoms less marked than usual; slight depression next morning.

55. Jan. 11, 1898; Airedale terrier; 0.22 g. cannabinol (as 31). No evident effect (60 m.), later transient depression, but no ataxia developed. Compare with 31.

56. Fox-terrier; 0.4 g. cannabinol (as 31). No effect (60 m.), later depression and unsteadiness but less than 32.

57. Jan. 25, 1898; Airedale terrier, 13,150 gms.; 0.21 g. cannabinol (as 31). Slight depression (60 m.), afterward sleepiness, unsteadiness, excited (5 h.).

58. Fox-terrier, 7980 gms.; 0.42 g. cannabinol (as 31). No effect (60 m.), later sleepiness, slight unsteadiness and depression.

59. Feb. 11, 1898; Airedale terrier; 0.16 g. third fraction cannabinol dissolved in .64 g. olive oil. Depression (30 m.) followed by sleep, no distinct unsteadiness, excited at times, vomited a little (4¼ h.); still depressed (5¼ h.).

60. Fox-terrier; 0.18 g. third fraction cannabinol dissolved in .64 g. olive oil. Depression (35 m.) and sleep, no ataxia observed but could not be induced to stand long; still depressed (5 h.).

61. Feb. 15, 1898; Airedale terrier; 0.16 g. second fraction cannabinol in .64 g. olive oil. Symptoms similar to 59.

62. Fox-terrier; 0.18 g. second fraction cannabinol in .64 g. olive oil. Slight depression and unsteadiness (2½ h.) but less marked than 60, vomited (5 h.).

63. Feb. 17, 1898; Airedale terrier; 0.16 g. first fraction cannabinol in .64 g. olive oil. Depression somewhat more marked than 61 but no unsteadiness, vomited slightly (3 h.).

64. Fox-terrier; 0.18 g. first fraction cannabinol in .64 g. olive oil. Some depression and slight unsteadiness, but doubtful if as marked as 62.

65. Feb. 22, 1898; Airedale terrier; 0.21 g. cannabinol distilled at atmospheric pressure, then heated 5 hours at boiling point. Slight depression and sleepiness, no ataxia observed; much better (5½ h.).

66. Fox-terrier; 0.23 g. cannabinol distilled at atmospheric pressure, then heated 5 hours at boiling point. Slight depression, no sleep; almost well (5½ h.).

67. Feb. 24, 1898; Airedale terrier; 2.1 g. cannabinol distilled at atmospheric pressure, then heated 5 hours at boiling point. Depression

and unsteadiness, but. symptoms not very marked, slept somewhat, vomited (3½ h., 4½ h.), slight improvement (6 h.).

68. Fox-terrier; 2.2 g. cannabinol distilled at atmospheric pressure, then heated 5 hours at boiling point. Depression and distinct unsteadiness, did not sleep; somewhat better (5½ h.).

69. Feb. 28, 1898; Fox-terrier; 0.43 g. acetyl-derivation of higher homologue of cannabinol. No effect (2½ h.).

70. March 1, 1898; Airedale terrier; 0.2 g. cannabinol distilled in vacuo. Depression, sleep and unsteadiness, more marked than 67; decided improvement (5½ h.).

71. Fox-terrier; 0.22 g. cannabinol distilled in vacuo. Distinct unsteadiness (60 m.), slight depression; symptoms similar to 68; much better (5½ h.).

72. March 3, 1898; Airedale terrier; 0.45 g. pitch dissolved in 1.5 g. olive oil containing some cannabinol. Slight depression and unsteadiness; much better (4½ h.).

73. Fox-terrier; 1.03 g. cannabinol regenerated from old acetyl compound. Slight depression and sleepiness, no obvious ataxia.

74. March 8, 1898; Airedale terrier; 0.06 g. morphin acetate in capsule. Vomited frothy mucous-like vomit (12 m., 14 m., 17 m.), marked depression, much worse than any previous observation, retching (22 m.), rapid breathing, quick pulse, head-nodding (40 m.), salivation (44 m., continued to 120 m.), still much depressed, constant moaning, slight myosis (130 m.), fall of temperature 1.1 degrees C., sleepiness, slight unsteadiness; improvement (4 h.), but still depressed (5½ h.).

75. Fox-terrier; 0.1 g. morphin acetate in capsule. No effect (20 m.), head nodding (30 m.), retching and vomiting of frothy colorless fluid (35 m., 38 m., 50 m., 55 m., 90 m., 105 m.), salivation, unsteadiness, depression (130 m.), not sleepy, salivation stopped (3¼ h.), fall of temperature 2.3 degrees C; could not be induced to stand up, somewhat better (4½ h.).

76. March 16, 1898; 0.93 g. olive oil extract of charas, containing about .2 to .25 g. soluble charas products. Slight depression and unsteadiness (60 m.), sleepiness, vomiting (160 m.), ataxia more marked, excited (3½ h.), slight improvement (5¾ h.).

77. Fox-terrier; 1.86 g. olive oil extract of charas, containing .4 to .5 g. soluble charas products. Sleepiness and depression (30 m.), distinct unsteadiness (60 m.), which became more marked later, vomited (105 m.); no obvious improvement (5¾ h.).

78. March 18, 1898; Fox-terrier, 8840 gms.; 0.15 g. extract cannab. indic. (B.P.) in pills (from London chemist). No effect (90 m.), afterward depression and marked ataxia, vomited (2½ h.).

79. March 22, 1898; Airedale terrier, 13,580 gms.; 1.03 g. partly (¾) saponified acetyl derivative of higher homologue of cannabinol. No distinct effect.

80. Fox-terrier; 0.35 g. oxycannabinol. No obvious effect.

81. March 25, 1898; Airedale terrier; 1.02 g. cannabinol. Depression, very distinct unsteadiness (60 m.), sleepiness, vomited (2 h., 3¼ h.), no distinct improvement (4¼ h.).

82. Fox-terrier; 0.99 g. cannabinol. No obvious effect (60 m.), depression (75 m.), vomiting (105 m., 115 m., 130 m., 135 m., 255 m.), slight unsteadiness (120 m.), symptoms increased; no improvement (4¼ h.).

83. March 30, 1898; Airedale terrier; 1 g. chloral hydrate in capsule. Sleepiness (15 m.), very slight ataxia, somewhat more marked (30 m.); fall of temperature 0.4 degrees C., apparently normal (4 h.).

84. Fox-terrier; 1 g. chloral hydrate in capsule. Sleepiness (15 m.), slight muscular weakness but no distinct ataxia; fall of temperature 0.4 degrees C., apparently normal (4 h.).

85. April 5, 1898; Airedale terrier; 0.5 g. chloralose in capsule. Slight depression and sleepiness, transient; fall of temperature 0.5 degrees C.

86. Fox-terrier; 0.0195 g. hyoscine hydrochlorid. Uneasiness (30 m.) followed by whining, dryness of the tongue, dilatation and less marked reaction of pupils to light, increased rapidity of heart beat (60 m.), improvement commenced (2 h.); no fall of temperature.

87. April 11, 1898; 0.21 g. cannabinol. Slight depression, sleepiness and unsteadiness, continued 6 hours.

88. Fox-terrier; 0.2 g. cannabinol. Slight depression (30 m.) but not much affected until (90 m.), became very unsteady, sleepiness, incontinence of urine, trembling, vomiting (2 h.); fall temp. 3 degrees C; most marked effect obtained with this dose.

89. English terrier, 7180 gms.; 0.15 g. cannabinol. Less reserved (20 m.), slight depression (30 m.), sleepiness chief symptom, no obvious ataxia; slight improvement (5 h.).

90. April 15, 1898; Airedale terrier; 0.2 g. cannabinol kept in sealed tube since Dec. 12, 1896. Slight depression and sleepiness (45 m.), became much more marked; unsteadiness developed, attention became impaired, vomited (5 h.), then improved.

91. English terrier; 0.14 g. cannabinol kept in sealed tube since Dec. 12, 1896. Slight depression and very distinct unsteadiness (30 m.), gradually increased until fell over every few steps, vomited (100 m., 104 m., 150 m., 200 m.), slept a little (3½ h.), much better but still markedly depressed (5 h.), temperature fell 0.5 degree C., then rose 1.2 degree C.

92. Fox-terrier; 0.39 g. cannabinol, through which oxygen has been passed 3 to 4 hours at 150 degrees C. Slightly depressed (45 m.), very slight unsteadiness (60 m.), became somewhat more marked, slight sleepiness; symptoms not severe but temperature fell 1.4 degrees C.

93. April 19, 1898; Airedale terrier, 12,840 gms.; 0.22 g. cannabinol (as in 90), subjected to oxygen for 6 hours at 150 to 160 degrees C. Slight depression and sleepiness (30 m.), increased, distinct unsteadiness; not much improved (6 h.).

94. English terrier; 0.16 g. cannabinol (as in 93). Depressed, restless (20 m.), sleepy (30 m.), slight unsteadiness (40 m.), gradually became worse, but not so bad as in 91; vomited (55 m., 115 m.), somewhat better (4½ h.), but no further improvement (5¾ h.).

95. Fox-terrier, 8270 gms.; 0.21 g. cannabinol (as in 90). Slight depression (30 m.), but not much affected during first hour, afterward much depressed, slight unsteadiness; no improvement (5¾ h.).

96. April 23, 1989; Fox-terrier; 0.19 g. cannabinol (as in 90). Asleep (30 m.), but no marked symptoms for three hours, then slight unsteadiness, which increased, distinct (6¼ h.).

97. Airedale terrier; 0.22 g. cannabinol through which CO_2 has been passed for 20 hours at 150 to 185 degrees C. Slight depression and sleepiness (30 m.) became more marked, unsteadiness (60 m.), vomited (105 m.); afterward improved but still under influence (6¼ h.).

98. English terrier; 0.2 g. cannabinol through which oxygen has been passed for 20 hours at 150 to 185 degrees C., pitchy appearance. Very slight depression and restlessness (30 m.) which quickly (1 h.) passed away; no ataxia.

99. April 27, 1898; English terrier, 7760 gms.; 0.2 g. tribrom-cannabinol. Depressed (60 m.), slight sleepiness but no distinct unsteadiness, apparently normal (4 h.).

100. Dec. 11, 1895; 2500 gms.; 3.5 g. charas given in mucilage (65 c.c.), chloroformed during injection. Vomited most of the substance (about 50 c.c.) after recovery from chloroform, depression, weakness, narcosis and death (4 h.); no characteristic macroscopic changes. *Experiments on cats.*

101. June 20, 1896; 2600 gms.; 0.15 g. cannabinol in meat. Sleepiness (90 m.), muscular weakness, marked ataxia, stupidity; commencing improvement (25 h.), complete recovery (44 h.).

102. May 26, 1896; 2700 gms., same cat; 0.27 cannabinol as pills with starch. Quiet (90 m.), restlessness and micturition, then salivation (3½ h.), muscular weakness and unsteadiness, anorexia; improvement (25 h.), almost well (28 h.).

103. June 2, 1896; 1.3 g. cannabinol in capsules. Tired, quiet (60 m.), salivation and unsteadiness (100 m.), marked ataxia, sleepiness, dilated pupils: improvement (30 h.), almost well (53 h.).

Experiments on rabbits. Substances were made into an emulsion with gum and injected through a catheter into the stomach.

104. Nov. 1, 1895; 1730 gms.; 0.895 g. impure (sesqui) terpene. Slight excitement.

105. Nov. 4, 1895; 1730 gms.; 0.895 g. charas with sodium bicarbonate. Slight excitement.

106. Nov. 5, 1895; 1730 gms.; 0.876 g. petroleum ether extract. Slight excitement.

107. Dec. 17, 1895; 1440 gms.; 1.44 g. charas. No distinct effect.

108. Jan. 16, 1896; 1500 gms.; 3 g. petroleum ether extract. Became quieter; number of heart beats and respiration, and temperature fell; death occurred on third day.

109. June 5, 1896; 1100 gms.; 2.2 g. cannabinol. Depression (60 m.), sleepiness, fall in pulse (252 to 100), respiration (142 to 18) and temperature (40.4 to 35.7 degree C.), diminished reflexes; improvement (20 h.), much better but not normal (29 h.).

110. June 10, 1896; 930 gms.; 2.2 g. charas. Quieter (90 m.), fall in pulse, respiration and temperature; died on fourth day, cold and marasmus.

111. April 5, 1898; 620 gms.; 2.3 g. cannabinol. Depressed, slight muscular weakness, sleepiness, fall in pulse, respiration and temperature; death, 3½ days.

Personal experiments. 112. Feb. 1, 1895; 0.1 g. cannabinol, taken about 2:45 P.M.

113. Feb. 8, 1985; 0.1 g. cannabinol in 0.05 c.c. alcohol and 20 c.c. water. Slight mental depression.

114. March 9, 1895; 0.5 c.c. monoterpene in 20 c.c. water. No effect.

115. March 10, 1896; 0.05 g. cannabinol in 0.1 c.c. alcohol and 20 c.c. water. No distinct effect for 4 hours, then feeling of dryness in mouth, pleasant tingling, slight unsteadiness, happiness, unpleasant visions on closing eyes, time relation not completely lost, feeling of tiredness but no marked tendency to sleep.

116. March 28, 1897; 0.05 g. cannabinol regenerated from acetyl compound. Taken at 8 P.M., retired to bed at 10:30 feeling a little tired,

slept soundly till 6 P.M., no distinct effect.

117. April 5, 1897; 0.05 g. cannabinol regenerated from acetyl compound. Taken at 10:30 A.M., slightly depressed in afternoon, no other effect.

118. April 5, 1897; 0.1 g. cannabinol regenerated from acetyl compound. Taken at 11 P.M., tired and sleepy in afternoon.

119. April 10, 1897; 0.2 g. cannabinol regenerated from acetyl compound. Taken at 1 P.M., slight dryness of mouth and paresthesia (160 m.) followed by sleepiness, depressed during evening, retired at 11:30.

120. April 13, 1897; 4 cannabinol tablets (a commercial preparation) = g. cannabinol. Taken at 5:08 P.M., feeling of lightness in head (5:55), dinner 6:00, afterward felt sleepy and slightly intoxicated; time relations altered but not annulled.

121. June 7, 1897; 0.2 g. cannabinol phosphate. Taken at 10:30 P.M., Retired at 12 M., no evident effect.

122. June 9, 1897; 0.4 g. cannabinol phosphate. No distinct action.

123. June 6, 1897; 0.8 g. cannabinol phosphate. Taken at 10:45 P.M., 11:40 very sleepy, retired, awoke at 7:20 A.M., feeling very sleepy, depressed all the morning.

124. March 17, 1898; 0.05 g. oily extract of charas, containing .013 g. soluble products. Dinner at 6:20, taken at 8:00, slight sleepiness and mental exhaustion followed.

125. March 18, 1898; 0.105 g. oily extract of charas, containing .013 g. soluble products. Taken at 6:25 P.M., dinner 6:50, 7:35 peculiar feeling of lightness in head, continued to work, 8:00 rather better, 11:00 retired feeling sleepy.

126. March 20, 1898; 0.016 g. (¼ grain) ext. cannab. Ind. (B. P.) pill. Tea 5 P.M;, slight indigestion, pill taken at 7:30, 10:30 no evident effect, 10:35 slight light-headedness, warmth of face and mental exhaustion, afterward fell asleep.

127. March 21, 1898; 0.14 g. partly (¾) saponified acetyl derivative of higher homologue of cannabinol. Taken at 5:30 P.M., no effect.

128. March 22, 1898; 0.1 g. third fraction cannabinol. Taken at 5:45 P.M., dinner 6:30, 8:25 feeling of lightness in head and mental exhaustion, continued working, effect passed off in about 30 m.

129. March 23, 1898; 0.1 g. second fraction cannabinol. Taken at 5:45 P.M., dinner 6:45, 7:20 no effect, 9:25 slight dryness of lips and lightness in head, seemed to pass off but worse again at 7:45, happy, have difficulty in reading, sleepy, 10:00 just awakened from a short nap, read a little but soon exhausted, 11:20 retired, 6:45 P.M., awoke, felt well.

130. March 24, 1898; 0.1 g. first fraction cannabinol. Taken at 5:45

P.M., dinner 6:45, 7:45 no effect, 7:50 feeling of slight dryness of lips and lightness of head, 8:00 somewhat more depressed, not working well, 8:45 working better. 10:00 still somewhat depressed, 11:30 retired but did not succeed in sleeping for some time.

131. March 25, 1898; 0.1 g. cannabinol (oldest). Taken at 5:45 P.M., dinner at 6:30, 7:30 peculiar light-headedness and dryness of the lips, 7:45 slightly unsteady, paresthesia in head and legs, heaviness of eyelids, no correct estimation of time, 9:30 awakened from short sleep, 10:00 rather better but unable to work, 10:30 retired, somewhat depressed the following morning.

132. March 27, 1898; 0.35 g. acetyl derivative of higher homologue of cannabinol. Taken at 7:30 P.M., no effect.

133. March 29, 1898; 0.05 g. cannabinol pill made 18 months ago. Taken at 5:50, dinner at 6:30, 8:30 unsteady symptoms, cannot work, estimation of time not so good, 9:15 worse, energyless, 10:30 went out for a few minutes, improved, 11:00 can read moderately well, but eyelids heavy.

134. March 30, 1898; 0.09 g. Merck's cannabinon. Taken at 5:45, dinner 6:30, 7:20 lightness in head, loss of time relation, happy, amused, pleasant tingling, etc.; sleepy, 8:00 lay down, slept till 10:30 then retired, awakened (7:00 A.M.) feeling dull and depressed, lasted the whole morning.

135. April 14, 1898; 0.05 g. opium. Taken at 9:00 P.M., 10:00 no obvious action, 10:05 slight heaviness of eyelids, very slightly tired, 10:20 rather better, 11:10 feel somewhat tired, head rather heavy, slight sense of "well-being," 12:00 still heaviness of eyes and tiredness of head but have worked fairly well last half hour, not sleepy; retired, soon fell asleep, awakened at 7:00 A.M. feeling well, pleasant sense of gravity, which continued most of morning; no constipation.

136. April 15, 1898; 0.1 g. cannabinol through which oxygen passed 3 to 5 hours at 150 to 160 degrees C. Taken at 5:45, dinner at 6:30, 9:15 slight visual indefiniteness, slight and transient paresthesia, afterward felt slight incapacity for work but no marked effects, 11:45 not sleepy but retired.

137. April 17, 1898; 0.05 g. cannabinol sealed up since Dec. 28, 1896. Tea 4:30, drug taken 5:45, 6:50 slight mental exhaustion and feeling of lightness in head, 7:20 rather sleepy, 8:00 trying to read but have little energy for anything, 9:00 condition same, no estimation of time, feeling of warmth in face and head, 10:00 sleepy, retired.

138. April 21, 1898; 0.065 g. same cannabinol treated with oxygen for 20 hours at 150 to 185 degrees C. Taken at 5:45, dinner 6:40, 8:05 slight feeling of lightness in head, 9:30 have been reading some time, at first had a little difficulty, now feel quite normal.

139. April 22, 1898; 0.05 g. same cannabinol treated with CO_2 for 20 hours at 150 to 185 degrees C. Taken at 5:50, dinner 6:30, 7:00 commencing light-headedness, 8:00 more distinct, a want of energy, 9:45 condition same, trying to read, 10:00 not able to do any work, 10:45, no improvement, retired.

140. April 24, 1898; 0.1 g. tribrom-cannabinol. Taken at 8:00 P.M., supper at 8:30, 9:30 slightly sleepy, 11:00 sleepy, no other peculiar effect of cannabinol, retired, slept till 6:45, depressed, suffered from mental exhaustion during three following days.

141. May 4, 1898; 0.065 g. oxycannabinol (as in 138) dissolved in oil. Taken at 5:45, dinner at 6:30. 7:15 went out for a walk, 8:15 arrived home, slightly tired, peculiar feeling in .eyes and head grew slightly worse and continued the whole evening, but was insufficient to prevent me writing; 11:10 retired, slept soundly, 6:40 A.M. got up, felt sleepy.

142. May 6, 1898; 0.1 g. charas (best). Taken at 5:45, tea at 4:30, dinner at 7:00, 7:00 slight effect in head, worked in garden, felt want of energy, 8:30 influence more marked, agreeable heaviness of eyelids, very little energy, 10:00 retired, condition same, slept well, depressed following morning.

143. May 12, 1898; 0.016 g. (¼ grain) ext. cannab. Indic (B. P.) in pill (cp. 126). Taken at 5:50, dinner at 6:30, 7:25 lightness of head, peculiar feeling about eyes, 7:50 pleasant tingling in face and feet, no other marked effect, reading fairly well, 8:40 tingling still present, unable to read with benefit, cannot calculate time very well, symptoms continued throughout evening, became sleepy but managed to do some copying. 12:30 retired, 7:30 got up feeling tired but soon well.

144. May 19, 1898; 2 c.c. sesqui terpene taken in weak mucilage. Taken at 12:45, lunch 1:10, 1:15 slightly listless and slight heaviness of head, which soon passed away.

THE DISPENSATORY

OF

THE UNITED STATES
OF AMERICA

TWENTIETH EDITION

THOROUGHLY REVISED, LARGELY REWRITTEN, AND BASED UPON
THE NINTH REVISION OF THE UNITED STATES PHARMA-
COPŒIA AND THE BRITISH PHARMACOPŒIA, 1914

BY

JOSEPH P. REMINGTON, Ph.M., F.C.S.

LATE PROFESSOR OF THEORY AND PRACTICE OF PHARMACY IN THE PHILADELPHIA COLLEGE
OF PHARMACY; CHAIRMAN OF THE COMMITTEE OF REVISION OF THE PHARMACOPŒIA
OF THE UNITED STATES OF AMERICA

HORATIO C. WOOD, Jr., M.D.

PROFESSOR OF PHARMACOLOGY AND THERAPEUTICS IN THE UNIVERSITY OF PENNSYLVANIA;
VICE-CHAIRMAN OF THE COMMITTEE OF REVISION OF THE PHARMACOPŒIA OF
THE UNITED STATES OF AMERICA

SAMUEL P. SADTLER, Ph.D., LL.D.

FORMER PROFESSOR OF CHEMISTRY IN THE PHILADELPHIA COLLEGE OF PHARMACY; MEM-
BER OF THE COMMITTEE OF REVISION OF THE PHARMACOPŒIA OF THE UNITED
STATES OF AMERICA

CHARLES H. LaWALL, Ph.M.

ASSOCIATE PROFESSOR OF THEORY AND PRACTICE OF PHARMACY IN THE PHILADELPHIA
COLLEGE OF PHARMACY; SECRETARY OF THE COMMITTEE OF REVISION OF THE
PHARMACOPŒIA OF THE UNITED STATES OF AMERICA

HENRY KRAEMER, Ph.G., Ph.D.

PROFESSOR OF BOTANY AND PHARMACOGNOSY IN THE UNIVERSITY OF MICHIGAN; MEMBER
OF THE COMMITTEE OF REVISION OF THE PHARMACOPŒIA OF THE UNITED STATES
OF AMERICA

JOHN F. ANDERSON, M.D.

DIRECTOR OF THE RESEARCH AND BIOLOGICAL LABORATORIES OF E. R. SQUIBB AND SONS,
MEMBER OF THE COMMITTEE OF REVISION OF THE PHARMACOPŒIA OF THE
UNITED STATES OF AMERICA

PHILADELPHIA AND LONDON
J. B. LIPPINCOTT COMPANY

The Dispensatory of the United States of America

BY JOSEPH P. REMINGTON, Ph.M., F.C.S., HORATIO C. WOOD, JR., M.D., ET AL.

CANNABIS. U.S. (Br.)

"The dried flowering tops of the pistillate plants of *Cannabis sativa* Linné, or of the variety *indica* Lamarck (Fam. *Moraceae*), freed from the thicker stems and large foliage leaves and without the presence or admixture of more than 10 percent of fruits or other foreign matter. Cannabis, made into a fluid extract in which *one hundred mils* represent *one hundred grams* of the drug, when assayed biologicaliy, produces incoordination when administered to dogs in a dose of not more than 0.03 mil of fluid extract per kilogram of body weight." *U.S.* "Indian Hemp consists of the dried flowering or fruiting tops of the pistillate plant of Cannabis sativa, *Linn.*, grown in India; from which the resin has not been removed." *Br.*

Cannabis Indicae, *Br.*; Hemp, Indian Hemp; Herba Cannabis Indicae; Chanvre, *Fr. Col.*; Chanvre de l'Inde, *Fr.*; Indischer Hanf, *G.*; Cañamo, *Sp.*

For many years the official *cannabis* was restricted to the drug which was used for centuries in India. The reason for this was that the Indian cannabis was more uniformly active. Recently the Indian Government has placed a high tax on every pound of the drug grown. The result has been that other markets have been sought and the hemp plant has been grown in other parts of Asia, Africa and America. While of course much of this material is not equal to that grown in India, the fact that it can be grown, as shown by experiments

Reprinted from *Dispensary of the United States of America.* 20th *Ed.* 1918, pp. 276–281.

in the United States (see Hamilton, *J. A. Ph. A.*, 1913, ii; 1915, iv, 389), of a very high quality has caused the framers of the U. S. Pharmacopoeia to permit the use of a cannabis, no matter where it may be grown, provided it comes up to the biological standard as given in the definition. Physiologically active cannabis is obtained at the present time not only from India, but Africa, Turkey, Turkestan, Asia Minor, Italy, Spain and the United States.

The *Cannabis sativa*, or hemp plant, is an annual, from four to eight feet or more in height, with an erect, branching, angular stem. The leaves are alternate or opposite, and digitate, with five to seven linear-lanceolate, coarsely serrated segments. The stipules are subulate. The flowers are axillary; the staminate in long branched, drooping racemes; the pistillate in erect, simple spikes. The stamens are five, with long pendulous anthers; the pistils two, with long, filiform, glandular stigmas. The fruit is ovate and one-seeded. The whole plant is covered with a fine pubescence, scarcely visible to the naked eye, and somewhat viscid to the touch. The hemp plant of India has been considered by some as a distinct species, and named *Cannabis indica*; but the most observant botanists, upon comparing it with the cultivated plant, have been unable to discover any specific difference. It is now, therefore, regarded merely as a variety, and is distinguished by the epithet *indica*. Pereira states that in the female plant the flowers are somewhat more crowded than in the common hemp, but that the male plants in the two varieties are in all respects the same.

C. sativa is a native of the Caucasus, Persia, and the hilly regions in Northern India. It is cultivated in many parts of Europe and Asia, and largely in our Western States. It is from the Indian variety exclusively that the medicine was formerly obtained, the heat of the climate in Hindostan apparently favoring the development of its active principle. H. C. Wood, many years ago, obtained a parcel of the male plant of *C. americana* (*C. sativa*) from Kentucky, made an alcoholic extract of the leaves and tops, and upon trying it on the system, found it effective in less than a grain, and, having inadvertently taken too large a dose, experienced effects which left no doubt of the powers of the medicine, and of the identity of its influence with that of the Indian plant. (*Proc. Am. Philos. Soc.*, vol. xi, p. 226.) The results obtained by H. C. Wood have been confirmed by a number of observers.

The fruits or "so-called" seeds, though not now official, have been used in medicine. They are from three to five millimeters long and about two millimeters broad, roundish-ovate, somewhat compressed, of a shining ash-gray color, and of a disagreeable, oily, sweetish taste. For a comprehensive monograph on the morphology of cannabis fruits, as well as their history and chemical composition, see Tschirch, *"Hand-buch der Pharmakognosie,"* p. 555. They yield by expression about 20 percent of a fixed oil, which has the drying property, and is used in the arts. They contain also uncrystallizable sugar and albumen and when rubbed with water form an emulsion, which may be used advantageously in inflammations of the mucous membrane, though without narcotic properties. The seeds are much used as food for birds, as they are fond of them. They are generally believed to be in no degree poisonous; but Michaud relates the case of a child in whom serious symptoms of narcotic poisoning occurred after taking a certain quantity of them. It is probable that some of the fruit eaten by the child was unripe, as in this state it would be more likely to partake of the peculiar qualities of the plant. (*Ann. Thér.*, 1860.)

In Hindostan, Persia, and other parts of the East, hemp has long been habitually employed as an intoxicating agent. The parts are the tops of the plant, and a resinous product obtained from it. *Bhang* is the selected, dried and powdered leaves. *Ganjah* or *gunjah* is the tops of the cultivated female plants, cut directly after flowering, and formed into round or flat bundles from two to four feet long by three inches in diameter. It is stated that in the province of Bengal great care is taken to eradicate the male plants from the fields before fertilization of the female, and that thereby the yield and quality of the resin is greatly increased. In Bombay this matter is commonly neglected, so that Bengal ganjah is much superior to Bombay ganjah. It is recognized in India that ganjah rapidly deteriorates on keeping, that which is one year old being not more than one-quarter as potent as the fresh drug, while two-year-old ganjah is practically inert and is required by the Indian government to be burned in the presence of excise officers. It is probable, however, that much old ganjah finds its way into the markets of the world.

All importations of ganjah or hemp from India should be made directly after the harvesting of the new crop in April or May, and the extract should be prepared at once and kept in hermetically sealed jars. There is on the surface of the plant a resinous exudation to which it owes its stickiness. According to Hooper (*P. J.*, 1909, lxxxi, 347) only small amounts of charas are raised in India, that which is being consumed there being mostly imported. The method of collection in Baluchistan is to gently rub the dried plant between carpets. The dust which comes off contains the active principle and is known as "rup." The second shaking produces an inferior variety, known as "tahgalim," and the third shaking is known as "ganja." In Nepal the plant is squeezed between the palms of the hands, and the resin scraped off from the hands. These balls, and also masses formed out of resin mechanically separated from the hemp plant are called *charas* or *churrus*. This is the *hashish* or *hasheesh* of the Arabs.

Hashish is also produced in considerable quantities in Persia by rolling and rubbing the flowers, stalks and leaves of hemp on rough woolen carpets and subsequently scraping off with a knife and making into balls or sticks the adherent resinous substance. The carpets are afterwards washed with water and the extract obtained by evaporation sold at a low price. The dose for smoking of the best hashish is said to be one-fourth to one grain (0.016–0.065 Gm.). The fanatics are affirmed to be generally hashish devotees.

The dealing in hashish in India is said to be a Government monopoly, and a very heavy license is required for the right to even purchase it in quantity. The importation of it into Egypt is so strongly interdicted that the mere possession of it is a penal offense; H. C. Wood found it, however, readily procurable. It is said to be brought into the country in pigs' bladders, in the Indo-European steamers, and thrown out at night during the passage into the Suez canal, to be picked up by the boats of confederates. Notwithstanding the Governmental interdiction, it is largely used by smoking in Egypt, as an intoxicant. The statement of W. E. Dixon (*B. M. J.*, Nov., 1899) that the inhalations of hemp smoke produce great exhilaration and cause muscular fatigue to disappear for the time being is undoubtedly correct, but his further belief that the habit is not apt to grow upon the hemp votary is more doubtful.

Momea or *mimea* is a hemp preparation said to be made in Tibet with human fat. From gunjah the Messrs. Smith, of Edinburgh, obtained a purer resin by the following process: Bruised ganjah is digested, first in successive portions of warm water, until the expressed liquid comes away colorless; and afterwards for two days, with a moderate heat, in a solution of sodium carbonate, containing one part of the salt for two of the dried herb. It is then expressed, washed, dried, and exhausted by percolation with alcohol. The tincture, after being agitated with milk of lime containing one part of the earth for twelve of the gunjah used, is filtered; the lime is precipitated by sulphuric acid; the filtered liquor is agitated with animal charcoal, and again filtered; most of the alcohol is distilled off, and to the residue twice its weight of water is added; the liquor is then allowed to evaporate gradually; and, finally, the resin is washed with fresh water until it ceases to impart a sour or bitter taste to the liquid, and is then dried in thin layers. Thus obtained, it retains the odor and taste of gunjah, which yields from 6 to 7 percent of it.

Properties.—Fresh hemp has a peculiar narcotic odor, which is said to be capable of producing vertigo, headache, and a species of intoxication. It is much less in the dried tops, which have a feeble bitterish taste. According to Royle, *churrus* is, when pure, of a blackish-gray, blackish-green, or dirty olive color, of a fragrant and narcotic odor, and a slightly warm, bitterish and acrid taste. Cannabis is officially described as "in dark green or greenish-brown and more or less agglutinated fragments, consisting of the short stems with their leaf-like bracts and pistillate flowers, some of the latter being replaced with more or less developed fruits; stems cylindrical, of varying length, not more than 3 mm. in diameter, longitudinally furrowed, light green to light brown, strigose-pubescent; leaves digitately compound; leaflets, when soaked in water and spread out, linear-lanceolate, nearly sessile, margin deeply serrate, bracts ovate, pubescent, each enclosing one or two pistillate flowers, or more or less developed fruits; calyx dark green, pubescent and somewhat folded around the ovary or fruit; styles two, filiform and pubescent; ovary with a single campylotropous ovule; fruit light green to light brown, broadly ellipsoidal, about 3.5 mm. in length, finely wrinkled and slightly reticulated; odor agreeably aromatic; taste characteristic. The powder is dark green, giving a strong effervescence on the addition of dilute hydrochloric acid; numerous sharp pointed fragments of upper portion of non-glandular hairs and fragments of bracts and leaves showing yellowish-brown laticiferous vessels, rosette aggregates of calcium oxalate from 0.005 to 0.025 mm. in diameter; non-glandular, with a very slender pointed apex and a considerably enlarged base containing, usually in the lumen, some calcium carbonate; glandular hairs of two kinds, one with a short, one-celled stalk and the other with a multicellular, long, tongue-shaped stalk, the glandular portion being globular and consisting of from eight to sixteen cells, fragments of fruits with palisade-like, non-lignified sclerenchymatous cells, walls yellowish-brown, finely porous, the lumina usually containing air; tissues of embryo and endosperm with numerous oil globules and aleurone grains, the latter from 0.005 to 0.01 mm. in diameter and consisting of large crystalloids and globoids. The yield of alcohol extractive is not less than 8 percent and the alcoholic solution is of a bright green color. Cannabis yields not more than 15 percent of ash." *U.S.*

The British Pharmacopoeia describes Indian cannabis as follows:

"In compressed, rough, dusky-green masses, consisting of the branched upper part of the stem, bearing leaves and pistillate flowers or fruits, matted together by a resinous secretion. Upper leaves simple, alternate, 1-3 partite; lower leaves opposite and digitate, consisting of five to seven linear-lanceolate leaflets with distantly serrate margins. Fruit one-seeded and supported by an ovate-lanceolate bract. Both leaves and bracts bear external oleo-resin glands and one-celled curved hairs, the bases of which are enlarged and contain cystoliths. Strong, characteristic odor; taste slight. When a mixture of ten grams of finely powdered Indian Hemp and one hundred millilitres of *alcohol* (90 percent) is shaken occasionally during twenty-four hours and then filtered, twenty millilitres of the filtrate, evaporated in a flat-bottomed dish, yield a residue weighing when dried at 100° C. (212° F.), not less than 0.250 gram. Ash not more than 15 percent." *Br.*

For a histological description of the leaf by A. R. L. Dohme, see *Proc. A. Ph. A.*, 1897, 569. The Cannabis of the market may consist of fruiting tops and stems and occasionally the staminate tops are admixed with it.

Hooper (*P. J.*, lxxxi, p. 80) describes a method for the chemical standardization of cannabis indica based upon its iodine value. He finds that the alcoholic extract of old samples has a lower iodine value than that from recent specimens, and there is more or less constancy of relation between the age and the iodine value.

For description of the U.S. method of physiological assay, see page 279.

Indian churrus or hasheesh is a hard resinous mass of a greenish-gray color, containing much gritty earth, and, as it occurs in Egypt, of a feeble, hemp-like odor and taste. Schlesinger found in the leaves a bitter substance, chlorophyll, green resinous extractive, coloring matter, gummy extract, extractive, albumen, lignin, and salts. The plant also contains volatile oil in very small proportion, which probably has narcotic properties. The resin obtained by T. & H. Smith of Edinburgh, in 1846, has been thought to be the active principle, and received the name of *cannabin*. By repeated distillation of the same portion of water from relatively large quantities of hemp renewed at each distillation, M. J. Personne obtained a volatile oil, of a stupefying odor, and an action on the system such as to dispose him to think that it was the active principle of the plant. As the water distilled was strongly alkaline, he supposed that his volatile principle might be a new alkaloid; but the alkaline reaction was found to depend on ammonia; and the liquid obtained proved to be a volatile oil, lighter than water, of a deep amber color, a strong odor of hemp, and composed of two distinct oils, one colorless, with the formula $C_{18}H_{20}$, the other a hydride of the first, $C_{18}H_{22}$, which was solid, and separates from alcohol in platelike crystals. For the former Personne proposes the name of *cannabene*. It is affirmed that when this is inhaled, or taken into the stomach, a singular excitement is felt throughout the system, followed by a depression, sometimes amounting to syncope, with hallucinations which are generally disagreeable, but an action on the whole slighter and more fugitive than that of the resin. The various substances of alkaloidal nature that have been described by different investigators as found in Indian hemp are now recognized as due to decomposition products of *choline*, which was identified as present by Jahns (*P.J.*, 1887, xvii, 1049). *Cannabin-*

don, $C_8H_{12}O$, is a dark red syrupy liquid obtained by Kobert (*Chem. Ztg.*, 1894, 741) from Cannabis Indica; it is soluble in alcohol, ether and oils; it is affirmed to be a narcotic in doses of from half a grain to two grains (0.032–0.13 Gm.). As a result of a reinvestigation of charras (churrus) from Indian hemp, Wood, Spivey, and Easterfield (*J. Chem. S.*, vol. lxix, 539) have found the following principles: (1) a *terpene*, boiling between 150° and 180° C. (302° and 356° F.); (2) a *sesquiterpene*, boiling at 258° to 259° C. (496.4°–498.2° F.); (3) a *crystalline paraffin* of probable formula $C_{29}H_{60}$, melting at 63.5° C. (146.3° F.); and (4) a *red oil*, boiling at 265° to 270° C. (509°–518° F.) under a pressure of 20 mm., to which they give the name *cannabinol*, and the formula $C_{18}H_{24}O_2$. This latter constituent they consider the only active ingredient. It is probably the same substance as the dark red syrup of Kobert, mentioned above under the name cannabindon. The authors found that cannabinol readily underwent superficial oxidation, at the same time losing its toxic activity. Famulener and Lyons (*A. Pharm.*, 1904) believe that the only reliable preparation of cannabis is a fluid extract made from the *fresh* drug. I. Ronx (*A. Pharm.*, 1887) has experimented upon extracts made by treating purified extract of hemp with petroleum benzin and ether. The ether extract produced insignificant results. The petroleum extract was excitant and convulsant. The alcoholic extract was a feeble narcotic. The resin "cannabin" of which *cannabinol* is the chief constituent, appears to be active. Frankel (*A. E. P. P.*, 1903, p. 266) claims to have isolated the active principle of hashish as a pure and chemically well defined body. It has the formula $C_{31}H_{30}O_2$, and is a phenol-aldehyde. It is of a pale yellow color and of a thick consistency. When heated it becomes quite fluid and distills at 0.5 mm. It oxidizes in the air, acquiring a brown tint. It responds to Millon's reaction, and can be acetylized, showing thus its phenol character. Frankel proposes that the name *cannabinol* be given to it and that the term *pseudocannabinol* be given to the inactive substance of Wood, Spivey and Easterfield.

Assay. —"Prepare a fluid extract and proceed as directed below." *U.S.*

Attempts have been made to apply physiological tests to the standardization of cannabis indica. Up to the present no means have been suggested for determining the relative potency of different samples of cannabis indica, the physiological test simply demonstrating that the drug possesses a certain indefinite amount of physiological action. This test is carried out upon dogs in the following manner: It is advisable to use the same animal for repeated tests, because the individual susceptibility of the dog varies so greatly, and the experimenter gradually learns the degree of reaction to be expected from a certain dog. A tincture of the specimen to be tested is either evaporated into a soft extract and given in the form of a pill or mixed with an inert absorbing powder and enclosed in a capsule; it must not be given hypodermically. The symptoms caused by cannabis indica in the dog recall those of alcoholism in the human being. There is at first a slight loss of control in the hind legs so that the animal staggers as he walks, later the ataxia becomes so marked that the dog is unable to stand up without leaning against some object, and about this time begins to show distinct drowsiness, and may eventually pass into a heavy sleep.

The details of assay as directed by the U.S. are as follows: "The assay of Cannabis and its preparations has been made a requirement and is based upon the fact that this drug produces certain symptoms of muscular incoordination. The method consists of ascertaining the dose of the preparation to be tested which will produce these symptoms of incoordination in dogs and then adjusting its strength by comparison with a standard preparation.

"*Dogs.*—The animals differ considerably in susceptibility to the drug and therefore it is best to make preliminary tests upon several dogs with average-sized doses and select from among them the animals which react easily to the drug. As a rule, fox terriers serve very well for the purpose, but any dog may prove satisfactory. It is best to provide at least two dogs for each assay, but if many samples are to be examined more dogs will be needed. The dogs should be at least one year old and in normal health and must be kept under the best sanitary conditions. They may be used repeatedly for the purpose but not at shorter intervals than three days. Each series of tests should be conducted by the same person, who should be perfectly familiar with the peculiarities of each animal in order that he may recognize more certainly deviations from the normal. While the tests are being made the animals should be kept in a perfectly quiet room, free from disturbance and separated so that they cannot see each other.

"*Preparation of the Drug.*—The drug may be given most conveniently in the form of the fluid extract which is administered in gelatin capsules, or the extract made into soft pills may be used; but whichever form is chosen the same should be used for both the standard and the preparation that is to be tested.

"Before administration the animal should not be fed for twenty-four hours in order to hasten absorption. The head of the animal being held, its mouth is opened and the capsule or pill is placed upon the back of the tongue. Usually the drug is easily swallowed when given in this way, but this may be facilitated by giving the animal a small amount of water to drink.

"*Assay.*—An average dose of the known or standard preparation is given to one of the dogs and a like dose of the preparation to be standardized is given the second dog. After one hour both dogs are observed very carefully for symptoms of muscular incoordination. The incoordination is manifested differently in different animals, but in small doses it shows itself most frequently in slight swaying, when the animal is standing quietly, or in some ataxia when it runs about. The observation should be made frequently during the second hour following the administration of the drug.

"The results obtained from the first test should be confirmed after an interval of not less than three days by repeating the administration, but reversing the order, that is, giving the known strength drug to the dog which received that of unknown strength before and *vice versa.*

"In subsequent tests which are carried out, the dose of the preparation of unknown strength is modified so as to produce similar symptoms to those produced by the standard. If the preparation to be tested is below the standard in strength, its dose must be increased, or if it is above strength its dose is lessened until equivalent doses of the two are found. Dogs may be used over long periods of time, even for some years, but occasionally they have to be discarded, as in some cases they seem to learn the effects of the drug and so refuse to stand up. A certain degree of tolerance is sometimes gained which necessitates larger doses.

"*Standard.*—As there is no chemical substance of definite

composition which can be adopted as a standard, a fluid extract of Cannabis or an extract which has been carefully prepared and suitably preserved may be utilized for this purpose. A standard fluid extract will produce incoordination when administered to dogs in the dose of 0.03 mil for each kilogram of body weight of dog. When administered in the form of the Extract a dose of 0.004 Gm. for each kilogram of body weight of dog should produce similar symptoms, and the requirement for a standard tincture is a dose of 0.3 mil for each kilogram of body weight of dog." *U.S. IX.*

Uses.—Aside from a slight local irritant effect the action of cannabis seems to be limited almost exclusively to the higher nerve centers. In man this is first manifested by a peculiar delirium which is accompanied with exaltation of the imaginative function and later by a remarkable loss of the sense of time. The delirium is often accompanied with motor weakness and diminished reflexes and generally followed by drowsiness. In the dog the earliest manifestation of the drug's action is a slight degree of restlessness which is soon followed by disturbances of equilibrium and later weakness of the legs and drowsiness.

Cannabis is used in medicine to relieve pain, to encourage sleep, and to soothe restlessness. Its action upon the nerve centers resembles opium, although much less certain, but it does not have the deleterious effect on the secretions. As a somnifacient it is rarely sufficient by itself, but may at times aid the hypnotic effect of other drugs. For its analgesic action it is used especially in pains of neuralgic origin, such as *migraine*, but is occasionally of service in other types. As a general nerve sedative it is used in *hysteria, mental depression, neurasthenia*, and the like. It has also been used in a number of other conditions, such as *tetanus* and *uterine hemorrhage*, but with less evidence of benefit. One of the great hindrances to the wider use of this drug is its extreme variability. Formerly many of the preparations of cannabis were inert before they left the manufacturers' hands, and the present requirements of the U.S.P. that the drug be tested upon dogs to insure its activity is an important step in the right direction. But even granted an active preparation when manufactured, so rapidly does the drug deteriorate that by the time the drug reaches the patient it has lost a large proportion of its activity. The only way of determining the dose of an individual preparation is to give it in ascending quantities until some effect is produced. The fluid extract is perhaps as useful a preparation as any; one may start with two or three minims of this three times a day, increasing one minim every dose until some effect is produced. According to C. R. Marshall (*L. L.*, 1897, i, also *J. A. M. A.*, Oct., 1898) the deterioration of cannabis is due to the oxidation of cannabinol, which he has found to act upon dogs and cats as the crude drug.

Dose, of cannabis, one to three grains (0.065—0.2 Gm.).

Official Prep.—Extractum Cannabis, *U.S.* (*Br.*);—Fluid extractum Cannabis, *U.S.*; Tinctura Cannabis (from Extract), *U.S.* (*Br.*); Collodium Sidicylici Composita (from fluid extract), *N. F.*; Tinctura Chlorali et Potassii Bromidi Composita (from Extract) *N.F.*

Marijuana

BY ROGER ADAMS, Ph.D.

The facts on marijuana which I shall present to you this evening comprise the results of the cooperative efforts of three laboratories—the chemical investigations at the University of Illinois, the pharmacology at Cornell Medical College under the direction of Dr. S. Loewe, and the clinical experiments at Welfare Island Hospital under the auspices of the Mayor's Committee on Marijuana and under the immediate direction of Dr. Samuel Allentuck. All three laboratories acquired their supplies of raw materials from Dr. H. J. Wollner of the Narcotics Laboratory of the Treasury Department, and received much encouragement and stimulation from him. Dr. J. R. Matchett of the same laboratory contributed significantly to the general problem by devising a method whereby a fraction of the red oil of hemp, containing a very high concentration of the active principle, could be obtained.

Cannabis sativa, more commonly called hemp, is of peculiar interest. It has been known for thousands of years as a product of commerce; the fiber of the plant for clothing and rope, the seeds for the oil they contain. The presence of an intoxicating principle in the resin of the plant has also long been recognized, since the physiological action of hemp preparations is mentioned in some of the earliest records available and is described in the first medical treatises. In the last two thousand years over four hundred articles have been

Reprinted from *Bulletin New York Academy of Medicine,* vol. 18, 1942, pp. 705-730.

published describing intoxicating characteristics and the effects on humans.[1]

The preparation of the hemp for consumption as an intoxicant varies in different countries and consequently several names, such as marijuana, charas, ganja, hashish, and others, have been adopted, each in a definite locality. It is significant that the same characteristic phenomenon from any of these products is observed in man when the doses are equated.

The clarification of the chemical and medical aspects of hemp extracts has been extraordinarily slow for a material known as long and as frequently as marijuana. The reasons have been several: the failure of chemists to isolate a pure active principle, the unsuccessful attempts of the pharmacologist to find an animal test which paralleled the activity in humans, and finally the lack of controlled clinical experiments.

The recorded medical literature is most confusing. The reports are contradictory, and the description of the drug varies from one which is habit-forming and which with constant use is as harmful to the system as morphine, to one which is almost completely innocuous with stimulation not far remote from that of alcohol. Spread of the use of marijuana in the United States has been due in part to its ready availability, since hemp grows wild in countless places all over the country. Newspaper articles have described marijuana smoking among school children, and magazine articles have carried vivid accounts of activies encountered in tea-pads—dens where marijuana is enjoyed by devotees. Marijuana has been accredited with precipitating premeditated criminal acts, of lowering morals and releasing inhibitions, and of serving as a stepping-stone to other drug addictions such as the use of heroin. Furthermore, the claim has been made that continued use of marijuana produces mental deterioration. A "Marijuana Bill" was passed by the United States Congress in 1934. For purposes of administration, marijuana is defined essentially as any part of the hemp plant or extract therefrom which induces somatic and psychic changes in man. The regulations and penalties in the bill for use and distribution of marijuana are as rigid as those imposed for the use and sale of morphine.

In the investigations which are to be described this evening, more quantitative data on the chemistry, pharmacology, and clinical aspects of marijuana has been gathered than hitherto have been available and present a foundation for the eventual complete understanding of this interesting natural product. The chemical investigations, an excellent résumé of which up to 1938 has been published by Blatt,[1] will be discussed first. Practically all of the chemical experiments which have been reported were performed on the resin present in hemp from various sources and the same general procedure for isolating the resin has been used by all investigators in this field. After extraction with an organic solvent, filtration of the solution thus obtained, removal of the solvent and vacuum distillation of the residue, a highly viscous, physiologically active oil results, red in color and boiling over a wide range. Fractionation of the oil leads to the concentration of the active components in the portion boiling from 180-190° (1 mm.) which is commonly known as "purified red oil." This purified red oil usually used in the chemical studies has been shown definitely to be a welter of closely related substances which are very difficult to separate from each other and which occur in varying proportions dependent on the sources of the hemp.

Between 1840 and 1895, most of the chemical investigations consisted in attempts to discover tests which would provide means of identifying a hemp extract. Numerous color reactions were reported, only one of which has received frequent application and until recently general acceptance. This is the so-called alkaline Beam test which is the purple color produced by treatment of a hemp extract with 5 percent methanolic potassium hydroxide.[3] From our chemical results and from an extensive investigation of agronomic varieties of hemp by Dr. Matchett[4] it can be concluded that this test is not indicative of a substance with marijuana activity.

In 1895 Wood, Spivey, and Easterfield[5] were able to isolate from "purified red oil" by means of a treatment with acetic anhydride, a crystalline acetate, which was removed from the residual oil and which could be purified in the normal way. Hydrolysis of this pure acetate resulted in a homogeneous viscous oil which these investigators called cannabinol. Until about a decade ago, when the fact was shown to be erroneous, cannabinol was accepted as the active principle of

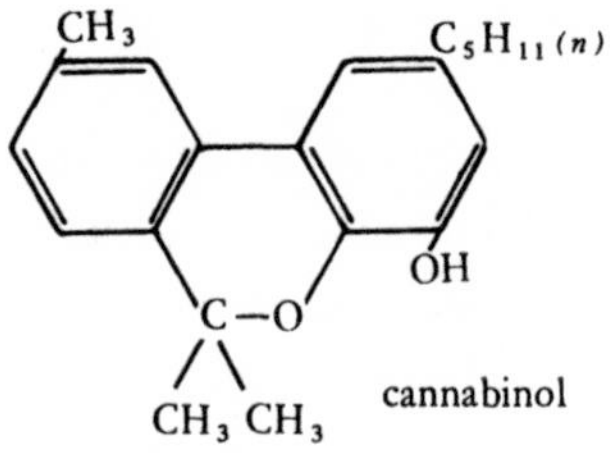

cannabinol

Cannabinol	M.P. °C.	Cannabidiol	M.P. °C.
$C_{21}H_{26}O_2$	75–76	$C_{21}H_{30}O_2$	66–67
p-Nitrobenzoate	165–166	*bis*-3,5-Dinitrobenzoate	106–107
m-Nitrobenzenesulfonate	127–129	*bis*-m-Nitrobenzenesulfonate .	119–120
Acetate	76–77	Oil	
3,5-Dinitrophenylurethan . . .	220–222	Oil	
Optically inactive		$[a]^{27}D$—125° (ethanol)	
No alkaline Beam test		Superb alkaline Beam test	
No marihuana activity		No marihuana activity	

CHART I

hemp. These same investigators performed preliminary experiments on the structure of the cannabinol molecule.
Further work on its chemistry was impeded by the fact that
in spite of many attempts in different laboratories the
isolation of cannabinol was not repeated until 1932. At that
time Cahn,[6] an English chemist, again obtained this compound and completed a series of brilliant researches from the
results of which he was able to establish the skeleton and the
substituents in the molecule but was unsuccessful in determining the orientation of all the groups.

It was with this background that the chemical experiments
were begun at the University of Illinois.* Attempts to isolate
cannabinol from the purified red oil of Minnesota wild hemp

* The experimental work of the series of researches at the University of
Illinois was performed by the following students: B. R. Baker, C. K.
Cain, J. H. Clark, Madison Hunt, Charles F. Jelinek, W. D. McPhee,
D. C. Pease, C. M. Smith, R. B. Wearn and Hans Wolff.

by the procedure described by Cahn failed. Consequently, attention was turned to attempts to isolate a phenolic product, the presence of which was established by qualitative tests. Of the numerous reagents employed, 3,5-dinitrobenzoyl chloride reacted to give a crystalline compound which was readily removed from the residual oil and purified. It proved to be a *bis*-ester, the hydrolysis of which by an appropriate method gave a new substance which was termed "cannabidiol" because of the presence of two phenolic groups.[7] It was isolated first as an oil but eventually was obtained as a crystalline solid. By developing a new procedure as a substitute for Cahn's method the isolation of cannabinol from this same oil was also accomplished, and for the first time cannabinol was induced to crystallize.[8] * The properties of cannabinol and cannabidiol are compared in Chart 1. Cahn's proposed formula for cannabinol is shown; his evidence for this structure was conclusive except for the positions of the hydroxyl and *n*-amyl groups.

The similarity in the empirical formulas of these two compounds is striking and led to the belief that these two sister substances must have structural formulas not too unrelated. The optical activity of cannabidiol suggested immediately the probability of partial hydrogenation of one aromatic nucleus in cannabinol and indeed the left one, since cannabidiol contains phenolic groups.

Although cannabidiol, like cannabinol, is physiologically inactive, the study of its structure and its reactions was most revealing. The results served to determine completely the structure of cannabinol and led to the formation of tetrahydrocannabinols, products of high marijuana potency which are probably active principles in the red oil of hemp.

The complicated and extensive chemical investigations on the structure of cannabidiol, on the synthesis of cannabinol, and on the preparation of tetrahydrocannabinol and synthetic analogs, will be presented in very brief form and only the more significant facts will be mentioned. The structure of cannabidiol[10] will be considered first with the pertinent

---

* Cannabidiol and cannabinol are the only pure compounds related by structure to the active constituents which have been isolated from hemp extracts. Claims have been made for the isolation of other compounds or their derivatives, but no detailed information is available and the results require confirmation.

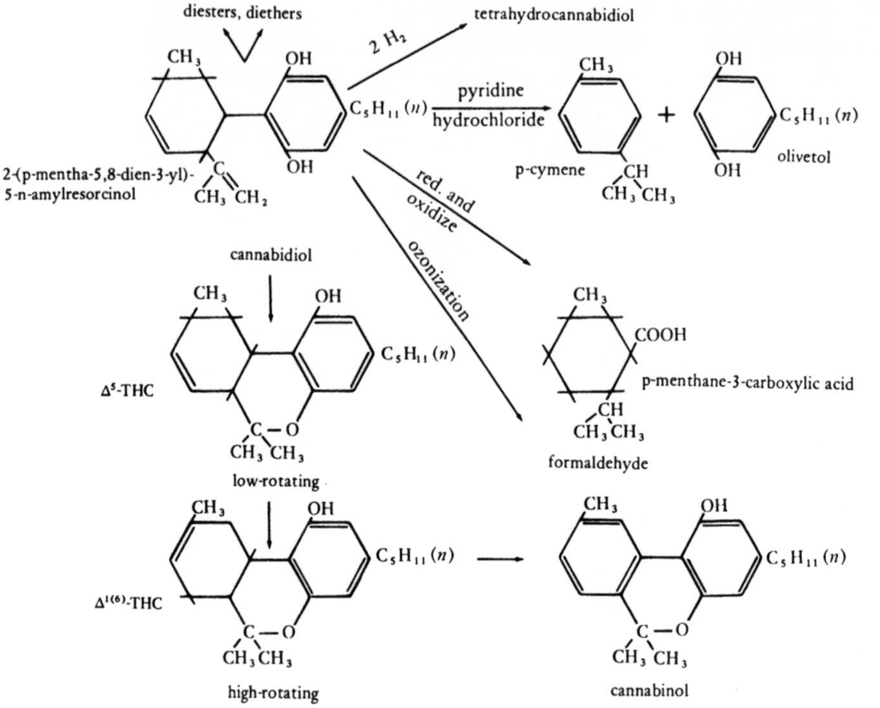

CHART II

reactions given in logical rather than chronological order.

Typical color tests indicated a phenol group, and formation of *bis*-esters and ethers the probable presence of two such groups. Catalytic reduction resulted in the absorption of two moles of hydrogen with formation of a molecule which still retained the two phenolic groups, thus leading to the deduction that two pyridine hydrochloride caused cleavage into *p*-cymene and olivetol (1,3-dihydroxy-5-*n*-amylbenzene) both of which were identified by comparison with authentic samples. This is convincing evidence that cannabidiol is composed of dihydrocymyl and olivetol residues. The positions of the linkage between these residues were determined next. Cannabidiol was first reduced to tetrahydrocannabidiol and then oxidized; menthane carboxylic acid was isolated, identical with a specimen obtained by synthesis from 1-menthol, thus demonstrating that the attachment of the dihydrocymyl residue was adjacent to the isopropyl grouping. From a comparison of the absorption spectra of various amyl resorcinols and of cannabidiol and its reduction product, the

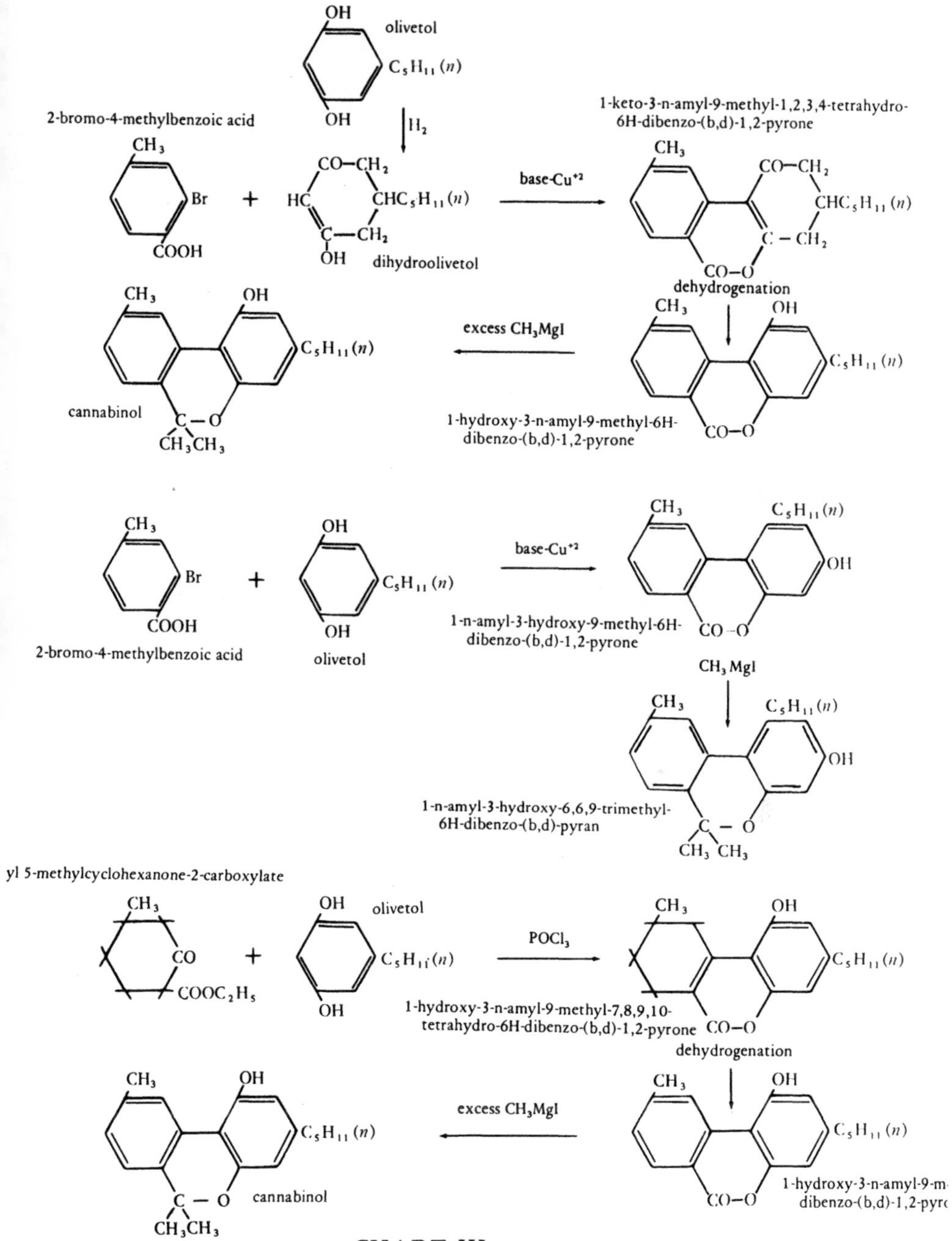

CHART III

dihydrocymyl was postulated as being attached to the olivetol between the hydroxyl groups. Direct chemical proof of this was accomplished by conversion of cannabidiol with

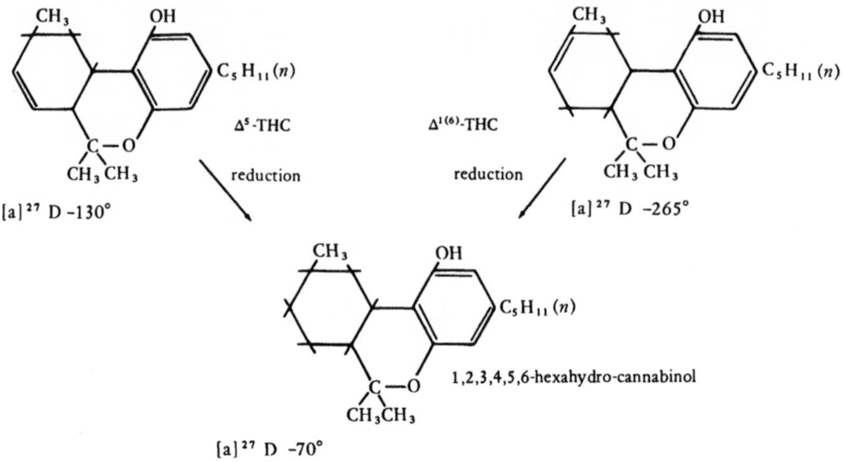

CHART IV

acidic reagents to tetrahydrocannabinol which, upon dehydrogenation, gave cannabinol. Cannabinol was shown to contain the linkage between the hydroxyls by synthesis of this molecule by an unequivocal method.

The structure of the cannabidiol molecule was thus established except for the orientation of the two aliphatic double bonds in the dihydrocymyl residue. One of these proved to be terminal, since ozonization of cannabidiol gave formaldehyde. This information, along with the fact that tetrahydrocannabinol was produced from cannabidiol through closure of a pyran ring, left no doubt that this terminal double bond must be present as an isopropenyl group. The location of the second double bond was determined only by indirect means. Since the arguments are rather involved, they will be omitted here and merely the positions assigned for the double bonds will be given. The tetrahydrocannabinol obtained in the isomerization of cannabidiol, varied in rotation dependent on the reagent used. Apparently two forms exist which were isolated as low-rotating and high-rotating isomers. In the low-rotating tetrahydrocannabinol, which presumably has the double bond in the same position as in cannabidiol, the double bond was deduced to be in the γ,δ-position between the unsubstituted carbons; in the high-rotating isomer, the double bond is probably substituted in the γ,δ-position which includes the ring carbon holding the methyl group.

The establishment of olivetol as a cleavage product of

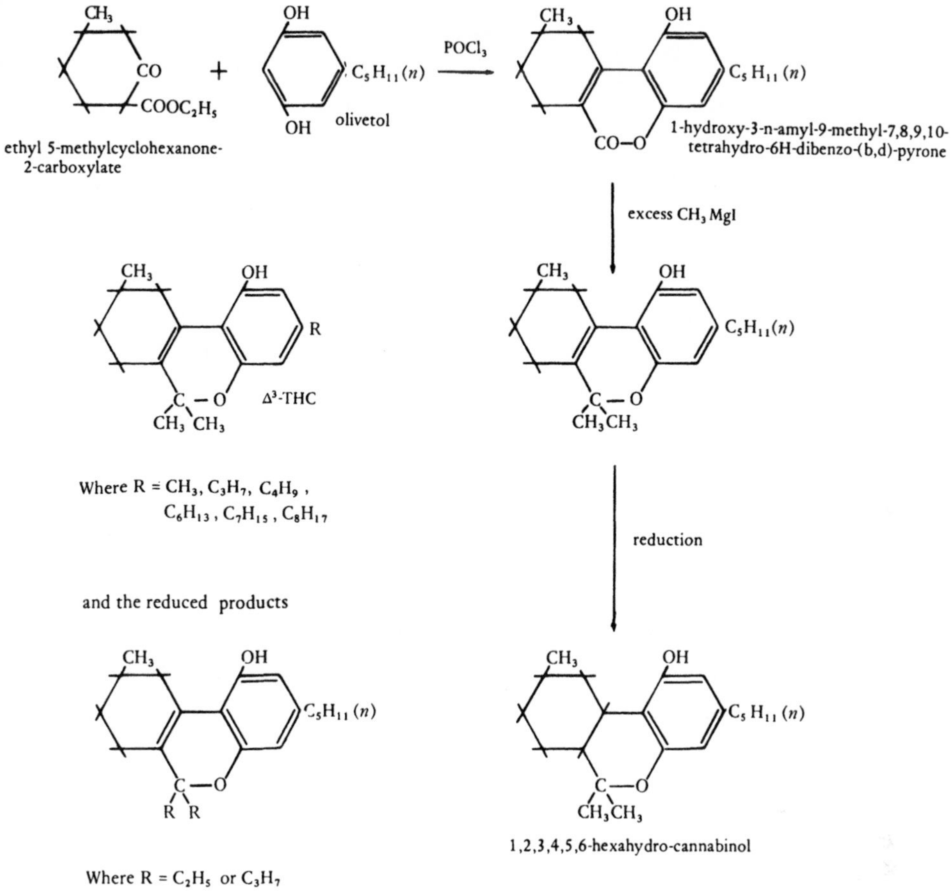

CHART V

cannabidiol revealed the probable orientation of the hydroxyl and *n*-amyl groups in cannabinol. This supposition was proven correct by the synthesis of cannabinol by two different methods[11] as shown in Chart III. The syntheses served also to prove that the position of the linkage of the two benzene rings is between the hydroxyl groups and thus confirmed a similar attachment of the rings in cannabidiol.

2-Bromo-4-methylbenzoic acid and dihydroolivetol condensed in the presence of alkali and a copper salt to 1-keto-3-*n*-amyl-9-methyl- 1,2,3,4-tetradydro-6-dibenzopyrone; dehydrogenation gave 1-hydroxy-3- *n*-amyl-9-methyl-6-dibenzopyrone which, with excess of methylmagnesium iodide, gave cannabinol, (1-hydroxy-3- *n*-amyl-6,6,9-trimethyl-6-dibenzopyran). An analogous condensation of 2-bromo-4-methyl-benzoic acid with olivetol, followed by treatment with methylmagnesium iodide, gave the isomeric cannabinol with the linkage between an hydroxyl and the *n*-amyl group. The second method consisted in condensation of ethyl 5-methyl-cyclohexanone- 2-carboxylate with olivetol in the presence of phosphorous oxychloride to give 1-hydroxy-3- *n*-amyl-9-methyl- 7,8,9,10-tetrahydro- 6-dibenzopyrone. Dehydrogenation to the corresponding 1-hydroxy-3- *n*-amyl-9-methyl-6-dibenzopyrone followed by treatment with methylmagnesium iodide gave cannabinol.

The disappointment accompanying the discovery that cannabidiol had no marijuana activity was more than compensated by the observation that both the low-rotating and high-rotating tetrahydrocannabinols possess very marked marijuana potency.[12]   These two substances, which were high-boiling oils, have not yet been induced to crystallize. All attempts to isolate solid crystalline derivatives have failed. The isomerization of cannabidiol required intensive study before procedures were found which resulted in products of constant rotation. Apparently, without very specific conditions, mixtures of low- and high-rotating forms are obtained which cannot be converted readily to a product of maximum rotation. Tetrahydrocannabinol of constant rotation $[a]^{27}$ D -265° can be produced conveniently from cannabidiol merely by heating the latter in benzene solution with a little toluene sulfonic acid until the reaction mixture exhibits no alkaline Beam test. This product was the principal one selected for pharmacological and clinical investigation.

The acetates of these tetrahydrocannabinols also had marijuana potency though less than that of the unacetylated compounds. By catalytic reduction all of the tetrahydrocannabinols of varying optical activity gave a hexahydrocannabinol of essentially the same optical activity. This product was physiologically active though less so than any of the tetrahydrocannabinols from which it was derived.

The typical marijuana activity manifested by the isomeric tetrahydrocannabinols constitutes ponderable evidence that the activity of the plant itself, and of extracts prepared therefrom, is due in large part to one or the other of these compounds, or both, and possibly also to their stereoisomers, of which a number are possible. Confirmation of this supposi-

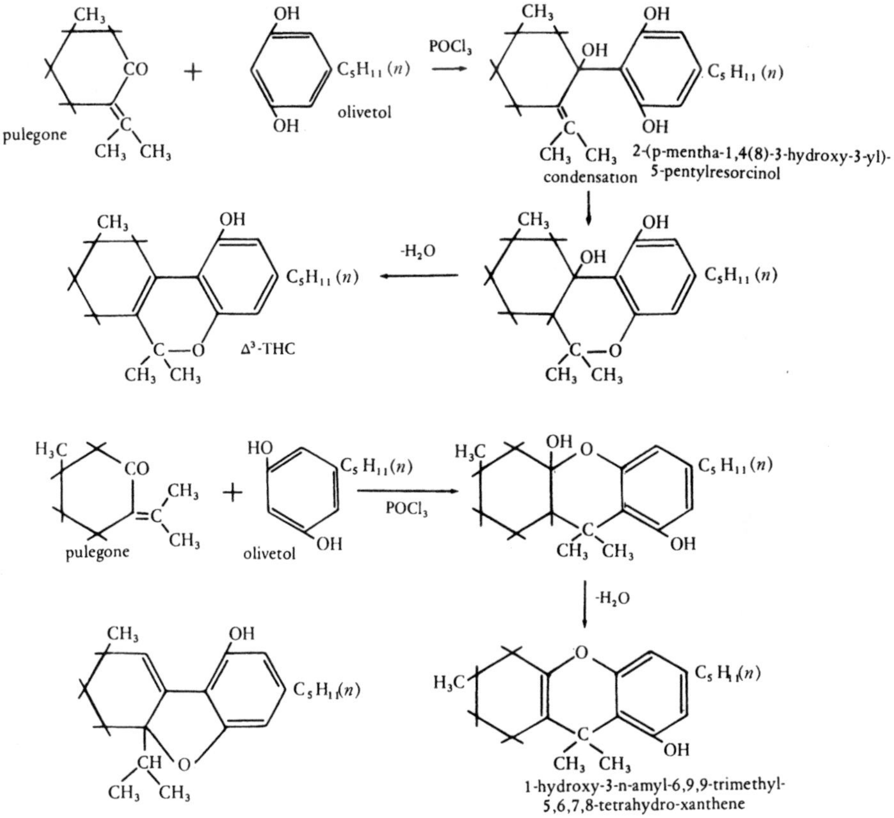

CHART VI   *See ref. 28.*

tion is available from an investigation by Wollner, Matchett, Levine and Loewe,[13] the results of which were published just recently. These authors have described the isolation from acetylated red oil of a tetrahydrocannabinol acetate of potency greater than than of either of the tetrahydrocannabinols prepared by isomerization of cannabidiol. Partition of the acetylated red oil was accomplished by selective absorption. Silica gel removed cannabidiol diacetate and unknown material from a benzene solution of the mixture; alumina adsorbed substances of lower rotation by two passages, first in carbon tetrachloride, then in pentane solution. The product was judged to be stereochemically homogeneous by failure to effect further separation through selective adsorption or by careful fractional distillation in a specially designed high-vacuum fractionating column. Hydrolysis of the acetate yielded a tetrahydrocannabinol whose structure was identified through analysis and dehydrogenation to cannabin-

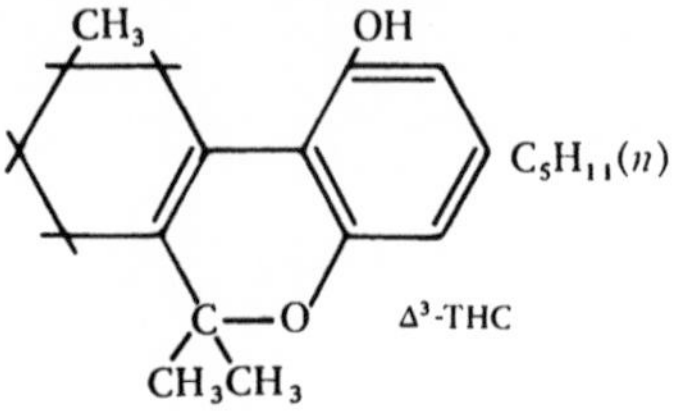

Δ^3-THC

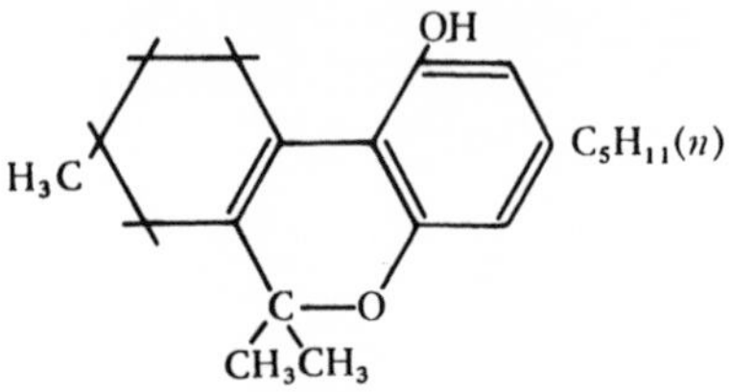

1-hydroxy-3-n-amyl-6,6,8-trimethyl-7,8,9,10-
tetrahydro-6H-dibenzo-(b,d)-pyran

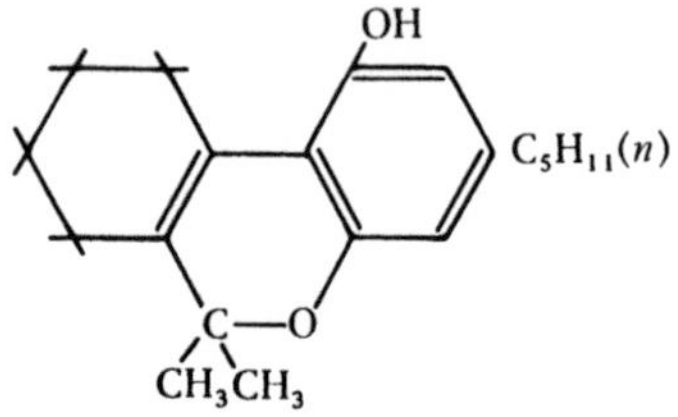

1-hydroxy-3-n-amyl-6,6-dimethyl-7,8,9,10-
tetrahydro-6H-dibenzo-(b,d)-pyran

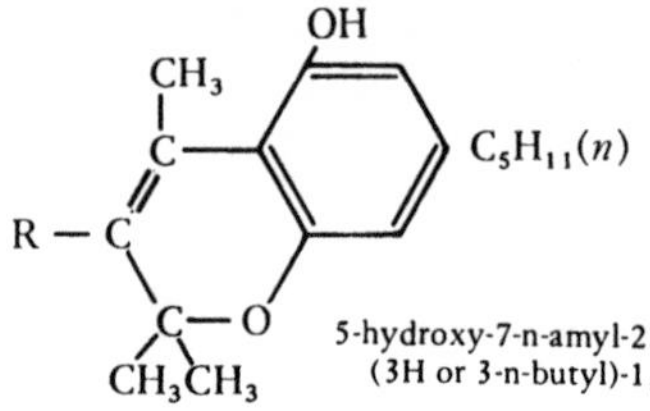

5-hydroxy-7-n-amyl-2,2,4-trimethyl-
(3H or 3-n-butyl)-1,2-benzopyran

R = H, C_4H_9

CHART VII

ol. Its potency was similar to the products prepared by
isomerization of cannabidiol. It would appear that rearrangement occurred during hydrolysis, since reacetylation failed to
restore either the optical rotation or physiological potency to
the original value.

With the discovery of the character of substances which
possess marijuana activity, attention was directed next to
attempts to synthesize compounds of similar activity. A very
satisfactory procedure was devised for obtaining an isomer of
the natural tetrahydrocannabinol with the double bond
conjugated to the benzene ring. It consisted in the condensation of ethyl 5-methylcyclohexanone-2-carboxylate with
olivetol to give 1-hydroxy-3-n-amyl-9-methyl-7,8,9,10-tetra-
hydro-6-dibenzopyrone which, with excess methylmagnesium
iodide, yielded 1-hydroxy-3-n-amyl,6,6,9-trimethyl-7,8,9,10-
tetrahydro-6-dibenzopyran.[14] The product proved to have
marijuana activity though only about one-tenth that of its
isomer, natural tetrahydrocannabinol. A series of several
closely related synthetic compounds was then prepared by
the same procedure using the same keto ester but homologs
of olivetol.[15] All of these products were reduced to the
corresponding hexahydro compounds.[16] The synthetic tetrahydrocannabinol was also modified by replacing the 6-methyl

groups by ethyl and propyl groups.[17] (Chart V.)

A provisional synthesis designed to obtain an optically active tetrahydrocannabinol was sought in the condensation of pulegone and olivetol.[17, 18] In the presence of phosphorous oxychloride, a product which analyzes for, and has the properties of tetrahydrocannabinol is formed. A possible mechanism by which such a reaction might take place is shown in Chart VI. The purity of the final product is by no means established. There is a possibility of contaminants formed by condensation of the two reactants to give a partially hydrogenated xanthane or a tetrahydrodibenzofuran, isomeric with tetrahydrocannabinol. Homologs in which the olivetol portion was substituted by other 1,3-dihydroxy-5-alkylbenzenes were synthesized.[16] The reduction product of each was prepared.

Finally in Chart VII are shown molecules in which the left-hand ring has been modified by removal or by change in the position of the methyl group.[17]

The pharmacological studies on hemp extracts have been equally as meager as the chemical investigations and in the long history of *Cannabis* preparations only three tests have been reported. Liataud[19] in 1844 observed that motor incoordination in the dog was a characteristic effect induced by marijuana preparations; Fraenkel[20] in 1903 interpreted this incoordination as a cataleptic condition. This was followed in 1928 by the observations of Gayer[21] that in various animals such as cats, rabbits, or dogs, intravenous injection of marijuana preparations in acetone solution induced corneal anesthesia which was characteristic of active fractions of the resin. In 1937, Munch and Mantz[22] reported no unequivocal effects when *Cannabis* preparations were administered to albino mice. On the other hand, Loewe[23] noted a definite increased depressant action when treated mice were given a hypnotic of the barbiturate series. Pernocton, butyl-bromo-allyl barbituric acid, gave the greatest enhancement of any of the drugs tested.

The Gayer corneal anesthesia test was developed further by Marx and Eckhardt[24] but neither these investigators nor Gayer himself went further than to designate that the corneal reflex was normal or abnormal. The corneal response was ascertained by tapping with von Frey hairs. Walton[25] took steps in a quantitative direction by counting the number of responses occasioned by tapping the cornea a given number of times and by plotting the results over the whole duration of the effect. By thus locating a definite maximum in the areflexia-versus-time curve of each experiment, quantitative comparisons were made possible by determining the ratios of doses producing equal maxima in different animals. Loewe[26] developed this procedure further by application of his method of "Bioassay by Approximation" to overcome as far as possible the large intra-individual and the large group variabilities which seem to be inherent in the reaction of all types of animals to marijuana preparations. His study of the Gayer test applied to the behavior of rabbits as test animals showed not only great inter-individual variations in sensitivity but also enormous intra-individual variations in the same animal. Using the same animal repeatedly, this investigator found a consistent decrease in sensitivity to one and the same dose. Therefore, even though the method of approximation was applied, the values of potency obtained by this method are not suitable for anything but qualitative purposes. Moreover, they do not parallel the dog-ataxia potencies of the same preparations, the divergence sometimes being tenfold. This indicates either that the Gayer test is not conclusive for quantitative measurements or else that an active principle other than that disclosed by the dog-ataxia test is present in red oil.

The "mouse sleep prolongation test" may be dismissed with merely a brief discussion. The *Cannabis* preparations, usually red oil, were administered by stomach tube. After a definite time, pernocton was injected intravenously at a level just above the threshold of hypnotic action. The synergistic effect of the *Cannabis* was measured by the period of suppression of the righting reflex averaged over all the animals of a single-dose group. This effect, though typical of red oil, could not be duplicated with the natural or synthetic tetrahydrocannabinols which had been shown definitely to have physiological activity in man. Pure cannabidiol, which is devoid of the marijuana effect upon man, showed the highest potency in this test and consequently the action from the red oil probably is due to its cannabidiol content.

The determination of the cataleptic condition in dogs reported by Fraenkel, as accepted in former editions of the United States Pharmacopoeia for bioassay of *Cannabis* extracts, was developed further by Walton[25] to attempt to make the effect the basis of a quantitative test. The arbitrary stages of intensity of effects were recognized; first a slight depression; second, a barely detectable ataxia; third, an obvious ataxia; fourth, a marked ataxia in which the animal frequently pitches forward and barely catches itself; fifth, inability to stand alone; sixth, inability to rise and plunge about. The ataxia is chiefly a static one and is manifested particularly by swaying movements. Intravenous doses of red oil dissolved in acetone always acted within half an hour. A similar intensity of effect by oral administration required five to seven times the dose. Walton employed for evaluating potency the procedure used in most bioassay methods, the comparison of test and standard doses of equal intensity of effect. By comparing the results at various levels of dosage and by repeating the procedure a considerable number of times, he obtained more accurate results than had hitherto been reported. About eight trials with the unknown on the same dog, calibrated in about six trials with the standard, were used. A single assay required about three weeks or more for completion.

Loewe applied his principle of "Bioassay by Approximation" to the ataxia test and has thus been able to obtain a more decisive method for comparison of active products. The procedure aims at obtaining from each one of an adequate number of calibrated dogs, several figures of comparison of a test dose with the calibration doses. These figures represent ratios of doses, the response to which is not quantitatively the same. They are used to approximate the true potency value from both sides. At the same time the degree of overlapping marks the range of variation and gives an idea of the inherent inaccuracy. An entire assay may in this way be performed in a single day and highly consistent results may be obtained. The maximum order of accuracy is 10 percent since this is the minimum of variation in the response of the same animal at different times. Since parallelism between the results of the dog-ataxia tests and the effects of different preparations on humans has been established, it may be concluded that the ataxia method as developed by Loewe represents a reliable index of potency.

Using this procedure as just outlined, the comparison of results on the various natural and synthetic products will be

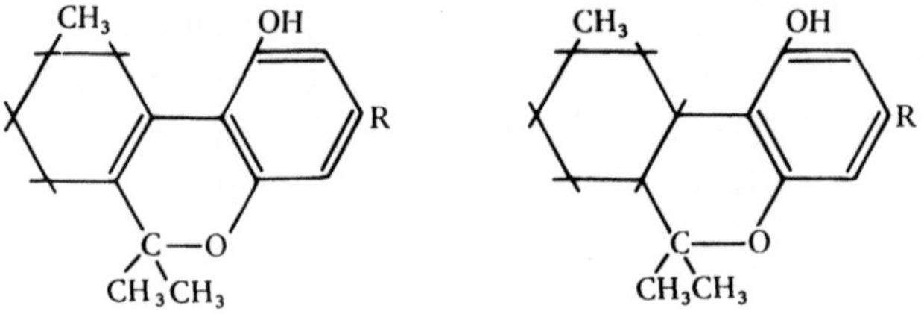

R = *n*-alkyl   Potency

	Tetrahydro	Hexahydro
CH_3	0.16 ± 0.03	below 0.04
C_3H_7	.40 ± .08	0.26 ± .04
C_4H_9	.37 ± .12	.37 ± .06
C_5H_{11}	standard 1.00	.51 ± .08
C_6H_{13}	1.82 ± 0.40	1.86 ± .37
C_7H_{15}	1.05 ± .15	0.83 ± .13
C_8H_{17}	0.66 ± .13	.24 ± .06

Tetrahydrocannabinol $[a]^{27}$D   Parke, Davis and Company
  $-265°$ 7.3   ± 0.89   Fluid Extract   0.060
  $-260°$ 7.8   ± .78   American Fluid Extracts
  $-240°$ 7.6   ± 1.1   thirty to forty different
  $-165°$ 9.3   ± 2.9   samples varied in
  $-160°$ 8.23 ± 2.17   potency   .003–0.130
  $-126°$ 6.5   ± 0.65   majority varied   .019– .052
  Hexahydrocannabinol   Purified red oil   1.24
  $-70°$ 3.0   ± 0.43   Highly purified red oil
                                               (Matchett)   4.33

CHART VIII

presented in charts. Each value given represents the result
obtained by the use of several dogs; three or four in the case
of low potency materials, ten to twenty or more for substances of higher potency.

In Chart VIII is shown a comparison of the potencies of
the series of products analogous to synthetic tetrahydrocannabinol. The latter was adopted as a standard. The corresponding hexahydro derivatives were also tested. It is observed that the modification of the alkyl group results in a
gradual increase in activity with increase in size until a

Pulegone Condensation Products

R = n-alkyl	Potency	
	Original products	Reduced products
C_3H_7	below 0.23	<0.20
C_4H_9	0.25 ± .10	< .15
C_5H_{11}	.58 ± .12	.64 ± 0.10
C_6H_{13}	1.22 ± .12	.78 ± .22
C_7H_{15}	1.15 ± .15	.83 ± .17
C_8H_{17}	1.37 ± .25	below .25
C_9H_{19}	below .20	. . . .

CHART IX

maximum is reached at the n-hexyl derivative. The point of maximum potency is the same in the hexahydro compounds, though all, with the exception of the n-hexyl, exhibit a decreased effect. There is also presented the potencies of tetrahydrocannabinols of different optical rotations all derived from cannabidiol, the potency of an average purified red oil and of a highly active portion of red oil obtained from it by extraordinarily careful fractionation. The increased activity of the optically active natural tetrahydrocannabinols is striking. The commercial cannabis fluid extracts are of very low and variable potency.

In Chart IX, the potency of products of questionable purity produced from pulegone and various olivetol homologs, together with their hydrogenated derivatives are shown. The maximum potency appears in the n-octyl molecule, and the values for the n-heptyl and n-octyl derivatives exceed those of the corresponding products synthesized by an unequivocal procedure.

Finally in Chart X, the activities of other analogs are shown. Each has an activity less than that of the molecule possessing methyl groups in the 6,6,9-positions.

Recognizing that the indulgence in marijuana in New York City has constituted a growing problem of major consequence involving psychiatric, medical, legal, sociological and civic aspects, a clinical study was undertaken by a committee appointed by Mayor LaGuardia and supported by funds

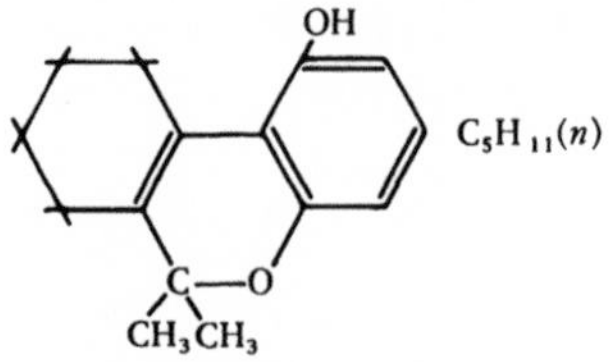

1-hydroxy-3-n-amyl-6,6-dimethyl-7,8,9,10-
tetrahydro-6H-dibenzo-(b,d)-pyran

0.126 ± 0.05

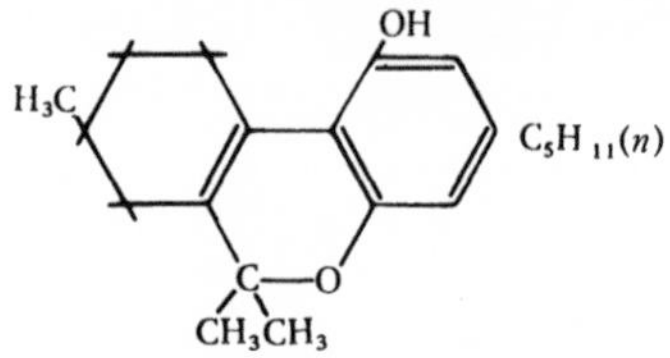

1-hydroxy-3-n-amyl-6,6, 8-trimethyl-7,8,9,10-
tetrahydro-6H-dibenzo-(b,d)-pyran

0.137 ± 0.01

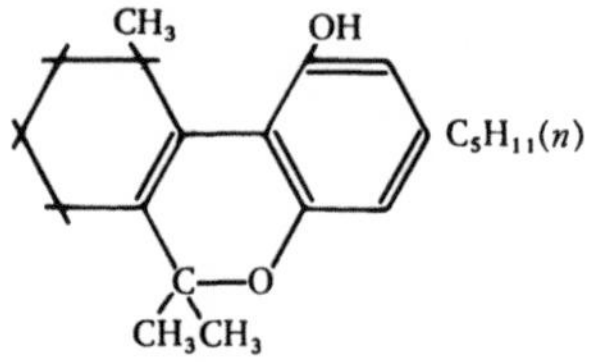

1-hydroxy-3-n-amyl-6,6,10-trimethyl-7,8,9,10-
tetrahydro-6H-dibenzo-(b,d)-pyran

0.25 ± 0.05

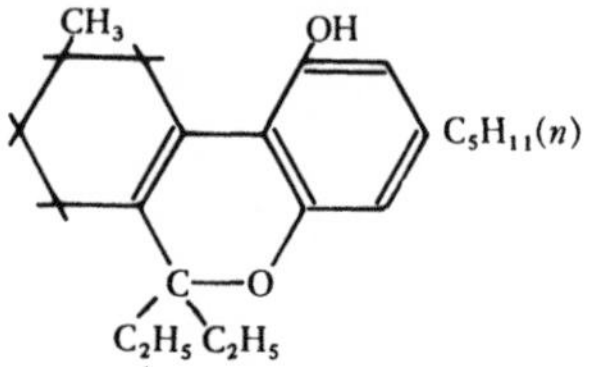

0.12 ±0.024
$(C_3H_7)(C_3H_7)$
0.04 ± 0.01

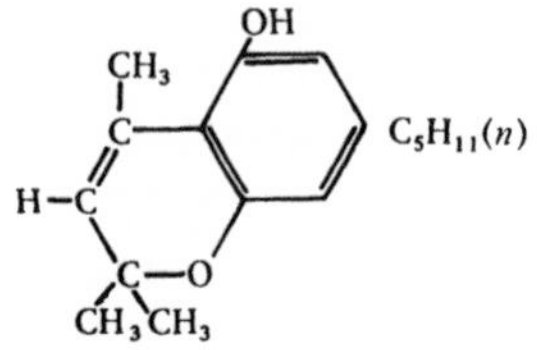

5-hydroxy-7-n-amyl-2,2,4-trimethyl-
3H-1,2-benzopyran
0.033 ± 0.010

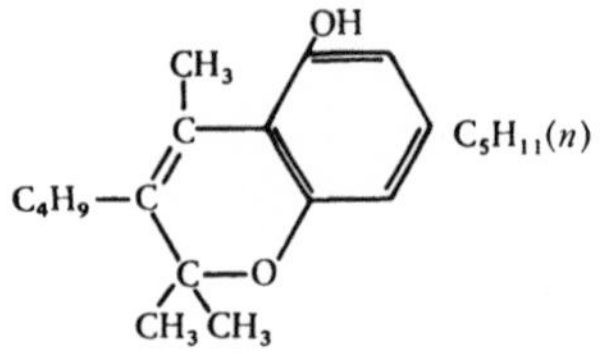

5-hydroxy-7-n-amyl-2,2,4-trimethyl-
3-n-butyl-1,2-benzopyran
0.04 ± 0.01

CHART X

allotted by several foundations. The primary objectives were
the determination of the mental and physical actions of marijuana on the kind of person resorting to its use and the
consequent social implications. Dr. Samuel Allentuck directed the clinical studies in a unit of the Welfare Island
Hospital, and the facts I am presenting have been summarized
from his report on the results.

An orientation group, the members of which were subjected to numerous and varied procedures, was used to
determine precisely which tests would best lend themselves
to the solution of the specific problems. From the results a
program was established which consisted in a systematic
study of a group of seventy-seven subjects ranging in age

from twenty-one to forty-five years and from borderline to superior in intelligence, all of them voluntary recruits from one prison population. About half had used marijuana previously. After a physical, neurological, and psychiatric examination, they were placed in one or more of five categories as to personality types—normal, antisocial, autistic, cyclothymic and epileptic. Each individual before and during the period of action of marijuana was interviewed at regular intervals throughout the day by various members of the staff. Possible subjective and objective phenomena resulting from use of the drug were discussed and elaborated upon in detail. Introspective reports were obtained in the absence of the drug, under pseudo-stimulation with placebos and during intoxication with marijuana or allied synthetics; analysis of the data was based on the most frequently mentioned phenomena. The patients were also subjected to periodic tests for blood pressure or pulse changes, pupillary changes, urinalyses, blood chemistries, hematological surveys, basal metabolic rates, electrocardiograms, arterial and venous pressure tracings and vital capacities. In addition, psychological examinations before and during the intoxication periods were carried out, including a wide variety of psychophysical, psychomotor and clinical tests.

The marijuana was supppplied in the form of a fluid concentrate which was desolvated and administered in the form of pills. Pure tetrahydrocannabinol was diluted with a little olive oil and placed in gelatin capsules holding 15 mg. of drug, the equivalent in physiological potency of one pill containing 300 mg. of crude solids from hemp. The 1-hydroxy-3-n-amyl,6,6,9-trimethyl-7,8,9,10-tetrahydro-6-dibenzopyran and its 3-n-hexyl homolog were administered in a similar manner using the equivalent doses which produced similar activity, namely, 120 mg. per capsule of the former and 60 mg. per capsule of the latter. It is significant that these relative amounts are practically identical with those observed by Loewe for obtaining identical effects in dog-ataxia tests.

The patients were started on two marijuana pills or on equated doses of tetrahydrocannabinol or the two synthetic analogs. The dose was increased by two pills at a time at intervals of two days unless toxic symptoms supervened. At the appearance of toxicity, the patient was returned to the physiological dose and this was increased one pill at a time. Thus the maximum tolerated dose for each individual was determined and at the same time approximately the threshold at which psychotic changes first appeared. Tetrahydrocannabinol and the synthetic compounds dissolved in olive oil were in some cases administered by intramuscular injection. Other clinical tests were made which involved intoxication from smoking marijuana cigarettes.

Barbiturates, cold showers and sweet candies were found to be efficacious in ameliorating any alarming physical or psychotic symptoms which developed following marijuana overdosage.

The detailed results of this carefully planned and executed clinical investigation, the first of its kind on record, must be left to the complete report when it is published. Merely the more significant findings which may prove of maximum value will be presented here. The crude drug in the form of concentrated marijuana extract, tetrahydrocannabinol derived from cannabidiol, and the two purely synthetic compounds, 1-hydroxy-3-*n*-amyl-6,6,9-trimethyl-7,8,9,10-tetrahydro-6-dibenzopyran and the corresponding 3-*n*-hexyl derivative elicited similar clinical and psychiatric phenomena upon the same subjects. The pharmacological action of these drugs somewhat resembles atropine and the psychiatric portrait, alcohol. The effects of marijuana do not vary qualitatively with the route of administration, whether ingested, injected or inhaled. By inhalation, however, they are more prompt in their appearance and disappearance; by ingestion they appear within one-half to one and one-half hours, reach their maximum in from three and one-half to five hours and disappear within seven hours.

The observed physical effects, one or more of which occur in each patient, are (a) elevation of the pulse rate, the increase being directly proportionate to the degree of intoxication; (b) elevation of the blood pressure; this varies with the individual and usually rises in direct proportion to the pulse; (c) injection of the conjunctival blood vessels which varies with the dose; (d) dilation of the pupils and sluggish reaction to light and in accommodation; vision for proximity, distance and color changes slightly; (e) circum oral tremors; tremulousness of the protruded tongue and the extremities; (f) dryness of the oral and pharyngeal mucous membranes;

(g) increased frequency with decreased amplitude of thoracic respiratory movements; (h) ataxia; (i) hyperreflexia. The observed psychiatric effects are (a) apprehension and anxiety, (b) euphoria, (c) loquaciousness, (d) lowering of inhibitions, (e) hunger and thirst, (f) feeling of being "high," (g) uncontrollable bursts of laughter or giggles, (h) drowsiness, languor, lassitude and a pleasant feeling of fatigue.

Clinical tests revealed that marijuana produces no significant changes in basal metabolic rates, blood chemistry, hematological picture, liver function, kidney function or cardiac electrical conduction. Marijuana delays somewhat gastric and intestinal motility as gauged by the Carlson apparatus and x-ray studies; it produces definite increase in the frequency of the alpha wave in electroencephalographic recordings thus indicating increased relaxation.

Other observations of a more general character were recorded. Tolerance for marijuana may be produced by repeated administration of subtoxic doses over a prolonged period of time. Thus the same dose elicited progressively fewer and milder symptoms. Marijuana is unlike opium derivatives in that it does not give rise to a biological dependence accompanied by withdrawal symptoms. Neither does it establish a strong craving as exists in tobacco smoking or in alcoholic indulgence. Follow-up of the subjects has failed to establish existence of any craving for the product. Many of the unpleasant physical symptoms previously mentioned appear only as a result of the administration of excessive doses of drug. It is no more of an aphrodisiac than alcohol.

Since all the clinical experiments at Welfare Island were conducted on volunteer prisoners, it was desirable for completeness or perhaps to satisfy my curiosity to obtain some results on subjects in another social class. As a consequence, I have conducted a dozen or more experiments using as test individuals chemists among whom were two members of the National Academy of Sciences and two high-ranking and very successful industrial chemists. In all cases very small doses, 15 mg. or 30 mg. of tetrahydrocannabinol, were administered about one hour before dinner. Each individual reacted differently with the possible exception of the observed stimulation of the appetite. They all recognized an intoxication which they described as in general like, but in detail different from that induced by alcohol. Thus, one industrial chemist who shows no outward change under the influence of alcohol, reported essentially no effect from 15 mg. except a mild stimulation of his desire for food. A 30 mg.-dose, however, to this same individual had a pronounced effect. Though he noticed no particular craving for food before dinner, as soon as he started eating he became particularly hungry and consumed a very large meal. He felt intoxicated and dissociated from his normal self, had a feeling of heaviness in his head and legs and reported a fogginess which he described as the inability to focus his eyes on more than a single object at a time. Since this man desired to get the effect of distorted time and space which is recorded as a frequent phenomenon associated with the marijuana user, he tried it a third time, taking 45 mg. The result was a ravenous hunger which was not satisfied after eating the equivalent of two hearty meals. A marked hypergeusia was also noted. The same fogginess appeared and heaviness in head and legs. During the conversation which took place among his five associates at the dinner table, he was able to comprehend a question but by the time the answer was given, which was immediately, he couldn't remember the question. In spite of the intoxication with the resulting phenomena, this subject had no difficulty in holding his own and then some in a poker game composed of expert players.

A second industrialist took 15 mg. at five o'clock in the afternoon and felt the first effects about 6:30 when he lost coordination in his fingers to the extent that he had to stop playing the violin, which he was doing at the time. Shortly thereafter he developed a tremendous appetite which was, if anything, sharpened by eating an enormous dinner and popcorn all through the evening. He had a mild lift about like a cocktail or two on an empty stomach and this and the hunger left about eleven o'clock.

A chemistry professor who took 30 mg. had a mildly increased appetite and reported feeling a bit fuzzy during his dinner, which resulted in difficulty in comprehending what his associates were saying. This was followed by sleepiness and lassitude until the effects of the drug disappeared two hours afterwards. The stimulation was only slight, which paralleled the effect of alcohol upon this man.

A fourth subject of high standing in university circles

wrote me in detail concerning his experience. I am quoting from his letter received two days after the experiment.

This is to report to you on the outcome of my trip conducted under the powerful guidance of the marijuana drops. I would be interested some time to know just how much of what specific material you gave me, but there is no question but that it gave me a most terrific wallop. In brief:

5:20 P.M. Took two capsules, went for short swim, had a highball and began to feel something beyond the mild glow from the drink about 6:15. By 6:30 felt bouncy in the knees, a little gay and foolish.

6:00-8:30 P.M. Very much in the fog. Had alternate waves of hilarity and depression. Sat in smoking compartment looking at myself in the mirror, writing notes on the experiment, and feeling very silly and stupid. Would feel the onset of a surge of hilarity and then break into a raucous, rippling laugh. This gaiety was not particularly pleasant, however, for throughout I felt wholly dissociated from myself, knew that I was at the mercy of the drug, and greatly resented this lack of control. The feeling was very different from that of being at one or another stage of intoxication, for I looked perfectly clear and normal and I could stand erect without swaying and execute motions with considerable precision. I could not, to my annoyance and as I was well aware, speak or write and think coherently. This bothered me particularly in the waves of depression, when my lips would feel very parched and salty and I would long to break the spell and regain my own consciousness. A very pressing and persistent sensation was that of extreme hunger, but I had sense enough to wait until the laughing spells were under control before going into the diner.

Here are a few excerpts from the log: "7:20. Not so good; for a few minutes I sat and looked at myself in a silly way. . . . This is *me* again. I very suddenly snapped out of it and am struggling back to normal. Lips are very dry. Maybe I'm not *quite* out of it. . . . The above is true. I am writing here in a serious vein—but quick, I must write that a minute or two ago I was sitting here in the men's lounge giggling at myself in the mirror and saying: This stuff does make you feel pretty gay (gay in the neese). Isn't that the damndest thing? [I knew the spelling was wrong but couldn't right it.] . . . 7:42. Yes, snapping out again. I just had a most jubilant laugh and feel another coming along. 7:45, not feeling laughy, feel like hell. This is really awful stuff. . . . 8:03. I feel like a fool. Lips bad. Want water, but I am terribly hungry and wish the experiment were over. I am thinking very much of eating, for I am very hungry. . . . 8:09. Nearly came out of it. It is awful. Helpless, awful feeling. Over, over, when will it be over? When can I eat? . . . 8:13. A fellow just came in to shave. Why now? Why not at this time of the evening EAT. . . . ha, ha. Now I have been silly. Looked silly. . . . ha, ha. Of all places to have this—the train. Bad, bad. Oh I feel like hell, salty lips . . ."

At 8:30 I devoured an enormous steak dinner with great rapidity and thoroughness, and left no trace of any of the fixings, even though I ordinarily do not eat ripe olives or salad, and although ordinary delicacy would keep me somewhat below the ten crackers I had with my cheese. The food tasted no better or worse than usual, and I had a dissociated feeling that my mouth was a purely mechanical guide for all that came its way, and wondered if mine was not very much the same as the "appetite" of a cat.

At 9:00 I felt myself coming out of the spell, and again at 9:15 I felt sane for a minute or two. A little later the sane periods began to predominate, and by 10 A.M. I was back again in control and could sit down and write out the details of a new natural product synthesis.

Thus ended the trip. I didn't sleep too well or too poorly, and the next morning I felt O.K. and had no hang-over.

It was an interesting experiment, but I can't write too enthusiastic an endorsement for this drug you fellows are synthesizing. The feeling of well-being would not, in my estimation, equal that from about three highballs, and the penalty seemed to me to be pretty severe. The outstanding impressions were the feeling of detachment from myself and the extreme hunger. Are these both associated with the same part of the molecule? If not, you might hydrogenate out some of the bad effects and thereby obtain a wonderful aperitif.

After the Welfare Island study of every phase of the action of marijuana and the synthetic drugs and after finding no discernible evidence of any permanent deleterious effects, either mental or physical, Dr. Allentuck considered the question of the possible therapeutic value of these substances. The potential availability of pure synthetics of standard potency invites such a study, for hitherto merely hemp extracts were accessible, the clinical activity of which must be determined for each batch of extracted material. Since the outstanding manifestation of the marijuana action is the euphoria which makes its user feel "high," consideration was given to its possible employment as a drug for individuals in various stages of mental depression as cyclothymics, involutionals, reactives, or those with organic conditions in which dysphoria is a dominant factor. The invariable characteristic of the drugs to stimulate the appetite, suggests they might be applicable in psychoneurosis in which a lack of desire for food exists. Many subjects show an alcohol-like picture of intoxication following the use of marijuana. The idea of using these drugs in the treatment of chronic alcoholic addiction was considered and preliminary experiments by Dr. Allentuck on private patients and colleagues were sufficiently encouraging to merit investigation on a larger scale and over a longer period of time.

The euphoria produced by marijuana is in many ways comparable to that achieved by the use of opium derivatives. This suggested the possibility of use in the treatment of opiate derivative addictions to eliminate or ameliorate the withdrawal symptoms commonly experienced during previously so-called "cures." To clarify this question Dr. Allentuck selected a series of cases among drug addicts undergoing treatment. One group of thirteen received 15 mg. of tetrahydrocannabinol orally three times daily at 5:00 A.M., 2:00 P.M., and 10:00 P.M. and a sterile hypodermic injection; another group of fourteen received the same treatment without the sterile injection. Subjective and objective findings were recorded. In general the consensus of subjective opinions favored the new treatment as compared to previous cures and the established routine taken by some of these patients. They felt happier, had a better appetite and wanted to return to activity sooner. These results served as a basis for further study of fifty cases in which quantitative criteria were employed.

Two groups of twenty subjects were selected, one group receiving the tetrahydrocannabinol up to a maximum of ten days and the others receiving none. Members of each group were observed throughout the day. Each morning they were interviewed and any complaints recorded on a chart. Thus an attempt was made to arrive at a quantitative comparison of the withdrawal symptoms. It was found that the tetrahydrocannabinol treatment was useful in alleviation or elimination of withdrawal symptoms and in diminishing or eliminating the accompanying discomfort which follows cessation of narcotic indulgence. Any withdrawal symptoms under the tetrahydrocannabinol treatment were of a mild character and occurred within the first three or four days following which the patients began to feel much better. The chief complaints were restlessness, headache and dryness of the throat. They had an increased appetite and desire for food which diminished or eliminated such withdrawal symptoms as nausea, diarrhea and perspiration. They felt physically stronger and showed psychomotor activity. The feeling of euphoria produced by the tetrahydrocannabinol helped in rehabilitating the physical condition and in facilitating social reorientation. An outstanding result is a subjective feeling of relaxation. The sleep induced by the drug likewise contributes to the general improvement in the patients' health. These results are in contrast to those from the use of Magendie's solution which produces in the patients contentment for the first three or four days, after which signs of marked discomfort or withdrawal effects appear. The patients after this treatment, upon their discharge were shaky and generally in poor physical condition. These preliminary results with tetrahydrocannabinol justify a more exhaustive study of its possibilities as a means of relieving the withdrawal symptoms in narcotic addicts.

With this brief picture of the results of the cooperative program before you, I may conclude by adding a few remarks about what may be expected from a continuation of the investigations under way. In the chemical field, repeated attempts to synthesize a tetrahydrocannabinol with a double bond in the γ, δ-position have failed. Just recently, however, a new approach has appeared and the results have progressed to the point where I am convinced it is merely a matter of time before the goal is reached. The physiological reaction of this product will allow a conclusion in regard to the relative importance of the position of the double bond in the alicyclic ring and of the optical activity in the tetrahydro-cannabinol molecule. Other synthetic molecules of a similar character, which are soluble in aqueous acids or bases and, therefore, perhaps suitable for intravenous injection, are being prepared. It is hoped also to clarify the significant groups and their orientation which induce marijuana activity. Thorough investigation of the constituents in red oil is necessary to complete the understanding of hemp extracts.

In pharmacology, there is still much to be done in cooperation with the chemist to elucidate in more detail relationship between activity and molecular structure. With pure chemical substances of marijuana activity, it will now be possible to determine experimentally what actions are exerted upon body functions other than those which have hitherto attracted attention. The relationship between the mechanism of ataxia action in the dog and the psychic action in man should be clarified. It has not yet been established that the structural differences between the various marijuana-active substances do not result in a relative prevalence toward ataxia effectiveness by some, psychic effectiveness by others.

In the clinical field, the practical application of these substances must be awaited with the usual necessary patience. The initial experiments of Dr. Allentuck make it appear likely that some use of this interesting drug or its synthetic equivalents will be discovered.

In all phases of this work just completed, the groundwork has been laid so that a wider interest should ensue, and significant contributions may be anticipated in the chemistry, pharmacology and clinical aspects of this class of substances.

REFERENCES

1. Brotteaux, P. *Hachich; herbe de folie et de rêve.* Paris, 1934.

2. Blatt, A. H. A critical survey of the literature dealing with the chemical constituents of Cannabis sativa, *J. Washington Acad. Sc.,*

1938, *28*:465.

3. Beam, W. A test for hashish, *Wellcome Trop. Research Lab. Report*, 1911, *4B*:25.

4. Wollner, H. J., Matchett, J. R., Levine, J. and Valaer, P. Report of the marihuana investigation, *J. Am. Pharm. A.*, 1938, *27*: 29.

— Matchett, J. R., Levine, J., Benjamin, L., Robinson, B. B. and Pope, O. A. Marihuana investigations, *ibid.*, 1940, *29*:399.

— Robinson, B. B. and Matchett, J. R. Marihuana investigations, *ibid.*, 1940, *29*:448.

5. Wood, T. B., Spivey, W. T. N. and Easterfield, T. H. Charas; the resin of Indian hemp, *J. Chem. Soc.*, 1896, *69*:539; and Cannabinol, *ibid.*, 1899, *75*:20.

6. Cahn, R. S. Cannabis indica resin, *J. Chem. Soc.*, 1930:286; 1931:630; 1932:1342; 1933:1400.

7. Adams, R., Hunt, M. and Clark, J. H. Structure of cannabidiol, a product isolated from the marihuana extract of Minnesota wild hemp, *J. Am. Chem. Soc.*, 1940, *62*:196.

8. Adams, R., Pease, D. C. and Clark, J. H. Isolation of cannabinol, cannabidiol and quebrachitol from red oil of Minnesota wild hemp, *J. Am. Chem. Soc.*, 1940, *62*:2194.

9. Jacob, A. and Todd, A. R. Cannabidiol and cannabol, constituents of Cannabis indica resin, *Nature*, 1940, *145*:350

Haagen-Smit *et al.* A physiologically active principle from Cannabis sativa (marihuana), *Science*, 1940, *91*:602.

Powell, G., Salmon, M., Bembry, T. H., and Walton, R. P. The active principle of marihuana, *ibid.*, 1941, *93*:522.

10. Adams, R. *et al.* Structure of cannabidiol, *J. Am. Chem. Soc.*, 1940, *62*:196; 732; 735; 1770; 2215; 2402; 2566; 1941, *63*:2209.

Jacob, A. and Todd, A. R. Isolation of cannabidiol from Egyptian hashish, *J. Chem. Soc.*, 1940, *1*:649.

11. Adams, R. *et al.* Structure of cannabinol, *J. Am. Chem. Soc.*, 1940, *62*:2197; 2201; 2204; 2208; 2401.

Bergel, F., Todd, A. R. and Work, T. S. Observations on the active principles of Cannabis indica resin, *Chem. & Ind.*, 1938, *16*:86.

Work, T. S., Bergel, F. and Todd, A. R. The active principle of Cannabis indica resin, *Biochem. J.*, 1939, *33*:123.

Todd, A. R. *et al.* Cannabis indica, *J. Chem. Soc.*, 1940:649; 1118; 1393; 1941:137.

Powell, G. and Bembry, T. H. Synthesis of cannabinol, *J. Am. Chem. Soc.*, 1940, *62*:2568.

12. Adams, R. *et al.* Conversion of cannabidiol to a product with marihuana activity, *J. Am. Chem. Soc.*, 1940, *62*:2245; 2402; 2566;

1941, *63*:2209.

Russell, P. B. *et al.* Cannabis indica: the relation between chemical constitution and hashish activity, *J. Chem. Soc.*, 1941 :169.

13. Wollner, H. J., Matchett, J. R., Levine, J. and Loewe, S. Isolation of a physiologically active tetrahydrocannabinol from Cannabis sativa resin, *J. Am. Chem. Soc.*, 1942, *64*:26.

14. Adams, R. and Baker, B. R. Structure of cannabidiol; a method of synthesis of a tetrahydrocannabinol which possesses marihuana activity, *J. Am. Chem. Soc.*, 1940, *62*: 2405.

Todd, A. R., *et al.*, Cannabis indica, *J. Chem. Soc.*, *1942: 1121; 1941: 137; 169.*

15. Adams, R., Loewe, S., Jelinek, C. and Wolff, H. Tetracannabinol homologs with marihuana activity, *J. Am. Chem. Soc.*, 1941, *63*:1971.

16. Adams, R., Loewe, S., Smith, C. M. and McPhee, W. D. Tetrahydrocannabinol homologs and analogs with marihuana activity, *J. Am. Chem. Soc.*, 1942, *64*:694.

17. Adams, R., Smith, C. M. and Loewe, S. Tetrahydrocannabinol homologs and analogs with marihuana activity, *J. Am. Chem. Soc.*, 1941, *63*:1973.

Bembry, T. H. and Powell, G. Compounds of the cannabinol type; synthesis of some compounds related to tetrahydrocannabinol, *ibid.*, 1941, *63*:2766.

18. Ghosh, R., Todd, A. R. and Wright, D. C. Cannabis indica; a new synthesis of cannabinol and of a product of hashish activity, *J. Chem. Soc.*, 1941:137.

19. Liataud. Mémoire sur l'histoire naturelle et les propriétés médicales du chanvre indien, *Compt. rend. Acad. d. sc.*, 1844, *18*:149.

20. Fraenkel, S. Chemie und Pharmakologie des Haschisch, *Arch. f. exper. Path. u. Pharm.*, 1903, *49*:266.

21. Gayer, H. Pharmakologische Wertbestimmung von orientalischem Haschisch und Herba cannabis indica, *Arch. f. exper. Path. u. Pharm.*, 1928, *129*:312.

22. Munch, J. C. and Mantz, H. W. *Pennsylvania Pharmacist*, July, 1937.

23. Loewe, S. Synergism of Cannabis and butyl-bromallyl-barbituric acid, *J. Am. Pharm. A.*, 1940, *29*:162.

24. Marx, H. and Eckhardt, G. Tierexperimentelle Untersuchungen über die Wirkung des Haschisch, *Arch. f. exper. Path. u. Pharm.*, 1933, *170*:395.

25. Walton, R. P., Martin, L. F. and Keller, J. H. Relative activity of various purified products obtained from American grown hashish, *J. Pharmacol. & Exper. Therap.*, 1938, *62*:239.

26. Loewe, S. Principle of "bioassay by approximation" and its application to the assay of marihuana (dog) and laxatives (monkey), *J. Pharmacol. & Exper. Therap.*, 1939, *66:*23, and Bioassay of laxatives on monkeys (rhesus) and on lower mammalians, *J. Am. Pharm. A.*, 1939, *28:*427.

27. Matchett, J. R. and Loewe, S. On the preparation of an extract having "marihuana-like" activity from the fruits of Cannabis sativa, *ibid.*, 1941, *30:*130.

28. Homologs were prepared in which the *n*-amyl group was substituted by C_3H_7, C_4H_9, C_6H_{13}, C_7H_{15}, C_8H_{17}, C_9H_{19}; the reduction product of each was also synthesized.

The Active Principles of Cannabis and the Pharmacology of the Cannabinols

BY S. LOEWE, Ph.D.

Today's status of the pharmacology of Cannabis, to be reported here as it has emerged from a fourteen year investigation,* part of which is as yet unpublished, contrasts sharply with the textbook presentations which even now often deal with the subject on the level of a-quarter-of-a-century-old knowledge. In fact, the pharmacological spectrum of the cannabis drug, formerly derived in part from misinterpreted actions of crude preparations of either Oriental (hashish) or American hemp (marijuana), has been classified and re-evaluated; botanical relations between the various "species" of Cannabis have been revised by aid of determinations of their content in active principles; the SAR† of the cannabis-active substances has been elucidated; a new class of chemical agents, comprising products of laboratory synthesis as well as of plant origin, has been opened up; and, last but not least, experimental and clinical investigation of the pure substances has turned a subject of merely toxicological interest into a source of therapeutic potentialities.

* The status of the Cannabis problem immediately before the discovery of the active principles (1938) is best surveyed in Walton's book and Blatt's chemical review. The literature from then on to 1942 will be found in Roger Adams' lecture and in the review which the author in 1941, contributed, upon the La Guardia Committee's invitation, to that committee's book published in 1944.

† "SAR" (relationship between chemical structure and biological activity) has found entrance into the American literature as a concise symbol suggested (Fed. Meetings, 6:352, 1947) for that phrase so difficult to compress into a brief expression, and will be used in that sense (Structure-Activity Relationship) hereinafter.

Originally published in German in *Arch. Exper. Path. u. Pharmakol.*, vol. 211, 1950, pp. 175–193. Translation courtesy of Dr. Carl C. Pfeiffer, New Jersey Bureau of Research in Neurology and Psychiatry, Princeton, New Jersey.

Chemistry of the   That the active substances are contained in the so-called
active principles   "Red Oil," a high-vacuum distillate from cannabis extracts,
of hemp.   had been known for many decades. Only in 1937 to 1942,
however, was it ascertained by the work of an American
research team[*] that the Red Oil consisted essentially of two
inactive substances, cannabinol ($C_{21}H_{26}O_2$; III) and cannabidiol ($C_{21}H_{30}O_2$; I), and a varying mixture of tetrahydrocannabinols ($C_{21}H_{30}O_2$; THC; II a, b, and c), the representatives of "cannabis activity."[†] The conclusion of this first
research phase was marked by a detailed description of the
first and apparently maximally potent natural agent, a THC
from Indian hemp resin, designated as charas tetrahydrocannabinol; its potency (P; cf. below) was 14.6.

Motor ataxia in the dog was the test reaction which served
as a guide in the procedures to isolate the active compounds.
It served to determine their content in the starting materials,
to fractionate the crude oils, and to assay the potency of the
purified substances. That the research plan resulted in success
is due to two circumstances, namely, the choice of the right
test response and its adaptability to quantitative purposes. It
is now evident that motor ataxia is the one action in
experimental animals which closely parallels psychic cannabis
action in man; although this action is not accessible to
evaluation by the customary biostatistical procedures because
of the excessive variation of inter-individual sensitivity of the
dog, a biostatistically adequate assay method could be developed by the introduction of a new principle of "intra-
individual potency comparison."

The history of the discovery of the cannabis-active substances is characterized by the following paradox. On the one
hand, those investigators who followed analytical procedures,
by employing tons of starting material, large-scale molecular

---

[*] H. J. Wollner, J. R. Matchett and J. Levine, Narcotics Laboratory,
U.S. Treasury Department, Washington, D. C.; Roger Adams, et al.,
Department of Chemistry, University of Illinois; and this author.

[†] This is the term to be employed hereinafter for the characteristic
psychic action and its equivalent in the animal experiment, which in
some countries are designated as "hashish action," in others as "marijuana action."

$C_5H_{11}(n)$

I cannabidiol

CH_3CH_2

inner
condensation

CH_3 OH

$C_5H_{11}(n)$

CH_3CH_3

II tetrahydrocannabinol (THC)

Identified isomers:

a. with double bond at 7,8, as shown
b. with double bond at 8,9
c. with double bond at 11,12 (synthetic THC)

CH_3 OH

$C_5H_{11}(n)$

CH_3CH_3

III cannabinol

CH_3 O

$C_5H_{11}(n)$

CH_3CH_3 OH

IV pulegon condensation product (hypothetical tetrahydroxanthane structure)

* *Ed. Note:* In the current chemical structural nomenclature, these formulae would be considerably changed. As an example, the pulegon condensation product would be shown as:

H_3C O

$C_5H_{11}(n)$

CH_3CH_3 OH

The "$-C_5H_{11}(n)$" is the normal amyl group, identical with "$-(CH_2)_4-CH_3$" found in the following review.

distillation, and chromatographic and elution methods rapidly got hold of numerous, obviously chemically pure active substances but were unable to identify them structurally, particularly since even today they foil all attempts at crystallization. On the other hand, the discoverer of the two inactive by-products predicted the structure of the plant principles without going into an analysis of any one of the natural agents. As early as 1930–33, Cahn in England had obtained cannabinol as a major component of the hashish resin formed as a surface excretion on Oriental hemp, and had identified it correctly except for minor inaccuracies in the positions of the hydroxyl and the amyl group. In 1939, Adams demonstrated it to be a 1-hydroxy-3-*n*-amyl-6,6,9-trimethyl-6-dibenzopyran and at the same time prepared it synthetically. Cannabidiol, of which hashish resin contains only minimal quantities, was discovered in 1940 by Adams in extracts from freshly harvested North American hemp as a similarly considerable part (33 percent) of the crude oil, identified as menthadienylolivetol, and synthesized. The chemical relationship between the two substances, their inactivity, and the age differences of the raw materials gave rise to the ingenious hypothesis that cannabidiol signified the starting material and cannabinol the end-product of a phytochemical conversion process and that the intermediates on the way of this process, namely, hydroaromatic cannabidiol-isomeric precursors of cannabinol, may be the searched-for active principles.

This was confirmed on various avenues of approach: (1) Adams, by intramolecular condensation of cannabidiol, obtained—depending on the process of isomerization employed—two such semi-synthetic tetrahydrocannabinols (II b and c), both of which Loewe found to be very markedly cannabis-active; the two isomers differ in optical rotation, position of the double-bond, and potency (7.3 and 8.2). (2) At once, the oily substances which Wollner and Loewe and their associates[5] had isolated from hashish and American hemp and found to be highly potent could now be identified as THC. (3) Soon, Adams mastered the difficult synthesis of another THC (IIa) from 5-methylcyclohexanon-2-carboxylate and olivetol, the much lower potency of which was from then on employed as standard (P = 1). (4) Part of the presumable processes which in nature create the active substances could be imitated *in vitro;* in an inactive cannabidiol synthesized by Adams, which had been irradiated with ultraviolet light, active substances could be demonstrated[4] in an amount which indicated that about 2 percent had been converted to THC.[2]

Like the synthetic cannabidiols, the completely synthetic THCs are racemates, whereas the natural and the semisynthetic THCs are laevorotatory. In 1942, Adams and his associates dissolved the synthetic rac. THC into its two optical isomers (rot. +152 and -114, respectively), and here, too, the *l*-isomer (P = 1.66) turned out to be superior to the *d*-isomer (P = 0.38).[8]

Stereo- and optical isomerism make possible a large number of isomeric THCs which differ in the spatial arrangement of the 9-methyl group and of the planes of the hydro-aromatic ring, and in the position of the double-bond in this ring. Probably all these isomers are cannabis-active, though they differ greatly in potency, and quite a number of them has been prepared from hemps of different origin.[4] The potency of fluid extracts from hemps of different origins also varies quite markedly. Botanically, however, it is noteworthy that on the one hand fluid extracts from hemp cultivated in Rumania, Manchuria, Italy, Tunis and climatically very different parts of U.S.A. were cannabis-active (P: max. 0.52 in Tunisian hemp, min. 0.003 in an American hemp).[4] On the other hand, a hemp grown from Oriental seeds on an experimental field near Washington, D.C., and re-seeded there for three subsequent years maintained its high potency.[4] It is therefore quite possible that the composition of the active fraction constitutes the only difference between various varieties of Cannabis sativa. American hemp appears to be characterized by THCs of P 6.0 to 7.3 and 8.0 to 9.5, which may be identical with Adams's semisynthetic THCs from cannabidiol. In Oriental hemp, THCs of P 12.0 to 14.6 occur, in which the position of the double-bond in the hydro-aromatic ring is as yet undefined and which have not yet been obtained from other hemps. At closer analysis, the cannabinol component of the hemp plant proved also to be cannabis-active; completely synthetic as well as natural, frequently re-crystallized cannabinols had the same potency of 0.04[9], which obviously is only of academic interest. The

Content of Cannabis in active substances.

hexahydrocannabinols are also active[4] and so are presumably the dihydrocannabinols† which can be assumed to be intermediate products in the conversion of THC to cannabinol; but none of these have as yet been demonstrated in hemp. In the plant, the cannabinols appear to occur in part as esters of aromatic acids.[17c]

The content in active substances is not limited to the "flowering tops of the male plant," but occurs in many parts of the plant; for example, even seedlings of a few centimeters in height[4] and seeds[6b] yielded active extracts.

Synthetic cannab- According to the preceding data, cannabinol and all reduc-
inols and Struc- tion products of its toluene ring can be considered to
ture-Activity embody cannabis activity, and, in view of the activity of the
Relationship parent substance, insignificant as it may be, it appears
(SAR) chemically and pharmacologically justified to designate the new class of chemicals as the class of cannabinols. After the gates had been opened by the disclosure of the natural agents and of synthetic procedures, the already mentioned representatives of the class were joined by many other compounds which served in our studies of SAR. Also to a team of British investigators[3, 4] who had already for quite a time devoted themselves to the problem of the Cannabis drugs, that gate opened up a field of successful and, in part, independent chemical research whose results, unfortunately, for reasons to be discussed below did not become serviceable to the comparative study of cannabis activity in its proper sense.

Information on SAR of the class was largely obtained by measurements of the ataxia potencies. It was demonstrated that the l-hydroxyl group is an important component of the phenol ring of the THCs; its effective blockade greatly diminishes activity.[3, 4] Also significant is the position of the substituents of this ring. For example, the 1-n-hexyl-3-hydroxy isomer of parahexyl,* the 3-n-hexyl homolog of the completely synthetic THC, has a P of only 0.05†; i.e., only one-fortieth that of the substance of comparison. The role of the hydro-aromatic ring was studied in many analogs of the "synthetic THC" (P = 1). Lack of the 9-methyl group brings P down to 0.13; its substitution by ethyl, to 0.22; transfer to position 10, to 0.25; to position 8, to 0.14; an additional methyl group in position 7, to 0.75, but in position 8, to 0.11; replacement of the 6, 6-methyls by ethyls reduces P to

0.12, by propyls to 0.04. All such alterations at the cyclohexene ring, as well as opening of the ring so as to leave in its place a 6-*n*-butyl and an 11-methyl group (P = 0.04), reducing it to an 11-methyl group 0.033) or replacing it by cycloheptan (0.21) reduce but do not completely abolish activity.

Not until the significance of the 3-alkyl side chain was studied were increases in potency observed. The changes of P with changes in the length and arrangement of this side chain are presented in condensed form in Figure 1. Essential facts on SAR are as follows: (1) Shortening of the 3-*n*-amyl chain decreases potency.[4] (2) Peak-effective, however, in the series of homologs of the "synth. THC" standard (Series A of Figure) is not this *n*-amyl compound, but its 3-*n*-hexyl homolog (parahexyl).[4] which is about twice as potent (1.8), yet far inferior to the natural THCs. The same relation repeats itself in the other homologous series (C, D; cf. below) having an unbranched side chain.[4] (3) Branching of the side chain can result in substances of far greater P, but in these series (E, F, and G[12-15]) peak potency is associated with a six- but not with a nine-C-atom side chain. (4) Optimum effectiveness was always found in side chains branched near to their "root"; for example, among the methyl-amyl isomers, P decreases consistently from the value 3.65 of the 1'-methylamyl-R (Series E) with transfer of the methyl group into position 2' (H; 1.58), into 3' (K; 1.25), and 4' (L; 1.14). (5) Methyl branching under otherwise equal conditions, appears to grant the greatest activity [compare in Series E 1'-methylamyl-R (3.65) with 1'-ethylbutyl-R (M; 1.68), and 1'-isopropyl-propyl-R (N; 3.18), and in Series G 1', 2'-dimethylbutyl-R (3.84) with 1'-ethyl-2'-methylpropyl-R (P; 3.40)]. (6) Double branching at the same C-atom appears not to offer any advantage over single branching (compare the two Series E and F). In contrast, two methyl branches at two adjoining positions 1' and 2' (Series G) result in representatives of outstanding potency which is only diminished by prolongation of the branched chain (Series P) or by addition of a third branch (Q).*

The role of the third (pyran) ring is illustrated by the observation that analogs of the hypothetical type IV, prepared from pulegon and appropriate resorcinol derivatives, are in tetra- as well as in hexa-hydrated from (Series C and D,

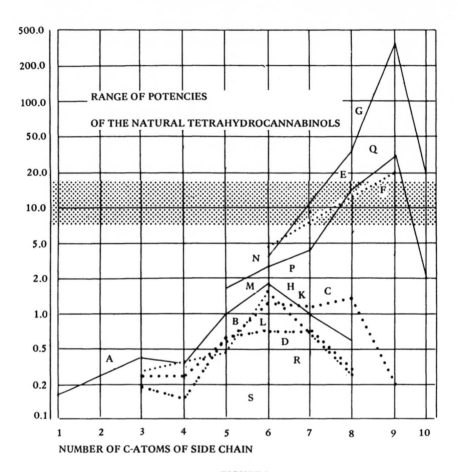

FIGURE I

Relationship between structure of the alkyl side chain and the ataxia potency of the cannabinols. — The majority of the 47 synthetic cannabinols represented in the figure are 1-hydroxy-3-alkyl isomers or homologs of synthetic tetrahydrocannabinol and these are designated, in the following legend, only by the structure of their 3-alkyl side chain. — A:————, 3-*n*-alkyl. — B: ········ , 3-*n*-alkyl (homologs of synthetic hexahydrocannabinol). — C: • • • • • • • • 3-*n*-alkyl (tetrahydrogenated pulegon condensation products). — D: ••• ••• ••• • , 3-*n*-alkyl (hexahydrogenated pulegon condensation products). — E: —————— , 3-(1′-methylalkyl). — F: ············ , 3-(1′,1′-dimethylalkyl). — G: —————— , 3-(1′,2′-dimethylalkyl). — H: 3-(2′-methylamyl). — K: 3-(3′-methylamyl). — L: 3-(4′-methylamyl). — M: 3-(1′-ethylbutyl). — N: 3-(1′-iso-propylpropyl). — P: 3-(1′-ethyl-2′-methylpropyl). — Q: 3-(1′,2′,4′-trimethyl-hexyl). — R: 3-(1′-methylhexyl), tetrahydrogenated pulegon condensation product. — S: 2-cyclohexyl-3-hydroxy. — For further details compare text.

respectively) approximately as potent as the corresponding cannabinols. These compounds may differ from the cannabinols in the mutual position of the two carbon-rings and in the structure of the heterocyclic ring. 1'-methylation appears not to increase potency in this series (cf. R).

Naturally, the problems of SAR are by no means consummated by the comparative bioassays of this scanty hundred of compounds hitherto studied. Many questions, among them that of the applicability of experiences in one series to other series, e.g., to homologs of the natural THCs, are still open. The role of the configuration of the 3-side-chain could certainly be further elucidated by the study of another hundred congeners; for example, substances have been synthesized in which the 3-alkyl chain is linked to the phenol ring by an ether linkage[16 - 17a]; if it were permissible to draw conclusions from the results of the Gayer test, a weak Cannabis activity would have to be ascribed to some of these ethers.[17a]

Only recently, in a study of 2-cyclohexyl-3-hydroxyl-6, 6, 9-trimethyl-7, 8, 9, 10-tetrahydro-dibenzopyran,[11] we found that cyclic arrangement of the side chain is superior to a straight and unbranched side chain (compare S in Figure 1; potencies of the corresponding n-alkyls are below the frame of the graph)—a finding which points to new possibilities.

The substances of the cannabinol class are viscous oils, some solid at room temperature, and extremely poorly water-soluble. Even in the best solvents for cannabinols (acetone, ethanol, glycols), certain representatives with long side chain dissolve only slowly and yield only colloidal solutions. Accordingly, all cannabinols are difficultly absorbed; even after intravenous injection, thirty to sixty minutes and often more elapse until peak effect is attained, and the peak effect persists for hours—even for five days, as was observed after a single medium-sized intravenous dose of the 1'-methylnonyl representative of Series E. Oral administration requires twenty to thirty times the intravenous dose, and subcutaneous administration hardly ever produces a demonstrable effect. Even after high doses, we were as yet unable to demonstrate urinary excretion of active substances.[18] In the blood, however, 1.6 to 10.5 percent of

Conditions of action of the Cannabinols

parahexyl given by vein were found circulating after two to three hours and 2.4 percent after eleven hours; the lungs of a dog contained 0.9 percent of a dose injected twenty hours before.[18] Probably because of these physicochemical characteristics of the compounds, the margin of safety is enormous; per kg body weight, the oral L.D.$_{50}$ of Charas THC in the mouse is more than two hundred thousand times the intravenous threshold dose for ataxia in the dog and more than forty thousand times the oral threshold dose for psychic action in man.[19]

The action spectrum of the cannabinols.

Not all the actions of crude hemp preparations or oil redistillates reported in the literature could be reproduced with pure active substances. At that, many of them are of minor importance at the present state of the Cannabis problem. This holds true, for instance, for the effects upon heart rate, respiration and pupil. Therefore, the following discussion will be limited to those, in part newly revealed, sections of the large action spectrum, which have been studied with the aid of pure substances.

1. Psychic Actions. Analysis of the psychic actions in man, still more so in animals, is a task as yet unsolved. Even with pure substances, neither the host of experimental psychologists of the LaGuardia Committee[20] nor the effects with a "battery of psychological tests" both elsewhere[22] and in test persons in our department[21] were capable of disclosing more than a large range of variation of all phenomena tested. Thus, the availability of numerous pure substances of the class has not as yet given impetus to the analysis of the unique "pleasure action," but a few experiences have been collected which deserve to be mentioned partly as modest beginnings, partly with a view to therapeutic aspects. For instance, both parahexyl[22] and compounds "RA 122" and "RA 125A"[21] were found to have no effect upon the normal human EEG or upon musical appreciation.[22b] Therapeutic effects of parahexyl have been reported in depressive states[23a] but in consideration of the negative experiences of Pond[23b] and of unpublished personal reports to the writer they are in urgent need of further verification. Charas THC has been extensively employed for "psychic relaxation" and is reported[24] to be equivalent to the customary barbiturates for purposes of narcoanalysis, narcocatharsis and narcosuggestion. The idea, however, that Cannabis and morphine may be comparable in euphorizing effects has not proved fruitful in its application to morphine withdrawal; withdrawal symptoms were neither shortened nor abated by parahexyl treatment.[25a] Noteworthy, though difficult to evaluate, are reports on psychiatric episodes, mostly in psychopaths, occurring in some instances under prolonged treatment with, and in other instances upon withdrawal of cannabis-active drugs.[25a-g]

2. *Cataleptic Effects.* They are never missing in the picture of the hemp "jag," always accompany the ataxia effects in the dog, and are produced by all ataxia-active pure substances.[4,19] They can be seen in many species of animals, and a catalepsy test has been described[19] which occasionally has been found quite serviceable.

3. *Ataxia Action.* This has gained ever-increasing prominence among all cannabis actions, as an experimental tool. It is not only highly serviceable,* but is closely correlated with psychic action. This has been confirmed for all those crude and pure products which have been both bioassayed by the writer and evaluated in man[20,24]; particularly good agreement was found between ataxia and psychic potencies of four cannabinols at the occasion of their especially careful and expert evaluation by Dr. L. Kubie. There are only vague notions about the locus and mechanism of the ataxia action.[4] In view of its outspoken parallelity to the psychic action, a close correlation in the mechanisms of the two actions has to be considered seriously. As a matter of course, final proof of both identity in mechanism and the quantitative parallelity can only be expected from an evaluation in man of all the compounds available.

4. *Central Stimulant Actions* were observed with all substances of the class. From medium degress of ataxia upward, dogs at times exhibit convulsive motor symptoms.[4, 19] They are possibly related to the compensatory counteractions against the disturbance in coordination; their frequency varies with the dog's individuality and strain. Indisputable and unique convulsions appear consistently after doses greater than twenty times the threshold ataxia dose after intravenous administration of the high-potent "RA 122" and dominate the picture of action of lethal doses. Mice often become pugnacious after medium doses of cannabinols.[19]

Vomiting occurs in dogs rather regularly and late, usually one to five hours after injection, following doses upward from a medium-effective intravenous dose. The emetic effect as well as the hyperexcitability of the scratch reflexes can probably be ascribed to a central stimulant action.[4, 19]

5. *Hypnotic Activity.* Elements of central nervous stimulation among the actions of hemp are of interest in view of the question of its soporific action. Probably cataleptic symptoms in man have often been interpreted as signs of a sedative action. In the dog, concomitance of catalepsy with higher degrees of ataxia which prevent upright posture results in a syndrome which might impress a superficial observer as sleep. In experiments with combinations of aqueous hemp extracts and hypnotics, Burgi believed he had demonstrated a hypnotic component of Cannabis action.[27] We were able to duplicate his observation with fluid extracts of hemp; they prolonged sleep duration in mice after a pernocton dose which is just enough to suppress the righting reflex. Sleep prolongation, in our experiments, was significant indeed, but only for this one hypnotic; however, even the consideration prolongation by a large dose of Cannabis equals no more than the effect producible by an additional 10 to 20 percent of the pernocton dose employed. Above all, however, a study of pure substances gave proof that this action is due not to any one of the cannabis-active components, but to the otherwise inert cannabidiol.[28] * Moreover, the natural as well as the synthetic cannabis-active substances lack any other indications of central nervous depressant action. Even in states of severest hypomotility and impairment of attention, up into the terminal phases of lethal effect, the animals, quite contrary to those under the influence of hypnotics, still respond, with frustraneous movements to moderate acoustic, tactile, or pain stimuli. This is in accordance with the characteristic criterion of Cannabis action both in dog and in man, namely, that the drugged individual can readily be diverted by environmental stimuli.[4]

6. *Corneal Areflexia.* Abolition of the wink reflex in rabbits after administration of hemp extracts or crude oils was discovered in 1928 by Gayer in Straub's laboratory and considered to be a faithful expression of Cannabis activity.[29] First of all, at closer analysis this systemic action has proved inappropriate for quantitative purposes because of the great

variation in inter- and intraindividual susceptibility. Only after a tedious search in a large stock of animals by way of numerous recalibrations can one find a number of individuals suitable to yield conclusive data in strictly intraindividual potency comparisons[4, 30] that there are two types of areflexia producing agents, namely, (a) ataxia-active THCs which lose neither in ataxia nor in areflexia activity by such oxidation, and (b) other extractives possessing little or no ataxia activity, but a marked areflexia activity which can be destroyed by oxidation. In the search for the as yet unidentified substances of this type (b), the Gayer test in its present[30] more complicated but more reliable form is thus the test reaction of its choice.

7. *Anticonvulsive Action.* It was only by the aid of the highly active synthetic cannabinol congeners and due to the methods elaborated in this laboratory by Goodman and Toman and associates[32] that the antiepileptic activity of cannabinols could be disclosed and specified. All cannabinols tested were effective. Their activity is of the type of anticonvulsant activity of diphenylhydantoin. Like this drug, they abolish the tonic hind leg extensor component in the pattern of supermaximal electroshock in rats and cats[33] (and presumably also in man[34]), whereas they prolong the duration of metrazol convulsions, modify their appearance and display a strong lethal synergism with metrazol.[33] The cannabinols differ from diphenylhydantoin and its congeners by exhibiting, in their maximum-potent representatives, much greater potency and, in reference to lethal effectiveness an incomparably greater margin of safety. When referred to psychic side effects, the therapeutic indices of the various agents vary considerably. In a preliminary experiment,[35] "RA 122" lacked the ability of diphenylhydantoin, discovered by Toman et al.,[36] to raise the threshold of the isolated nerve preparation for electrical stimulation and to prevent the repetitive discharge elicitable by immersion of the nerve in neutral isotonic phosphate solution; it is true that, in view of the minimal water-solubility of the cannabinols, the result is inconclusive.

Alteration of the electroshock pattern points to anti-grand mal activity, suppression of metrazol convulsions to anti-petit mal activity.[32] Accordingly, clinical experiments were undertaken with some of the agents. A first series[37] in diphenylhydantoin-refractory grand-mal epileptics proved noteworthy effectiveness and absence of psychic side effects when "RA 122" was given orally for several months in daily doses of one mg or less, or the weaker isomer, "RA 125A," in somewhat higher dosage. A second series[38] consisted of five institutionalized children with severe grand-mal epilepsy and mental underdevelopment, in whom daily doses of 0.13 gm phenobarbital combined with 0.3 gm diphenylhydantoin or 0.2 gm Mesantoin had proved inadequate. "RA 122," in daily doses of 1.2 to 1.8 mg, was in three children "at least as effective" as prior therapy; the fourth became almost free from attacks and the fifth completely free. Following transfer to 4 mg of "RA 125A," the attacks remained infrequent in one patient, the other one suffered exacerbations. The first patient had a brief paranoid episode, similar to others he had repeatedly experienced prior to the cannabinol therapy. In contrast to their ineffectiveness upon the normal EEG the cannabinols normalized the EEG of grand-mal patients.

The protective activity of cannabinols against electroshock and grand-mal attacks is of theoretical interest in view of the apparent absence of structural relationship between the cannabinols and the antiepileptics from the classes of hydantoins, barbiturates and oxazolidinediones. The practical evaluation of cannabinols as antiepileptics, notwithstanding their superior potency and persistence of action, will largely depend upon the problems of their side effects which will be discussed below.

8. Analgesic Action. It was probably the conceivable tendency to compare every euphorizing drug with. morphine regarding anodynic properties, which brought British investigators to take up anesthesia tests and to ascertain the intravenously injected hashish extracts were somewhat effective, and that some cannabinols of the 1-hydroxy-3-alkyl-R and one of the 2-alkyl-3-hydroxy-R type were considerably effective (see Table 1). Using a modification, introduced in this department by Nickerson, of the customary methods of rat-tail heat stimulation which had also been employed in the afore-mentioned studies, we observed an even greater effectiveness in two other cannabinols.

9. Lethal Action. As already mentioned, large doses are required for a lethal effect, which are not always available and are not easy to administer because of the poor solubility of the substances. Data for quite a number of older preparations (previous to 1947) have been presented previously.[4, 19] Only some particularly illustrative observations need be reported here. The values of intravenous L.D.$_{50}$ in the mouse[4] indicate that the lethal toxicity of pure substances is markedly lower than that of the crude preparations. The necessity of employing solvents such as propylene glycol, which are by no means indifferent, and the minimal water-solubility of the drugs are probably responsible for the poor reproducibility of the lethal-dose values. Such shortcomings are less important than the experience that the lethal mechanism of the same substance can be different with different routes of administration. The late death of dogs after oral administration of parahexyl is associated with profuse intestinal hemorrhage, after intravenous injection with severe pulmonary edema. In contrast, incomparably smaller intravenous doses of "RA 122," which is ataxia-effective even in doses of a few micrograms, cause death associated with convulsions within a few hours, obviously owing to some primary central nervous mechanism. This suggests the interpretation that the lethal effect of the lower-potent cannabis-active substances is due to non-specific mechanisms and that only that of the high-potent agents originates from a mechanism more closely related to the main activity, which in the low-potent substances is masked or outdone by non-specific toxicity.

10. Habituation. The clinical authors of the La Guardia Committee's report, on the basis of observations in chronically marihuana-smoking prisoners, deemed the danger of habituation negligible.[20] This has evoked a vehement controversy.[40] The most lucid answer to the problem of hemp habituation will be found with Goodman and Gilman.[41] Conclusive animal experiments are not available. For its curiosity value, the "beginner's habituation" may be mentioned: The more than one hundred fifty dogs from the writer's twenty-six hundred bioassay experiments, some of which had been tested twice per week for many years, almost invariably exhibited a certain decrease in sensitivity during the period of the three to four initial experiments, and from then on maintained a rather constant susceptibility. This habituation was the more pronounced, the less the individual's postural behavior was dominated by tenseness. Accordingly, the apparent decrease in susceptibility seems to be due to the "learning" of postural responses compensating for the ataxic incoordination, at the mercy of which the individual finds itself quite helpless during its first experiences in ataxia. All other intraindividual variations in susceptibility, as they developed over long periods, were completely irregular, varied in intensity, and consisted in increases as well as decreases; in bitches, they were not without relation to sex cycles and pregnancy, for which reason all assays were conducted in males.

Interrelation between different cannabinol actions. It has been repeatedly emphasized above that up to now all observations have pointed to an even quantitatively close relation between the psychic and the ataxia activity. The ratio between psychic potency in man and ataxia potency in dogs of an individual substance is a constant which varies very little in the entire class. Contrariwise, it has been demonstrated above that neither of these two activities has a constant relationship to lethal activity.

That the corneal areflexia action is not correlated with the ataxia action, is evidenced by the fact that in crude hemp products the two activities can be dissociated by oxidation. It is true that not only the unknown cannabis-inactive substances disclosed by that procedure, but also ataxia-active cannabinol possess areflexia activity. However, the potency ratio between the two activities varies from substance in a wide range, as has been shown earlier[4] for a series of cannabinols and is confirmed in Table 1 in nine, partly new substances. A similar inconstancy of the potency ratios is also evident when analgesia and ataxia activity are compared (Table 1, column 5).

The relation between antiepileptic (anti-electroshock) and ataxia activity is also marked by a certain though lesser inconstancy of the potency ratios (Table 1, column 4). Here, however, the results should be evaluated with greater reserve. For the electroshock experiments, for better comparability of the cannabinols with other antiepileptics, were performed after oral administration of aqueous, lecithin-homogenized emulsions of oily drug solutions, whereas the potency values for ataxia and all other actions were determined after intravenous administration. Since in these comparisons numerator and denominator of the potency ratio originate from experiments with different routes of administration, it is possible that inequality of the ratios is due to differences in absorption, distribution and detoxification. A comparison of the E.D.$_{50}$ values for corneal areflexia of the British investigators with the writer's ataxia values indicates that in some cannabinols the areflexia dose is smaller than the ataxia dose. That makes it tempting to base all evaluation upon the Gayer test which, superficially judged, is more convenient than the ataxia test. For SAR studies and for the assay of cannabis activity of crude preparations and unknown mixtures, this must be urgently discouraged because the potency ratios are so inconstant. Quite inversely, the analgesic dose of all cannabinols and the anti-electroshock dose of some are high as compared with the ataxia dose. In such substances, each of the two therapeutic effects may be obtained only at the price of considerable psychic side effects. Were such an unfavorable potency ratio common to all cannabinols, the outlook would be small indeed that further search could reveal other substances of the class more devoid of these side effects. The inconstancy of the ratios leaves the possibility open that there are cannabinols of a greater therapeutic index both for analgesia and for epilepsy therapy. Actually, available experience already teaches that in clinically equieffective doses the only two cannabinols which have as yet undergone clinical examination are not equally liable to produce psychic side effects: "RA 122" not only exerted greater therapeutic action than "RA 125A" but also had a smaller incidence of psychic Cannabis effects. That the two substances differ clinically with regard to the risk of side effects agrees with the fact that the experimental potency ratios of different cannabinols differ; that "RA 122" has fewer side effects than "RA 125A" is contrary to what one would have expected according to the size of the two potency ratios and may thus indicate that ratios of experimental potency values which are obtained after administration by different routes are not the last word on this subject.

Theoretically, the dissociation between psychic activity on the one hand and analgesia, corneal areflexia and antiepileptic activity on the other hand, as demonstrated by the inconstancy of the respective potency ratios, is probably an indication that the actions compared must be ascribed to different reactive groups or, more generally expressed, to different parts of the total configuration of the same drug molecule.

Summary.   1. This review attempts to present some evidence for the proemial statement that our knowledge of the cannabis drugs has undergone a striking change.

2. After a report on the isolation of the natural Cannabis agents and their identification as tetrahydrocannabinols, their subsequently studied synthetic isomers and analogs are surveyed and some data are reported on the structure-activity relationship in this new class of chemicals, the cannabinols.

3. The pharmacology of the cannabis-active substances, as revised with the aid of a study of the pure substances, is briefly presented, and examples are given for the decisive elucidation obtained by the study of the most recent, highest-potent synthetic agents, the potency of which was found to be up to seventy times the average and up to thirty-five times the maximum potency of natural tetrahydrocannabinols.

4. Some details and therapeutic trials of the psychic cannabis action are reported.

5. The significance of the ataxia action in the dog, which appears to parallel closely the psychic action in man, for identification and bioassay of cannabis-active compounds is illustrated and, contrariwise, the corneal areflexia in the rabbit is discussed as a quite detached property of some of the hemp products and congeners, which is only of very limited usefulness.

6. The old question of the hypnotic activity of the Cannabis drugs is answered in the negative from a study of the pure substances; closest to hypnotic activity is the practically insignificant, very limited capability of crude preparations to prolong the hypnotic action of certain barbiturates, an activity which is absent in the pure cannabis-active substances and embodied only in an otherwise inert by-product, cannabidiol.

7. The analgesic activity of cannabinols, only recently disclosed and not yet tested for its practical applicability, is briefly discussed.

8. In their anticonvulsant activity, also an only recently discovered property, the cannabinols are demonstrated to be closely related to diphenyl-hydantoin, according to both

experimental criteria and clinical experiences; the most potent synthetic congener of the cannabinols appears to possess more than one hundred fifty times the anti-grand mal potency of diphenyl-hydantoin.

9. The problem of the therapeutic indices of the five major actions and that of their mutual relations in the roles of main and side actions are dealt with on the basis of experimental data; the potency ratios hitherto established do not preclude the possibility that continued search of the new class of compounds will lead to congeners having a still greater margin of antiepileptic effectiveness than the as yet best examined "RA 122," and perhaps also to congeners having an adequate therapeutic index of analgesic activity.

10. Contributions are presented to the problems of habituation and of the mechanism of the lethal action; as a menace of habituation, addiction and tolerance the cannabis-active drugs appear to rank lowest among the narcotics, and according to the margin of safety some of them rank uppermost among all drugs.

TABLE 1

1	2	3	4	5
		Potency Ratios P/P'[b] P': ataxia; P:		
	ataxia potency[a]	corneal areflexia	anticonvulsant potency	analgesia
1-hydroxy-3-alkyls:				
1. n-amyl (synth. THC)	$1,4^4$	1,18	—	3,33
2. n-amyl (Charas-THC)	$14,6^5$	0.15^{30}	0,08	$0,41^d$
3. n-hexyl (Parahexyl)	$1,82^4$	1,0	1,0	1,0
4. 4'-methylamyl (isohexyl)	$1,14^{13}$	0,16	—	—
5. n-heptyl	$1,05^4$	1,73	—	—
6. 1'-methylheptyl	$16,4^{13}$	1,33	—	0,067
7. 1',2'-dimethylheptyl (RA 125A)	$60,0^e$	—	1,67	—
8. 1',2'-dimethylheptyl (RA 122)	$512,0^{14}$	—	0,40	—
3-hydroxy-2-alkyls:				
9. n-hexyl	$0,028^e$	8,6	—	71,4
10. n-heptyl	$0,010^e$	48,5	—	—
11. cyclohexyl	$0,074^e$	10,1	—	—
	Mean:	8,0	0,79	15,2
	s.e.:	15,6	0,70	28,0
	% s.e.f:	195%	89%	184%

* The details underlying the figures of the Table will be published separately; for the present purpose of demonstrating the inconstancy of the P/P'-ratios the details can be dispensed with. — a: All values referred to synth. THC. — b: All

\

REFERENCES

1. Walton: Marihuana. Philadelphia—London 1938.

2. Blatt: J. Washington Acad. Sci. **28**, 465 (1938).

3. Adams: Harvey Lectures, Ser. **37**, 168 (1941–42).

4. Loewe: Studies on the Pharmacology of Marihuana. In: The Marihuana Problem in the City of New York. Lancaster 1944.

5. Wollner, Matchett, Levine & Loewe: Jour. Amer. Chem Soc. **64**, 26 (1942).

6a. Loewe: Jour. Amer. Pharmaceut. Ass. **28**, 427 (1939).

6b. Matchett & Loewe: ibid. **30**, 130 (1941).

6c. Loewe: Science **106**, 89 (1947).

7. Levine: Jour. Amer. Chem. Soc. **66**, 1868 (1944).

8. Adams, Smith & Loewe: ibid. **64**, 2087 (1942).

9. Loewe: Science **102**, 615 (1945).

10. Madinaveitia, Russell & Todd: Jour. Chem. Soc. **1942**, 628.

11. Avison, Morrison & Parkes: ibid. **1949**, 952.

12. Adams, Chen. & Loewe: Jour Amer. Chem. Soc. **67**, 1534 (1945).

13. Adams, Aycock & Loewe: ibid. **70**, 662 (1948).

14. Adams, Mackenzie & Loewe: ibid. **664**.

15. Adams, Harfenist & Loewe: ibid. **71**, 1624 (1949).

16. Alles, Icke & Feigen: ibid. **64**, 2031 (1942).

17a. Bergel, Morrison, Rinderknecht, Todd, MacDonald & Woolfe: Jour Chem. Soc. **1943**, 286.

17b. Bergel & Wagner: Ann. d. Chem. **482**, 55 (1930).

18. Loewe: Jour. Pharmacol. and Exper. Therap. **86**, 294 (1946).

19. Loewe: ibid. **88**, 154 (1946).

20. The Mayor's Committee on Marihuana, Clin. Study in: The

---

values referred to Parahexyl. — c: = Anti-electroshock potency, according to unpublished experiments of Dr. E. A. Swinyard. — d: This value results from the author's own experiments (analgesia comparisons after oral administration), whereas all other values of this column are calculated from the analgesia doses which Avison c.s.[11] determined after intravenous injection. Hence this value is not directly comparable with the other values of this column, but this is of no significance for the overall outcome. — e: Loewe, unpublished. — f: s.e. as percentage of mean.

Marihuana Problem in the City of New York. Lancaster, 1944.

21. Davis: Unpublished.

22a. Williams, Himmelsbach, Wikler, Ruble & Lloyd: Publ. Health Reports 61, 1059 (1946).

22b. Aldrich: ibid. 59, 431 (1944).

23a. Stockings: Brit. Med. J. 1947, 918.

23b. Pond: J. Neurol. 11, 271 (1948).

24. Kubie & Margolin: Psychosomat. Med. 7, 147 (1945).

25a. Himmelsbach: South. Med. J. 37, 26 (1944).

25b. Fraser: Lancet 1949, 747.

25c. Chopra, Chopra & Chopra: Indian J. Med. Res. 30, 1 (1942).

25d. Marcovitz & Myers: War Medicine 6, 382 (1944).

25e. Bromberg: J. Am. M. A. 113, 4 (1949).

25f. Reichard: Fed. Probationer, Oct.-Dec. 1946, 15.

25g. Allentuck & Bowman: Amer. J. Psychiat. 99, 248 (1942).

26. Loewe: Federation Proc. 6, 352 (1947).

27. Gisel: Z. f. exper. Path. u. Ther. 18, 1 (1916). Burgi: (German). med. Wschr. 1924, Nr. 45.

28. Loewe: J. Amer. Pharm. A. 29, 162 (1940).

29. Gayer: Arch. exper. Path. u. Pharmakol. 129, 312 (1929).

30. Loewe: J. Pharmacol. and Exper. Therap. 84, 78 (1945).

31. Alles, Haagen-Smit, Feigen & Dendliker: ibid. 76, 21 (1942).

32. Goodman & Toman: Proc. First Nat. Med Chemistry Symp. of the Amer. Chem. Soc. 1948, June 17-19, 93; Toman & Goodman: Physiol. Rev. 28, 141 (1948); Goodman, Toman & Swinyard: Arch. Internat. de Pharmacodynamie 78, 144 (1949).

33. Loewe & Goodman: Federation Proc. 6, 352 (1947).

34. Toman, Loewe & Goodman: Arch. Neurol. a. Psychiat. 58, 312 (1947).

35. J. E. P. Toman: Personliche Mitteilung.

36. Toman, Greenhalgh, Carlson & Bjorkman: Federation Proc. 8, 284 (1949).

37. Belknap, Ramsey & Loewe: Unpublished.

38. Davis & Ramsey: Federation Proc. 8, 284 (1949).

39. Davies, Raventos & Walpole: Brit. J. Pharmacol. and Chemotherapy 1, 113 (1946).

40. Bouquet: Jour. Amer. Med. Ass. 124, 1010 (1944). Bowman: 125, 376 (1944); (editorial) 127, 1129 (1945); Walton: 128, 383 (1945); Bowman: 899. Anslinger: 1187; Marcovitz: 129, 387 (1946);

41. Goodman & Gilman: The Pharmacological Basis of Therapeutics, New York, 2nd edition.

Recent Developments in Cannabis Chemistry

BY ALEXANDER T. SHULGIN, Ph.D.

The marijuana plant *Cannabis sativa* contains a bewildering **Introduction** array of organic chemicals. As is true with other botanic species, there are representatives of almost all chemical classes present, including mono- and sesquiterpenes, carbohydrates, aromatics, and a variety of nitrogenous compounds. Interest in the study of this plant has centered primarily on the resinous fraction, as it is this material that is invested with the pharmacological activity that is peculiar to the plant. This resin is secreted by the female plant as a protective agent during seed ripening, although it can be found as a microscopic exudate through the aerial portions of plants of either sex. The pure resin, hashish or charas, is the most potent fraction of the plant, and has served as the source material for most of the chemical studies.

The family of chemicals that has been isolated from this source has been referred to as the cannabinoid group. It is unique amongst psychotropic materials from plants in that there are no alkaloids present. The fraction is totally nitrogen-free. Rather, the set of compounds can be considered as analogs of the parent compound cannabinol (I), a fusion product of terpene and a substituted resorcinol. Beyond the scope of this present review are such questions as the distribution of these compounds within the plant, the botanic variability resulting from geographic distribution, the diversity of pharmacological action assignable to the several

Reprinted from *Journal of Psychedelic Drugs*, vol. II, no. 1, 1971.

distinct compounds present, and the various preparations and customs of administration. This presentation will be limited to chemical structure and synthesis, with only passing comments on the topics of biosynthesis and human use.

Early Structural Studies   A brief review of the early analytical and synthetic studies in the area of cannabis chemistry is necessary as a background for the discussion of recent developments. Cannabinol (I) was the first compound isolated from the resin of *Cannabis sativa* as a pure chemical substance. Its synthesis established the carbon skeleton that is common to the entire

Fig. 1

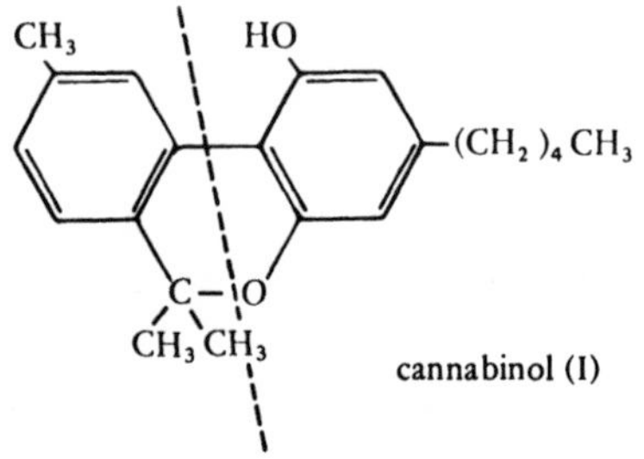

cannabinol (I)

group of cannabinoids. This 21-carbon system can be best described as an amalgamation of a 10-carbon monoterpene and 5-amylresorcinol (olivetol). The terpene half is shown to the left of the dotted line above. In cannabinol, it is completely aromatic and represents a molecule of cymene. In all of the remaining cannabinoids isolated from the native resin it is found in a partially hydrogenated state, usually with a single double bond remaining. The resorcinol moiety, olivetol, is the portion that is represented to the right of the dotted line. It is to be found as an invariable component of all the constituents of the resin, although as will be described below, it often appears as the corresponding carboxylic acid, olivetolic acid. Synthetic variations on the amyl group have proved to be one of the most rewarding series of studies in this area of chemistry, and represents most of the structure-activity investigations that have been pursued. This early synthetic work will be described only briefly, for it has involved analogs of tetrahydrocannabinol which display the terpene double bond in an unnatural position. The most recent chemical advances represent syntheses of the exact natural products, and these will be the body of this discussion.

A brief comment is desirable concerning the various modes of ring numbering that have been employed in this area. Four separate and distinct methods can be found in the chemical literature. Each has a virtue over the others, but each carries with it limitations. These complications arise from the fact that, in many of the cannabinoids present in the natural resin, the oxygen-containing ring (the pyran ring in the cannabinol above) is not present. These materials as isolated are dihydroxybiphenyls, with no heterocyclic ring.

The first of these numbering systems was introduced by Todd in England. It considers these substances best referred to as variously substituted pyrans. Thus the base numbers are

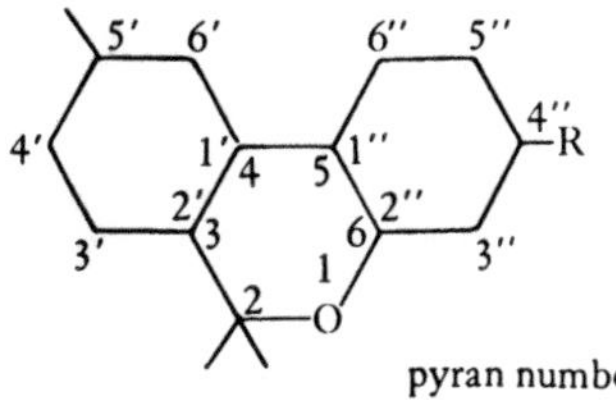

Fig. 2

pyran numbering

assigned to the pyran ring, and the 4,5-bond between the two remaining rings defines the 1-position of each. The first of these, the "prime" set, is applied to the terpene ring and proceeds clockwise. The second, or "double prime" set, refers to the aromatic ring and proceeds counterclockwise. Thus the carbon atoms common to the pyran ring are numbered one and two in each case.

A related numbering system is one that employs the Chemical Abstracts convention. Here these substances are considered as substituted dibenzopyrans, and are numbered

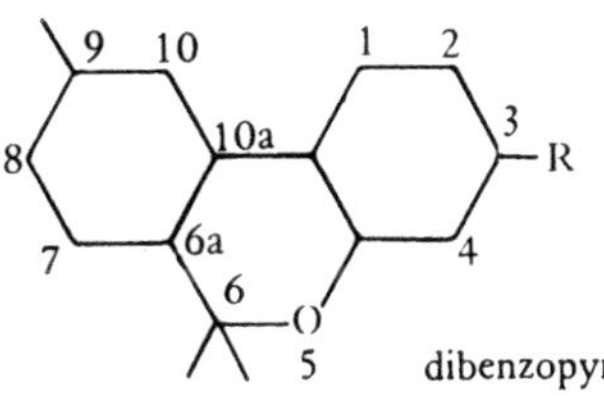

Fig. 3

dibenzopyran numbering

starting with the first unfused position of the aromatic ring. The obvious disadvantage of both of these systems is that the numbering must be totally changed in those isomers in which the central pyran ring is open.

To compensate for this latter limitation, a biphenyl numbering system has come into usage, primarily in Europe.

Fig. 4

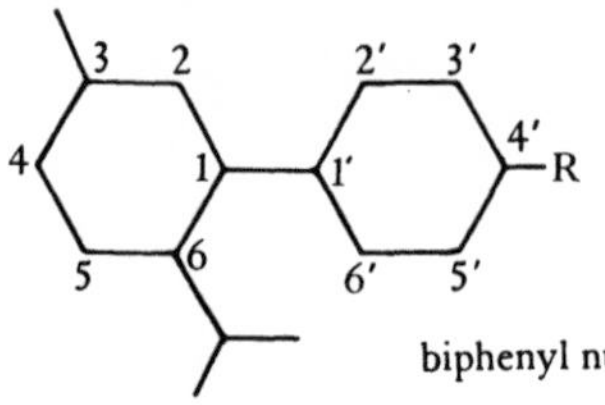

biphenyl numbering

Here, the various substitution positions are sequentially numbered from the central carbon bond of biphenyl. The terpene ring is fundamental, and the aromatic ring commands the prime numbers. The advantages of this system are reciprocal to those mentioned above. The open ring compounds are easily numbered, but there is no general convention that extends to modifications that include the pyran ring. Note should be made of the fact that the course of numbers in the terpene ring is opposite to that of the other systems.

Most broadly used today is a numbering system that recognizes both the terpene nature and the aromatic nature of the two different parts of the molecule. Thus the terpene is numbered in a manner that is conventional for it, i.e., from the ring carbon that carries the branched methyl group. This is in turn numbered seven, and the remaining three carbons

Fig. 5

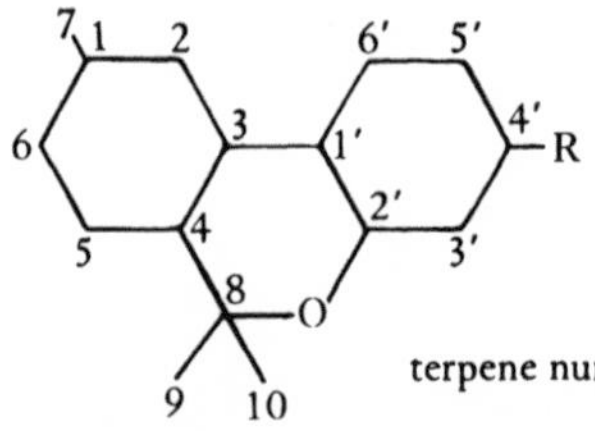

terpene numbering

of the isopropyl group are then numbered sequentially. The aromatic ring assignments are straightforward. The overwhelming advantage here is that this numbering system is applicable whether the center ring is open or closed, and further it can be extended to new compounds that may be isolated as long as they can be represented as a combination of a terpene and an aromatic ring. The only exception is in the instance that the terpene portion is an open chain. Examples of this are known, and their numbering system will be mentioned later.

A brief discussion of the early synthetic efforts in this area is informative, as it provides the only systematic correlation between chemical structure and biological activity. Early in these chemical studies, at about the time of World War II, two compounds were isolated from the red oil fraction of cannabis. One was an optically active tetrahydrocannabinol which carried a double bond in the terpene ring. The other was the open-ring counterpart; it contained two phenolic groups and two double bonds. It was also optically active,

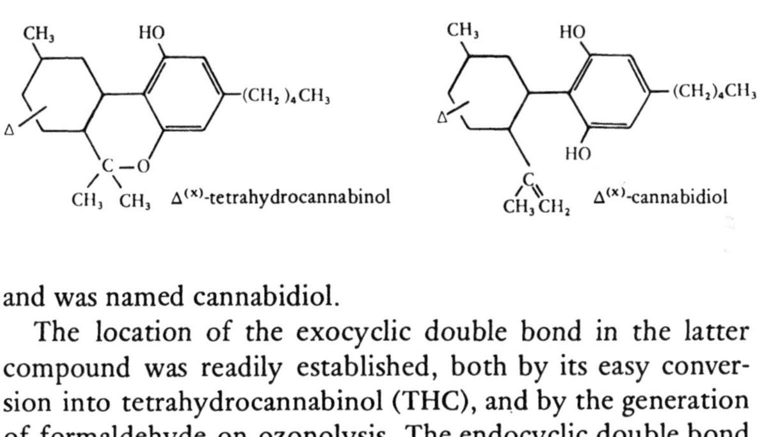

Fig. 6

$\Delta^{(x)}$-tetrahydrocannabinol $\Delta^{(x)}$-cannabidiol

and was named cannabidiol.

The location of the exocyclic double bond in the latter compound was readily established, both by its easy conversion into tetrahydrocannabinol (THC), and by the generation of formaldehyde on ozonolysis. The endocyclic double bond proved to be extremely difficult to locate. It was known not to be in conjugation either with the exocyclic counterpart of with the aromatic ring. This still left three possibilities, the Δ^1, the Δ^5, and the $\Delta^{1\,(6)}$-THCs.

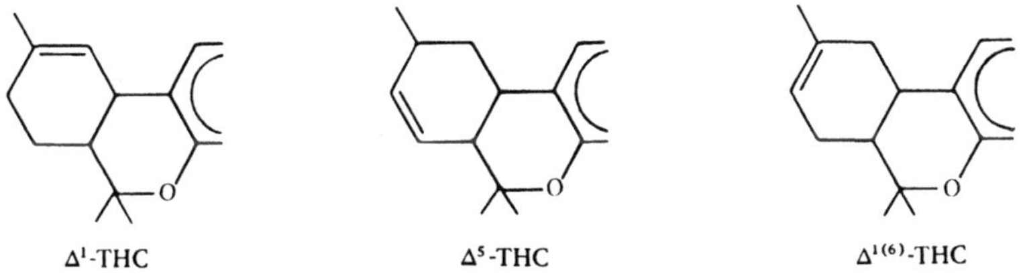

Fig. 7

Δ^1-THC Δ^5-THC $\Delta^{1(6)}$-THC

Although this problem has only recently been solved, during the period of these initial isolations and characterizations, synthetic explorations were numerous. As two generally different synthetic methods were employed, and two different biological assays as well, it is quite difficult to interrelate these studies. The first of the tetrahydrocannabinol syntheses was that of Todd and co-workers in England. Their scheme consisted in the fusion of a terpene such as pulegone with olivetol, thus producing the three ring product. Pharmacological evaluations were made employing

Fig. 8

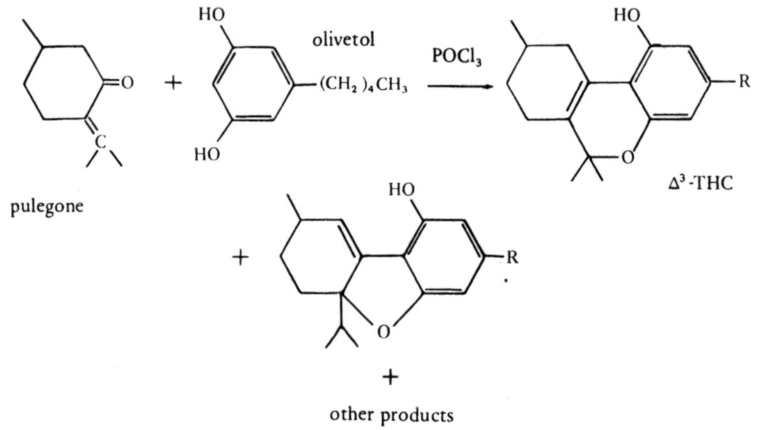

rabbit corneal areflexia; unfortunately there are no available correlations between this response and human intoxicative potency. Two serious complications have appeared in this approach. The pulegone employed has been shown to be of uncertain optical purity, thus leading to optically active products of inconsistent composition. Further, the actual nature of the condensation leads to structural isomers. This was due in part to the contamination of pulegone as isolated from natural sources with isopulegone, and in part to a sensitivity to the specific nature of the condensation agent.

A more satisfactory scheme was developed by Adams and his co-workers at Illinois. In this process a completely synthetic keto-ester was condensed with olivetol, and the resulting lactone converted in a separate step to the gem-dimethyl product. Again, as with the pulegone synthesis above, the unnatural Δ^3 isomer of THC was the principle

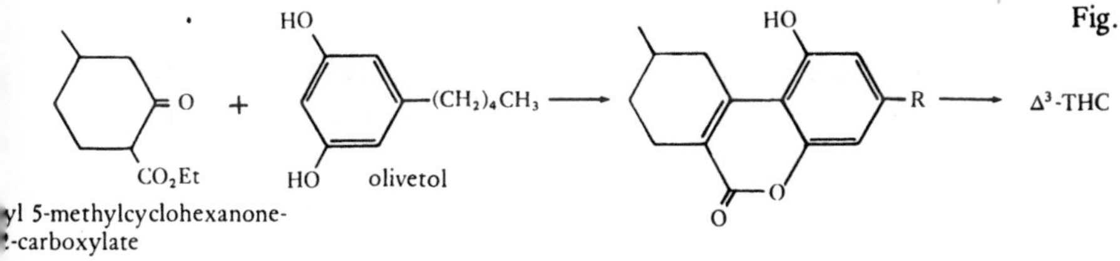

Fig. 9

ethyl 5-methylcyclohexanone-
2-carboxylate

product. This, and related homologs, were titrated pharmacologically by dog ataxia assay. They were found to be
qualitatively similar although quantitatively less active than
natural THC isolated from the red oil. This unnatural but
reproducibly available isomer was taken as a reference standard for an extensive study of structural modifications.

A complete review of these studies would be out of place
in a presentation designed to emphasize recent developments.
Comment should be made, however, on the importance of
the amyl group on the aromatic ring. It was found that, in
the straight chain series, a maximum activity was observed at
the 6-carbon (hexyl) substitution. This material was about
twice as active as the reference amyl compound in the ataxia
analysis, and has undergone extensive clinical study under the
name of Synhexyl or Pyrahexyl. The replacement of the
straight chain with one branched at the alpha- carbon, led to
the alpha-methylhexyl counterpart, with the increase of
potency of a full order of magnitude. The studies that have
resulted in the development of alpha, beta- dimethyl analogs,
have led to the dimethylheptyl-analog, a compound known as
DMHP or Adams' nine-carbon compound. It is yet a full

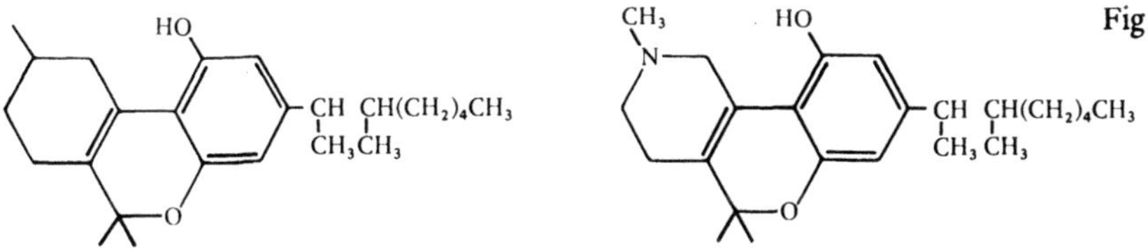

Fig. 10

Adams' 9-carbon compound

Pars' nitrogen analog

order of magnitude more potent than the methyl hexyl
material mentioned above, i.e., five hundred times more
potent than the reference Δ^3-THC. Its activity has been
confirmed in human subjects, and just recently the tedious

task of its separation into the eight possible isomers has been reported by Aaron. Quite recently a nitrogen analog of this compound has been prepared by Pars, and appears also to be biologically active.

Recent Chemical Analyses In recent years, immense strides have been made in the area of the chemistry of the cannabinoids of *C. sativa*. The development of sophisticated spectroscopic instruments, particularly in nuclear magnetic resonance, has settled the question of the exact isomeric configuration of the elusive double bond in the terpene ring, and has established the stereoconfiguration about the 3,4-position. The principle isomer present in the red oil is Δ^1-tetrahydrocannabinol, II, in which the 3,4-hydrogens are oriented trans- to one another. The open-ring counterpart to Δ^1-THC is consequently Δ^1-3,4-trans-cannabidiol (III). It has been reported that the $\Delta^{1(6)}$-isomer of THC (IV) is also present in the

Fig. 11

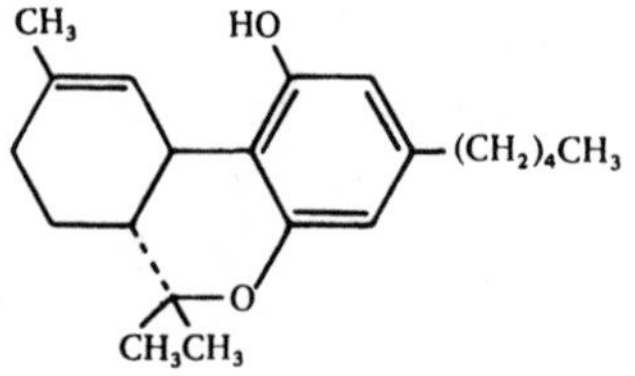

Δ^1-3,4-trans-tetrahydrocannabinol (II) 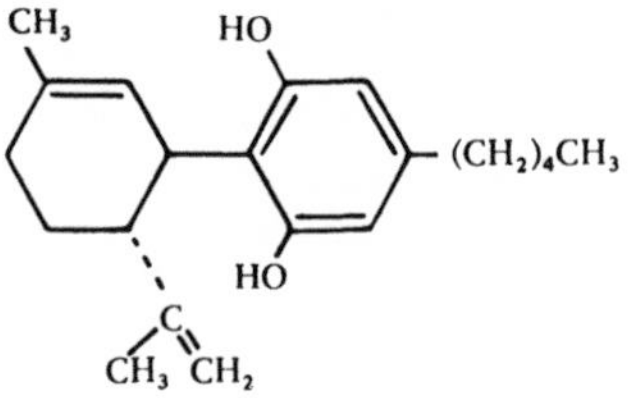 Δ^1-3,4-trans-cannabidiol (III)

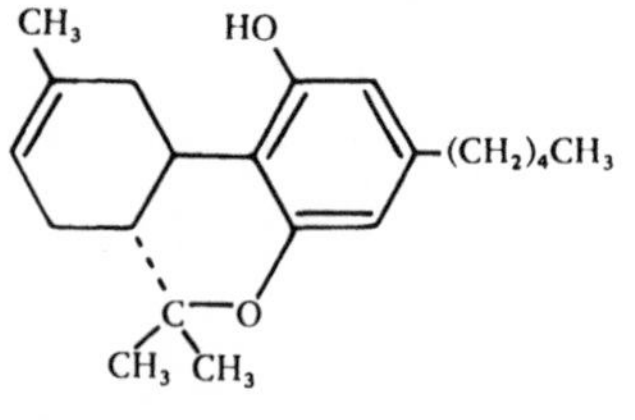

$\Delta^{1(6)}$-trans-tetrahydrocannabinol (IV)

native resin, but this is uncertain as it could have arisen as an artifact of isolation.

None of these fine structural assignments could have been possible, however, without the development of elegant methods of fractionation and isomer separation concurrently with the instrument techniques. The procedures of column and thin layer chromatography have made possible not only the isolation of characterizable amounts of isomerically pure materials, but have led to the discovery of a host of

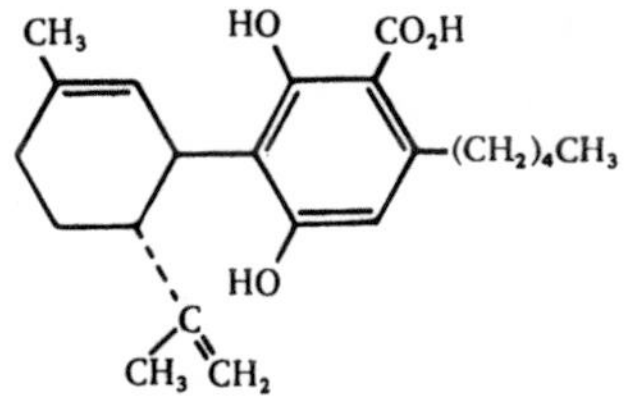

cannabidiolic acid (V)

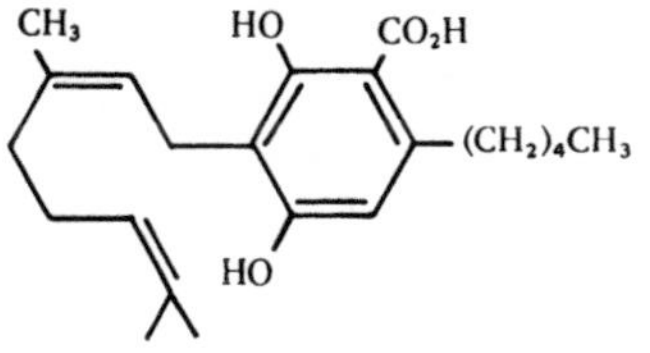

cannabigerolic acid (VI)

Fig. 12

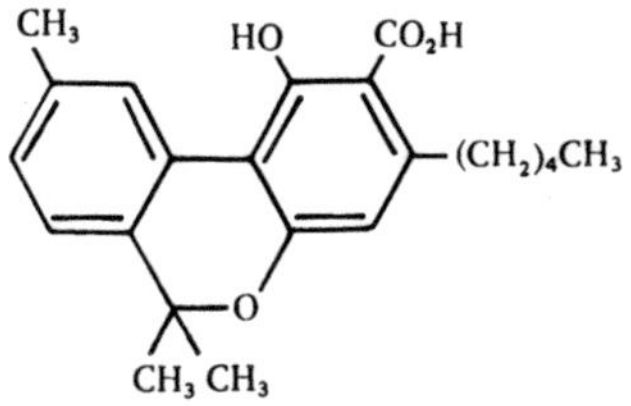

cannabinolic acid (VII)

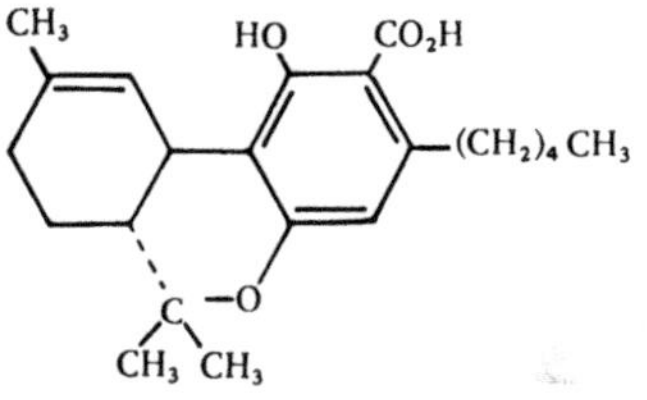

Δ^1-3,4-trans-THC acid (VIII)

additional chemicals that had heretofore been unknown.

An acidic fraction has long been known to be present in the red oil of *C. sativa*. Some ten years ago an acid was isolated which proved to be, after structural correction for the now-known location of the endocyclic double bond of Δ^1-THC, the benzoic acid that corresponds to III, i.e., cannabidiolic acid, V. This material corresponds to cannabidiol both in the double bond location and in the trans-configuration about the 3,4-bond. The presence of this and other acidic materials in the resins isolated from marijuana grown in the colder northern latitudes suggests their roles as biosynthetic presursors to the more neutral aromatic, active, fractions. Careful chromatographic separation of this acidic fraction into individual components has afforded three more aromatic carboxylic acids. These are cannabigerolic acid (VI) that upon decarboxylation could yield cannabigerol (*v.i.*), cannabinolic acid (VII) which can give rise to cannabinol (I), and Δ^1-3,4-trans-tetrahydrocannabinolic acid (VIII) which can be converted to, and which may well be argued as being a normal biosynthetic precursor to, Δ^1 THC. The possible roles of these acids as biological intermediates which could lead to the neutral (phenolic) cannabinoids, will be discussed below.

In the chromatographic analysis of the less plentiful components of the resinous fraction of *C. sativa* several

additional phenolic components have been isolated and assigned tentative chemical structures.

A one-ring resorcinol has been separated that, upon spectroscopic analysis, appeared to be the simple fusion of an
open-chain terpene and olivetol. This material, cannabigerol
(IX) has had its structure proven by synthesis. The fusion of
this terpene with olivetolic acid would then give rise to the
above-mentioned acid, cannabigerolic acid (VI). This type of
open-ring terpene compound presents yet another numbering

Fig. 13

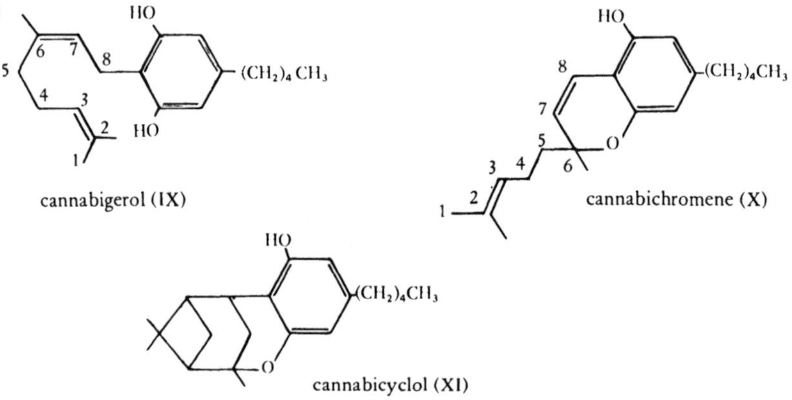

cannabigerol (IX)

cannabichromene (X)

cannabicyclol (XI)

system, being determined by the eight-carbon chain attached
to the olivetol nucleus. The numbering by convention starts
at the distal end of the chain, as shown in IX and X.

Two additional phenolic components have recently been
described. Cannabichromene, X, is an open-chain benzopyran
containing a carbon system closely related to the material
cannabigerol but with heterocyclic ring closure. A phenol
named cannabicyclol (XI) has also been isolated which,
lacking any unsaturation whatsoever, has been assigned the
structure shown. These two hypothetical structures lack
support from synthetic studies. These fusions of terpenes and
aromatics have suggested several of the resent synthetic
approaches into this area, and also provide the basis of
biosynthetic paths, to be discussed.

Recent
Chemical
Syntheses
An expected correlary to the establishment of the tools of
structural analysis of *C. sativa,* was their use in the development and evaluation of synthetic techniques. It must be
noted that, in this same period of time—the last four years or

so—no less than six separate and mutually confirmatory syntheses within this family of compounds have appeared in the chemical literature. Three of these represent modifications of the olivetol ring providing the basis for the construction of the terpenacious half of the cannabinoid molecule. The remaining three syntheses employ the reactivity of the resorcinol system itself and, in effect, bring a terpene into reaction with it.

The first of these procedures can be illustrated by the general reaction between citral and the lithio-derivative of the dimethyl ether of olivetol. The first description of this reaction was advanced by Mechoulam and Gaoni. The coupling product shown undergoes an internal rearrangement to yield the trans- isomer of the dimethyl ether of cannabidiol. Demethylation leads to cannabidiol itself, and cyclization provides a mixture of the Δ^1 and the $\Delta^{1(6)}$ -isomers of THC. The over-all yield in this procedure is small.

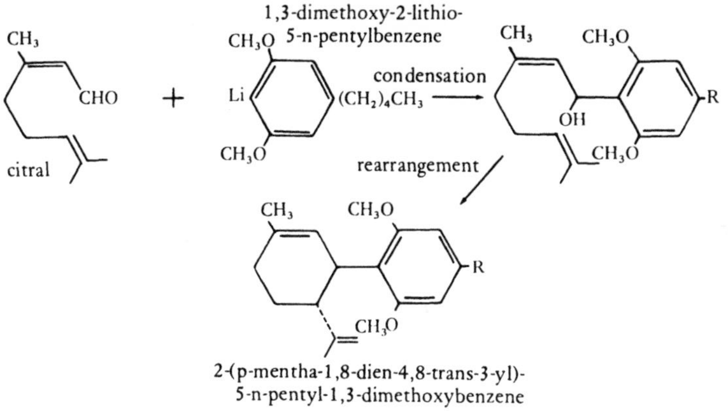

Fig. 14

2-(p-mentha-1,8-dien-4,8-trans-3-yl)-
5-n-pentyl-1,3-dimethoxybenzene

Taylor, Lenard and Shvo have confirmed this reaction scheme and have found that the $\Delta^{1(6)}$ -trans isomer of THC to be a principle product. They did obtain after chromatographic separation, a reasonable yield of the Δ^1 -THC isomer. Very recent modifications of the procedure of Taylor have been investigated by Gaoni and Mechoulam, in which they use BF_3 rather than HCl as the condensation agent between the terpene and olivetol. They have observed a 20 percent yield of the stereo-specifically proper isomer of Δ^1 -THC. The details of these most recent studies have not yet been published.

Two more syntheses have been described which employ

modifications of the olivetol molecule. Both effect the construction of the terpene ring through some form of the Diels-Alder reaction, but the necessary intermediates are derived in different ways.

In one of these processes, the diene is attached to the olivetol nucleus, between the two oxygen functions. This

Fig. 15

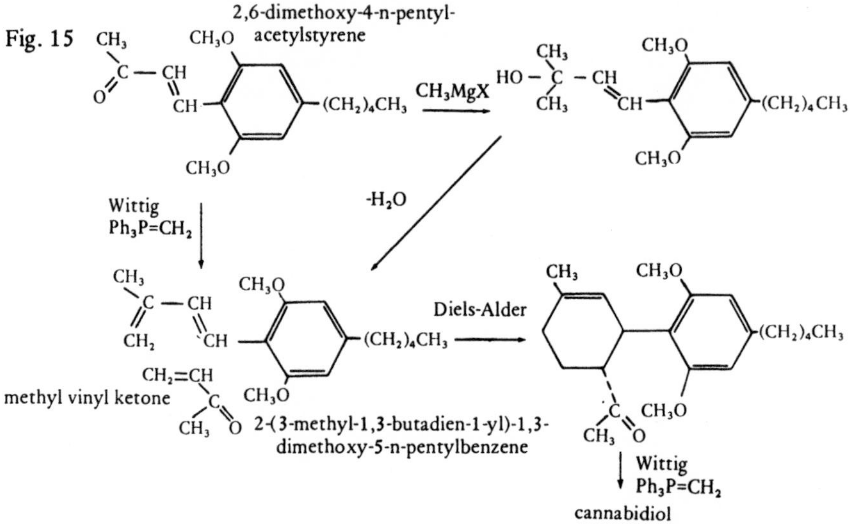

diene has been obtained through two separate procedures. In one, Korte, Dlugosch, and Claussen converted the appropriate ketonic intermediate directly to the diene through a Wittig reaction. In the other, Kochi and Matsui dehydrated the carbinol that resulted from a Grignard reaction on this ketone. In both cases, they achieved an identical diene that cyclized readily with methyl vinyl ketone. This reaction led to a stereo-specifically correct bicyclic methyl ketone which, upon a Wittig methylene replacement, led to the dimethyl ether of cannabidiol. The yields are poor, but both the stereo-configuration and the double-bond location are correct for the natural orientation.

The other Diels-Alder synthesis involves a scheme in which the dieneophyle is itself attached to the olivetol nucleus. Here either the cinnamic acid or the corresponding methyl ketone is employed as a condensing agent with isoprene. Korte, Hackel and Sieper have reported this reaction with the styryl methyl ketone and have found that the isoprene orientation is proper. After the necessary Wittig reaction,

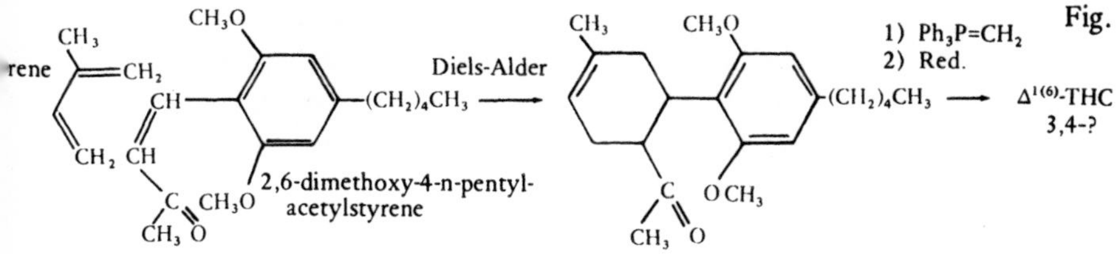

Fig. 16

they found that the resulting $\Delta^{1(6)}$-cannabidiol did not have an assignable configuration about the 3,4-bond. A modification of this approach has been described by Jen, Hughes and Smith in which, through the employment of the free cinnamic acid itself, a product is obtained that is not only

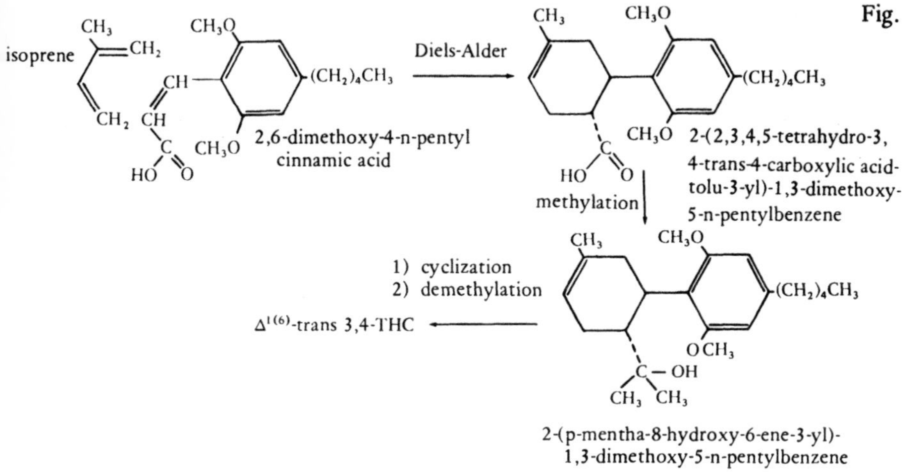

Fig. 17

properly oriented with regard to the isoprene molecule, but is also appropriately trans- about the eventual 3,4-terpene bond. This carboxylic acid has been resolved into its optical isomers. These separate enantiomorphs have been appropriately methylated, cyclized, and finally demethylated to provide both the natural and the unnatural optical isomers of $\Delta^{1(6)}$-THC. In neither of these reactions is the yield good, and it is only in the second example that the appropriate stereoconfiguration is obtained. This must be isomerized at an additional expense in yield, to the natural Δ^1-isomer.

The three remaining synthetic procedures all employ olivetol as a free resorcinol, not protected or activated in any manner. The first of these examples represents a complete

construction of the terpene ring through synthetic procedures, but the last two involve reactions with natural or
near-natural terpenes, and so might cast light on those
biosynthetic pathways actually effected in the plant in the *in
vivo* production of these cannabinoids.

Fahrenholtz, Lurie and Kierstead have reported the
syntheses of both the Δ^1- and the $\Delta^{1\,(6)}$-3,4-trans-tetra-
hydrocannabinol through a synthetic process that represents
a complete construction of the terpene ring. The condensation of olivetol with acetoglutarate yields a cyclic product, a
benzopyran. This lactone is converted to a three-ring system
which carries a ketonic group at the one-location of the
terpene ring. This lactone carries a 3,4-double bond, but it

Fig. 18

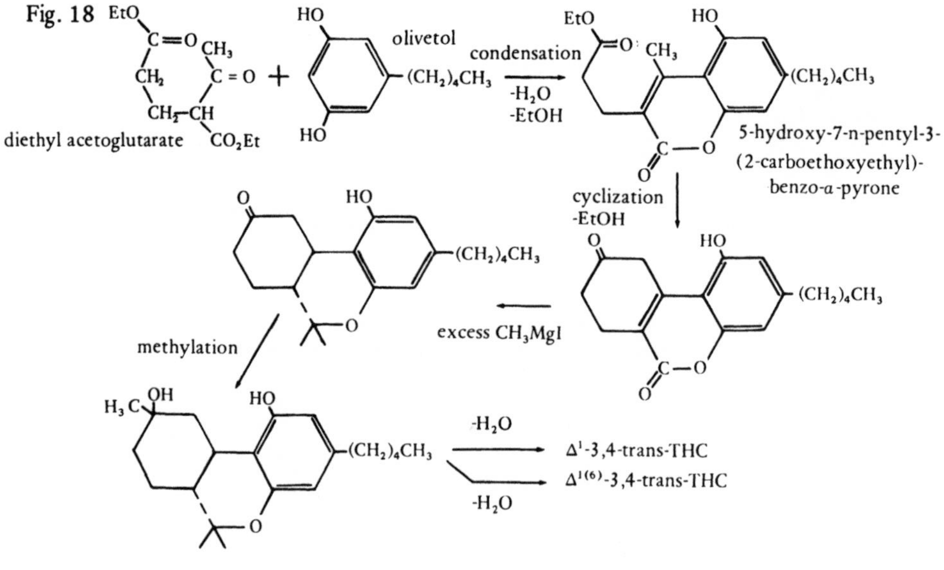

diethyl acetoglutarate

olivetol condensation
-H₂O
-EtOH

5-hydroxy-7-n-pentyl-3-
(2-carboethoxyethyl)-
benzo-a-pyrone

cyclization
-EtOH

excess CH₃MgI

methylation

-H₂O

-H₂O

Δ^1-3,4-trans-THC

$\Delta^{1(6)}$-3,4-trans-THC

can be converted through appropriate protection and methylation, to the 2,3- conjugated counterpart with a geminal
methylation. The resulting (trans) cyclohexanone is easily
methylated and dehydrated to a mixture of THC's which can
be separated chromatographically. The stereoconfiguration is
correct but the over-all yields are poor.

Mechoulam, Braun and Gaoni have reported a total synthesis that starts from the readily available terpene, pinene.
This is oxidized to the allyl alcohol, verbinol, and then
condensed with olivetol to produce a heroic mixture of

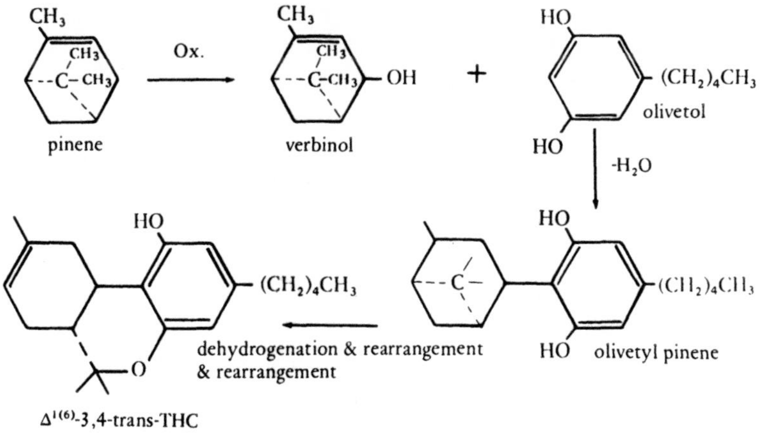

Fig. 19

$\Delta^{1(6)}$-3,4-trans-THC

products. Olivetyl pinene can be chromatographically separated, and converted into the $\Delta^{1\ (6)}$-THC product, which
can in turn be isomerized and so converted into the natural
Δ^1-counterpart. In this reaction both the stereo-specificity
and the absolute optical configuration can be controlled, but
the necessary separations again limit the procedure to the
preparation of only small amounts of end-products.

The most recent synthesis in this area has been reported by
Petrzilka, Haefliger, Sikemeier, Ohloff and Eschenmoser.
They have described the reaction between unsubstantiated
olivetol and the easily synthesized terpenol (+)-trans-p-men-
thadien-2,8-ol. This leads directly to the stereospecifically

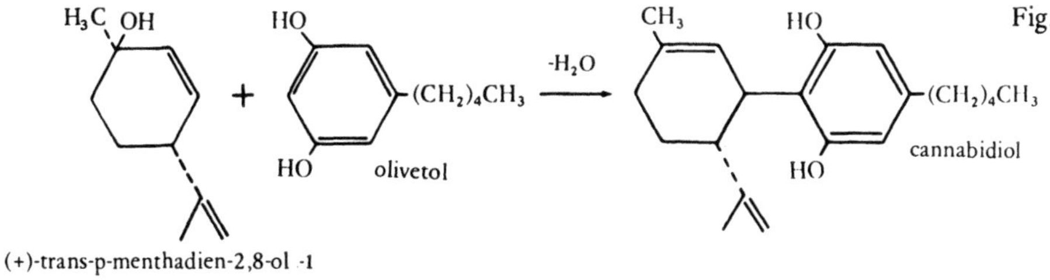

Fig. 20

(+)-trans-p-menthadien-2,8-ol -1

correct isomer of cannabidiol. The yields are quite good (ca.
25 percent) and the general process suggests an easy entry to
the study of structural isomers that carry the naturally
correct optical and stereo-configurations.

From the onset of this review it has been emphasized that **Biosynthetic**
the entire family of the cannabinoids can be considered as a **Considerations**
combination of the structures of a terpene and a resorcinol.
In fact, many of the recently evolved syntheses within this

family have employed just such a combination, with chemical modifications as might be dictated by the reaction conditions. It has been mentioned that the several carboxylic acid components of the resin may serve as precursors to this family. This is supported by the observation that in the colder climates, in the Northern regions which provide shorter growing periods and generally cooler conditions, the marijuana that is harvested is known to be more raw, to contain a greater percentage of acidic components, and to be less biologically active.

Mechoulam and Gaoni have presented an argument that not only olivetol but olivetolic acid may serve as the condensing moiety for the terpene component. It can be argued that geranol, upon appropriate activation, could con-

Fig. 21

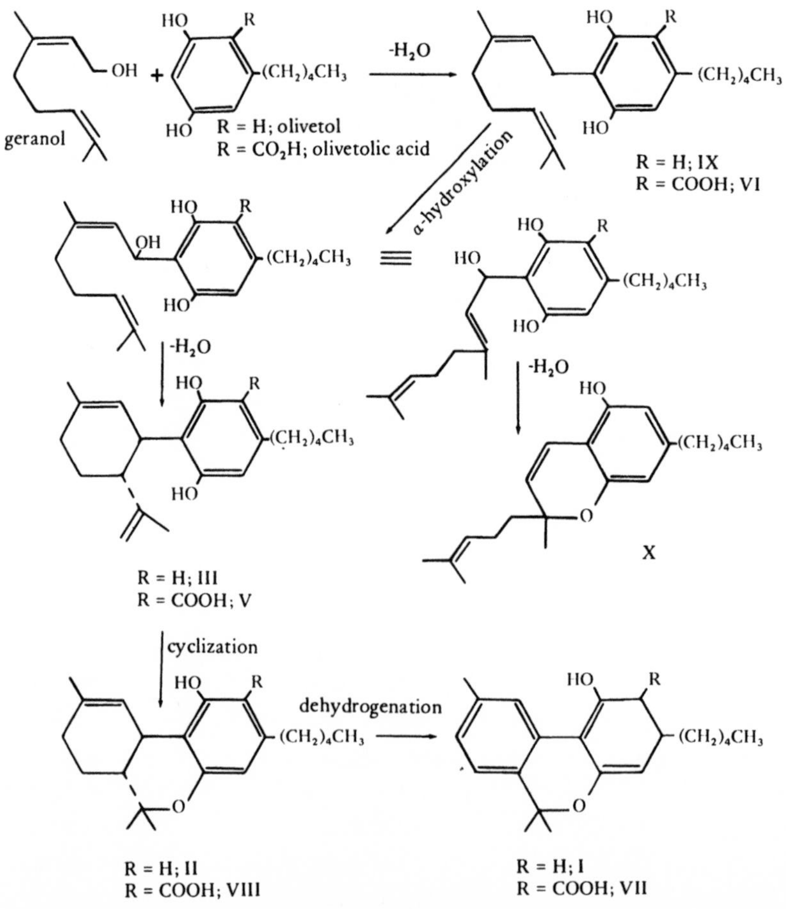

geranol

R = H; olivetol
R = CO_2H; olivetolic acid

$-H_2O$

α-hydroxylation

R = H; IX
R = COOH; VI

$-H_2O$

$-H_2O$

R = H; III
R = COOH; V

X

cyclization

dehydrogenation

R = H; II
R = COOH; VIII

R = H; I
R = COOH; VII

dense with olivetol or with olivetolic acid to yield cannabigerol. This reaction has been achieved *in vitro*. This compound can then undergo an alpha-oxidation to yield cannabidiol through hydroxy elimination, or cannabichromene through addition. The remaining components of the cannabis resin are then explainable by appropriate steps of cyclization, dehydrogenation, and decarboxylation. These transformations are outlined in the flow diagram in which chemicals known to be present are numbered in accordance with their presentation above. The one material of established structure missing from this scheme is the $\Delta^{1\ (6)}$-3,4-trans-THC, IV. It can be readily prepared in the laboratory by the acid-catalysed isomerization of the Δ^1-counterpart, and such a conversion could certainly occur in the intact plant.

Until recently the only laws that pertained to the posses- **Legal** sion and the use of marijuana were contained in the Federal **Considerations** Marijuana Tax Act of 1937, and the many state laws which were based primarily on it. All of these were concerned with the plant and its components. The exact wording of the California Narcotic Act, Health and Safety Code, is as follows:

> 1103.1 "Marijuana" as used in this division means all parts of the plant Cannabis sativa L. (commonly known as marijuana), whether growing or not; the seeds thereof, the resin extracted from any part of such a plant; and every compound, manufacture, salt, derivative, mixture, or preparation of such plant, its seeds or resin.

Although not explicitly stated, it has been accepted that the term "all parts of the plant" should be limited to those materials that are presumably capable of producing biological action similar to that of the entire plant. Such obvious components as chlorophyll and water, ubiquitous to the plant world, were excluded. Until recently chemicals such as tetrahydrocannabinol or cannabidiol could only have arisen from the plant and therefore were covered in this statute. The question as to whether a material might have been synthetically produced was moot, because until recently there had been no successful syntheses of these compounds. The recent syntheses of tetrahydrocannabinol and its congeners, coupled with the appearance through illicit channels of materials claimed to be synthetic "THC," has reopened the question as to whether a totally synthetic component of the plant should legally be considered the same as an isolated component of the plant.

This question was tacitly answered by recent modifications of the dangerous drugs section of the Federal Food, Drug, and Cosmetic Act, an entirely separate law. This section was designed to control the improper distribution of dangerous drugs. In 1968 the law was amended with the following insertion:

> Listing of drugs defined in section 201 (v) of the Act [shall be amended to include] synthetic equivalents of the substances contained in the plant, or in the resinous extracts of *Cannabis* sp. and/or synthetic substances, derivatives, and their isomers with similar chemical structure and activity such as the following:
> Δ^1 –cis– or trans–tetrahydrocannabinol, and their optical isomers,
> Δ^6 –cis– or trans–tetrahydrocannabinol, and their optical isomers,
> $\Delta^{3,4}$ tetrahydrocannabinol, and its optical isomers.

It is recognized in this amendment that the nomenclature of these substances has not been internationally standardized and it is the specific compounds (and their racemic combinations) that are specified, regardless of the numerical designation employed. As these ten specific compounds are handled by a separate law, they are considered synthetic substances and not materials of plant origin. Whether the terms "isomers with similar chemical structure and activity" will probably prove to be worthless for similarity between things, unless specified in detail, is a matter of individual opinion.

Because of these distinctions, it will be the responsibility of the legal authorities not only to demonstrate that a contraband drug is tetrahydrocannabinol, but also to determine its origin. Since the two laws define two completely different tetrahydrocannabinols (synthetic or natural), they cannot be applied in the same instance. The tasks of identification are thus multiplied several-fold by the necessity of identifying trace congeners present in the seized sample, for if these contaminants were not detectable the origin could not be established.

Although there have been many recent reports of the appearance of synthetic tetrahydrocannabinol in the illicit drug trade (as "Synthetic THC"), as of the present time these all appear to be false. The complexity of the currently reported syntheses of tetrahydrocannabinol makes it seem unlikely that a synthetic material, as a pure single isomer, could be inexpensively made. It would seem that this recent legislation might work hardships on legitimate investigators rather than on the enterprising amateur chemist.

As has been shown, marijuana contains a wealth of **Future Research** complex organic molecules, many of which have structures that are now well defined. Further it is known to present a complex spectrum of pharmacological properties in the human subject. It is certainly possible that some of these properties can eventually be assigned specifically to some of these compounds. Only within the last year has the first such experiment been attempted, in which an isolated component, Δ^1-tetrahydrocannabinol, has been studied in clinical experiments. It has been shown to account in part for the intoxicative properties of total marijuana.

The chemical and physical tools needed to implement an extensive research program in this area are now at hand, and the only remaining difficulties to a proper study of marijuana are administrative. There is obviously much pharmacological potential in *Cannabis sativa*. It is axiomatic that when this is revealed and appreciated, there will be valid contributions to the science of medicine.

THE SPREAD OF MARIHUANA USE IN AMERICA*
Culture Contact, Differential Association, and Subcultural Diffusion

MEXICO
↓

SOUTHWESTERN U.S.
(introduced about 1910 by Mexican laborers; becomes established among Mexican-Americans; sporadic cowboy use, but doesn't become established there)
↓

NEW ORLEANS
(introduced by Negroes, via Mexican-Americans, by 1920)
↓

URBAN NEGRO LOWER CLASS, SOUTH & NORTH
(well established by mid-1920's; rapid spread begins about 1931)

NEGRO JAZZ MUSICIANS** & NEGRO FANS (simultaneously with other Negroes, as above)
↓

WHITE JAZZ MUSICIANS & WHITE FANS (some by mid-1920's, esp. in Chicago, rapid spread among white musicians in mid-1930's, but not among fans until "hipsters" of early 1940's and "beat" fans from about 1948 onward)

WHITE LOWER CLASS IN RACIALLY MIXED NEIGHBORHOODS (some by mid-1930's, but mostly since late 1940's)

NON-MUSICIAN WHITE ENTERTAINERS (some by early 1930's; mainly nightclub & stripper subcultures—incl. criminals & prostitutes assoc. with those industries —but also some movie, circus, & legit theatre people)

"BEATS" GENERALLY
(by 1950; incl. the minority not especially devoted to jazz)

WHITE MIDDLE- & UPPER-CLASS PSEUDO-BOHEMIANS (late 1950's; *Playboy* types, e.g., sportscar set, "hippy" ad. copywriters)

WHITE "ETHNIC," "FOLK," & "ROCK" TEENAGERS, FOLKSY-ARTSY CIRCLES (late 1950's onward—to the "hippies" of mid-1960)

WHITE COLLEGE STUDENTS (some by 1950, rapid spread since 1960) → WHITE MIDDLE- & UPPER-CLASS HIGH SCHOOL STUDENTS (mainly since 1961)

---

*This chart derives to a small extent from printed sources (e.g., Mezz Mezzrow's *Really the Blues*), but is based mainly on information given me by present and former marihuana users of long standing (three of whom were smoking marihuana in the 1920's).

**The earliest of many jazz records whose titles refer to marihuana is Louis Armstrong's *Muggles* (OK 8703), recorded December 7, 1929. ("Muggles" is an obsolete argot term for marihuana.) The titles of three earlier jazz records refer to other drugs: Josie Miles's *Pipe Dream Blues* (1924), Duke Ellington's *Hop Head* (1927), and Victoria Spivey's *Dope Head Blues* (1927). I take these from Charles Delaunay's *New Hot Discography* (New York: Criterion Music Corp., 1948), but have not been able to check through Brian Rust's later and fuller discography.

References to marihuana also occur in the lyrics, but not the titles, of other jazz records, e.g., Bessie Smith's *Gimme a Pigfoot* (1933) and Joe Marsala's *Salty Mama Blues* (1940).

***Innumerable post-1960 references to marihuana can be found in recordings by white "folk" and "rock" singers (Bob Dylan, the Rolling Stones, *et al.*).

From Ned Polsky's *Hustlers, Beats & Others* (Garden City, N.Y.: Doubleday & Co.; paperback ed. Anchor Books, 1969).

416

VI

SOCIAL ORIGINS OF
THE MARIJUANA LAWS

Dr. David Musto debunks the myth of "Horrible Harry" Anslinger. He depicts the former head of the Federal Bureau of Narcotics more as a "reluctant dragon," representing an equivocating Federal Government that caved in to racist fears of Mexican migrant workers.

The prohibition of marijuana was promoted and facilitated by certain doctors and resisted by the pharmaceutical industry and others of the medical profession.

The byzantine mosaic of events leading up to that strange hearing is explored. Then, the American Medical Association representative strongly favored the retention of marijuana for use as a medicine. The house liberals, still smarting from the AMA's blocking of national health insurance's inclusion in the Social Security Act, raked him over the coals as being an obstructionist to the good health of the country.

The National Institute of Health's pharmacology expert testified that prolonged marijuana use could lead to insanity. The NIH medical expert said that marijuana could produce a frenzy that might result in violence.

A nationally known addiction specialist described marijuana to be worse than opium.

This well-researched paper chronicles the timeless nature of bigotry and the all-too-easy bureaucratic acquiescence to this evil.

TREASURY DEPARTMENT

ORIGINAL
Value Two (2) Cents

UNITED STATES INTERNAL REVENUE

ORDER FORM FOR MARIHUANA, OR COMPOUNDS, MANUFACTURES, SALTS, DERIVATIVES, MIXTURES, OR PREPARATIONS UNDER THE MARIHUANA TAX ACT OF 1937.

MARIHUANA ORDER FORM NUMBER	DATE ISSUED BY COLLECTOR:	19

TO: _____ ,

_____ , _____ .

Sir:

Application having been presented and transfer tax in the amount of $ _____ having been paid, as evidenced by transfer tax stamps affixed to the original hereof in accordance with the provisions of the Marihuana Tax Act of 1937 and regulations issued thereunder, you are authorized, in so far as the provisions of that Act and the regulations issued thereunder are concerned, to transfer to _____ to be delivered to him in person or consigned to him at _____ , _____ , _____ , a quantity of marihuana not to exceed _____ ounces in the form of the following products:

ITEM	NAME OF PRODUCT OR PREPARATION	QUANTITY
1		
2		
3		
4		

Signed: _____ , Collector,

By _____

NOTE: Not valid to authorize a transfer of marihuana unless signed by the collector and the full amount of transfer stamps indicated above are affixed to the original copy.

The 1937 Marijuana Tax Act

BY DAVID F. MUSTO, M.D.

Social reformers successfully initiated federal restrictions on cannabis, along with alcohol, opiates, cocaine, and chloral hydrate in the first decade of this century. The Pure Food and Drug Act of 1906 required that any quantity of cannabis, as well as several other dangerous substances, be clearly marked on the label of any drug or food sold to the public.[1] Early drafts of federal antinarcotic legislation which finally emerged as the Harrison Act in 1914 also repeatedly listed the drug along with opiates and cocaine (for example, H.R. 25,241 61st Cong., Second Session [1910] which was prepared and endorsed by the State Department and introduced April 30, 1910). Cannabis, however, never survived the legislative gauntlet, probably because of the pharmaceutical industry's opposition. At that time, and for at least a decade longer, the drug trades did not see any reason why a substance used chiefly in corn plasters, veterinary medicine, and other non-intoxicating forms of medicaments should be so severely restricted in its use and sale. Not even the reformers claimed, in the pre-World War I hearings and debates over a federal antinarcotic act, that cannabis was a problem of any major significance in the United States.

Dr. Hamilton Wright, a State Department official who from 1908 to 1914 coordinated the domestic and international aspects of the federal antinarcotic campaign, wanted cannabis to be included in drug abuse legislation chiefly

Reprinted from *Archives of General Psychiatry*, vol. 26, February 1972, pp. 101–108.

because of his belief in a hydraulic model of drug appetites. He reasoned, along with numerous other experts, that if one dangerous drug was effectively prohibited, the addict's depraved desires would switch to another substance more easily available. He felt, therefore, that cannabis should be prohibited in anticipation of the habitual user's shift from opiates and cocaine to hashish. The narcotic reformer's task, then, was to prohibit and control as many dangerous and seductive substances as possible at one time.

Although congressional hearings rarely heard any witnesses defend opiates or cocaine, those against including cannabis in federal legislation spoke more openly. In January 1911 hearings were held on a federal antinarcotic law before the House Ways and Means Committee. The National Wholesale Druggists' Association (NWDA) representative protested, in addition to other aspects of the proposed legislation, the inclusion of cannabis alongside opiates and cocaine. Charles A. West, chairman of the NWDA Legislative Committee, complained that "cannabis is not what may be called a habit-forming drug."[2] Albert Plaut, representing the New York City pharmaceutical firm of Lehn & Fink, objected to including "insignificant articles, the habit-forming quality of which is more than doubtful."[2] In particular he objected to the inclusion of cannabis; he attributed its reputation more to literary fiction, such as the description of hashish in *The Count of Monte Cristo*, than to informed opinion. "Cannabis brought into this country," Plaut explained, "is used almost altogether for the manufacture of corn cures and in veterinary practice. As a habit-forming drug its use is almost nil.[2] When questioned as to whether cannabis might be taken by those whose regular supply of opiates or cocaine is restricted, Plaut responded that the effects of cannabis were so different from those of opiates and cocaine that he would not expect an addict to find cannabis attractive.[2]

The drug industry's complaints received stern rebuttals but no one denied that cannabis constituted at that time a very small part of drug abuse. Arguments for inclusion rested on the belief of such authorities as Dr. Alexander Lambert, of Bellevue Hospital and later President of the American Medical Association, that some of his patients were habitual users of cannabis and that, therefore, the drug was habit-forming.[2] One of the most stirring attacks on cannabis came from a comrade of Dr. Lambert, the lay proprietor of a profitable hospital for addiction treatment, Charles B. Towns. Towns's chief fame arose from his popularization of a supposed cure for the cravings of drug-users, but he made an active sideline out of appearing before committees of inquiry and drafting model legislation to combat the evils of drug abuse. He was an impressive witness in 1911, nearing the peak of his fame as one of mankind's benefactors.[3] He took a very uncompromising attitude toward drug use:

> To my mind it is inexcusable for a man to say that there is no habit from the use of that drug. There is no drug in the Pharmacopoeia today that would produce the pleasurable sensations you would get from cannabis, no not one—absolutely not a drug in the Pharmacopoeia today, and of all the drugs on earth I would certainly put that on the list.

The "Father of the Pure Food Law," Dr. Harvey Washington Wiley of the Department of Agriculture, was no less adamant than Towns. Dr. Wiley favored prohibition of the drugs listed in the proposed legislation but if regulation was all he could get, he would settle for that. To his mind the list of drugs was too short and it should have included not only acetanilid, antipyrene, and phenacetin, but also alcohol and caffeine. Dr. Wiley declared alcohol to have no medicinal value and caffeine to be a habit-forming drug, sold indiscriminately even to children in cola and other drinks. The only value he saw to habit-forming painkillers was to permit an easy death; a patient who had a chance for recovery would be better off without them since he might establish a habit which could never be broken.[2]

While most spokesmen for the drug trades opposed federal regulation of cannabis, one distinguished member favored its control and most of the other provisions of the new legislation: Dr. William Jay Schieffelin of New York, like Dr. Lambert, was prominent in the nation's social and political life as well as in his profession as the president of a wholesale drug house. He moved with the progressive and reform spirit of the era and was, therefore, somewhat separated from the rank and file as regards the acceptable burdens antinarcotic legislation would place on the drug trade. Schieffelin believed cannabis was "used only to a slight extent in this country," but he had heard that there was a demand for it in the "Syrian colony in New York" where he thought it was smoked like prepared opium. He concluded, "The evil is minute but it ought to be included in the bill."

Cannabis was not included, though, and except for the Pure Food and Drug Act's provision as to labeling, no federal regulatory law was enacted until 1937. (By 1931 regulations under the Food and Drug Act had limited the importation of cannabis except for medical purposes.) Meanwhile the two contrasting attitudes toward cannabis remained pretty much the same: the reformers feared its use; the drug industry, which used it in rather minor preparations, felt less concern about possible misuse and opposed its regulation. Both sides seemed to agree that cannabis was not as threatening as other drugs and that its inclusion in regulatory laws would be for the purpose of anticipating its popularity once opiates and cocaine were brought under control.

Complaints about cannabis continued to come to the attention of the federal government, although without the frequency or insistence which was to occur in the 1930s. In preparation for the First Hague Conference, which led to the Hague Convention (1912) for the control of the world's narcotic traffic, one of the American delegates, Henry J. Finger of the California Board of Pharmacy, wished to draw particular attention to the dangers of cannabis. Many Californians, particularly in San Francisco, were frightened by the "large influx of Hindoos ... demanding cannabis indica" who were initiating "the whites into their habit."[5] Finger wanted the world traffic in cannabis to be controlled.[5] The United States delegation, of which Dr. Wright was a member, gladly adopted Finger's goal, but did not find the Hague Conference favorably disposed to include cannabis in the Hague Convention. The best the United States could accomplish at this time was the adoption of a recommendation that nations look into the character of the drug and see whether it merited regulation[6] Agreement that international traffic in cannabis should be regulated did not come until the Second Geneva Convention in 1925.[7]

Domestic concern over cannabis seemed to originate in the Southwest and to begin increasing after the First World War. In 1919 the crucial Supreme Court decision outlawing addiction-maintenance for pleasure or comfort led to national restrictions on physicians, druggists, and other outlets for drugs believed to be responsible for America's many addicts. Such a time was also appropriate for control of other dangerous substances. Of course, alcohol was outlawed for convivial consumption when the 18th Amendment became effective in January 1920. Cannabis also ought to be controlled, argued the Governor of Louisiana and the president of Louisiana's Board of Health. Their contact with "mariguana" had elements which would become familiar in the 1930s. A white, twenty-one-year-old musician in New Orleans had been arrested for forging a physician's signature in order to get some "marihuana" imported from Mexico. The musician said the substance was taken to "make you feel good," but the dangers of this substance were clear to Dr. Oscar Dowling and Governor John M. Parker. Dr. Dowling, who was also a member of and later chairman of the American Medical Association's Board of Trustees, warned the Governor that marihuana was "a powerful narcotic, causing exhilaration, intoxication, delirious hallucinations, and its subsequent actions, drowsiness and stupor."[8] He also urgently requested of the Surgeon-General of the Public Health Service that the federal government take "some action" to control the traffic in marihuana.[9] The Surgeon-General replied that he was in complete agreement with Dr. Dowling's concern.[10] Shortly thereafter Governor Parker claimed in a letter to Prohibition Commissioner John F. Kramer that "two people were killed a few days ago by the smoking of this drug, which seems to make them go crazy and wild" and he expressed his surprise that there were no restrictions against marihuana.[11] But the troubles the government was already having with enforcement of the Harrison Act may not have encouraged addition of more drugs for control.

Yet, the United States continued to press for international control of cannabis, as well as of other drugs. International drug control, if obtained, would have solved much of the American problem since opiates, coca leaves, and some cannabis were imported. The cool reception other nations gave the American proposals to control cannabis did not discourage the American delegation, but rather added one

International Control of Cannabis: 1911-1925

more proof of international perfidy. Since the earliest stir-
rings of an international campaign by the United States,
American diplomats believed that other nations, some of
whom received considerable revenue from the narcotic traffic, used various stratagems to discourage or nullify American
efforts. That foreign governments should also oppose the
inclusion of cannabis in a schedule of controlled drugs was
almost a confirmation of the wisdom of controlling the
cannabis market.

The United States, having started the antinarcotic campaign which resulted in the Hague Opium Convention of
1912, lost its premier role during the 1920s. The League of
Nations assumed responsibility for the Hague Convention
from the government of the Netherlands, a transfer which the
United States would not recognize. Although the intricate
formalities by which the State Department avoided any
appearance of "recognizing" the League were certainly effective in achieving their goal, such actions also lost the United
States its leadership in the world antinarcotic movement.

Repeatedly the League tried to involve the United States
in planning for the international control of narcotics. While
the United States maintained meticulously distant relations
with the League's Advisory Committee on the Traffic in
Opium and Other Dangerous Drugs, American cooperation
did emerge. These hopeful signs were reversed, however, by
the walkout of the American delegation, led by the chairman
of the House Committee on Foreign Affairs, from the Second
Geneva Opium Conference in February 1925.[12]

The delegates' exit was based on righteous indignation at
the weak will of other nations: they left behind an opportunity to sign the first Convention which sought to bring the
cannabis traffic between nations under international supervision.

Five years would pass before the United States would
again sit in such an international meeting.

Rising Domestic   Fear of cannabis, or as it was beginning to be known,
Fear of Cannabis: marihuana, was minor throughout most of the nation in the
1920-1934   1920s. Nevertheless, it still concerned the federal government. For example, in January 1929 Congress authorized
two narcotic farms to be operated by the Public Health

Service largely for the treatment of addicted federal prisoners. The law specifically defined "habit-forming narcotic drug" to include "Indian Hemp" and made habitual cannabis users, along with opium addicts, eligible for treatment.[13] Although there seems to have been almost no transfer of cannabis users to the two "farms," later known as the Lexington and Fort Worth Hospitals, it is significant that congressional worry about cannabis continued after passage of the Pure Food and Drug Act and clearly was present before the Federal Bureau of Narcotics (FBN) was established in 1930.

In certain areas of the United States, however, the fear of marihuana was more intense. These areas mostly coincided with concentration of Mexican immigrants who tended to use marihuana as a drug of entertainment or relaxation. During the decade, Mexican immigration, legal and illegal, rapidly increased into the region from Louisiana to California and up to Colorado and Utah. Mexicans were useful in the United States as farm laborers, and as the economic boom continued they received inducements to travel to the Midwest and the North where jobs in factories and sugar beet fields were available.[14]

Although employers welcomed them in the 1920s, Mexicans were also feared as a locus of crime and deviant social behavior. By the mid-1920s horrible crimes were attributed to marihuana and its Mexican purveyors. Legal and medical officers in New Orleans began studies on the evil, and within a few years published articles claiming that many of the region's crimes could be traced to marihuana. They implicated it particularly in the most severe crimes, for they believed it to be a sexual stimulant which removed civilized inhibitions.[15] As a result, requests were made to include marihuana in the federal law which controlled similar substances, the Harrison Narcotic Act.[16]

When the great Depression settled over America, the Mexicans, who had been welcomed by at least a fraction of the communities in which they lived, became an unwelcome surplus in regions devastated by unemployment. Considered a dangerous minority which should be induced to return to Mexico by whatever means seemed appropriate, they dwelt in isolated living groups. A contemporary writer described their mood in 1930, the first year of the Depression.

A . . . factor in decreasing Mexican immigration is
what officials call "the fear of God." It may be
indefinite, but it is very real; and the quality is standard
all the way from California to Texas.

And that *fear* hovers over every Mexican Colony in
the Southwest is a fact that all who come in contact
with them can readily attest. They fear examination by
the border patrol when they travel; they fear arrest;
they fear jail; they fear deportation; and whereas they
used to write inviting their friends, they now urge them
not to come.[17]

Naturally, cotton, fruit, and vegetable growers in the
Southwest and sugar beet farmers in Colorado, Michigan,
Montana, and the Northwest favored further immigration. On
the other hand, the American Federation of Labor under-
standably favored strict bars against foreign labor. But
another group which worked for an end to Mexican immigration as energetically as those with economic interests did so
for social reasons, afraid that mixture with an "inferior race"
was causing "race suicide." Citizens anxious to preserve what
they believed valuable in American life banded together into
"Allied Patriotic Societies," "Key Men of America," or the
group which united many of these associations, the "American Coalition" whose goal was to "Keep America American."[18] One of the prominent members of the American
Coalition, C. M. Goethe of Sacramento, saw marihuana and
the problem of Mexican migrants as closely connected (*New
York Times*, Sept. 15, 1935, section IV, p. 9):

Marihuana, perhaps now the most insidious of our
narcotics, is a direct by-product of unrestricted Mexican
immigration. Easily grown, it has been asserted that it
has recently been planted between rows in a California
penitentiary garden. Mexican peddlers have been caught
distributing sample marihuana cigarettes to school children. Bills for our quota against Mexico have been
blocked mysteriously in every Congress since the 1924
Quota Act. Our nation has more than enough laborers.

Southwest police and prosecuting attorneys likewise raised
a continual protest to the federal government about the

Mexican's use of the weed (H. J. Anslinger, oral communication, June 30, 1970).

In 1934, a U.S. marshal in Tulsa, Oklahoma, wrote to the FBN, describing marihuana as a most dangerous and crime-causing drug which gave its users the feeling that they had "superman and superwoman" powers.[19] Newspapers occasionally headlined the weed as a cause of horrible crimes. For example, in 1933 the *New York Mirror* presented an article in its Sunday supplement on "Loco Weed, Breeder of Madness and Crime." That same year Dr. Walter Bromberg, a respected researcher, informed a meeting of the American Psychiatric Association that some authors had estimated the number of marihuana smokers in the southern states to be one out of four.[20] Dr. Bromberg, who did not subscribe to the alarm over marihuana displayed by some writers, nevertheless told of its spread from the South to the large cities and to New York, "where its use is widespread."[20] He noted that marihuana's inclusion in the Harrison Narcotic Act had been requested. Although denying that crimes were directly and simply caused by marihuana and asserting that it was something like alcohol in its effect, nevertheless, on the basis of good physiological and psychological studies of cannabis, he was persuaded that it was "a primary stimulus to the impulsive life with direct expression in the motor field."[20] Marihuana "releases inhibitions and restraints imposed by society and allows individuals to act out their drives openly," and "acts as a sexual stimulant," particularly to "overt homosexuals."[20]

Dr. Bromberg's description of marihuana in 1933 differed in quality from the writings, for example, of New Orleans' Prosecuting Attorney who, in 1931 fearfully portrayed "Marihuana as a Developer of Criminals."[21] Yet, Dr. Bromberg's statements would not have calmed the apprehensive. Furthermore, neither the New Orleans studies, which began at least in the late 1920s nor Dr. Bromberg's research can be ascribed to any "campaign" by the FBN for a federal marihuana law. It is reasonable to assume that in the first few years of the 1930s, marihuana was known among police departments and civic leaders, particularly those connected with Mexican immigrants and even among scientific investigators as a drug with dangerous propensities. This situation led naturally to pressure on the federal government to take

"some action" against marihuana. What was the attitude of
the new Federal Bureau of Narcotics to the growing concern
over marihuana?

The Decision to   During its first few years, the FBN, as judged from its
Seek a Federal   annual reports, minimized the marihuana problem and felt
Anti-marihuana
Law: that control should be vested in the state governments. The
1935-1937 report published in 1932 commented that:

> This abuse of the drug is noted among the Latin-
> American or Spanish-speaking population. The sale of
> cannabis cigarettes occurs to a considerable degree in
> States along the Mexican border and in cities of the
> Southwest and West, as well as in New York City and, in
> fact, wherever there are settlements of Latin Americans.
> A great deal of public interest has been aroused by
> newspaper articles appearing from time to time on the
> evils of the abuse of marihuana, or Indian hemp, and
> more attention has been focused upon specific cases
> reported of the abuse of the drug than would otherwise
> have been the case. This publicity tends to magnify the
> extent of the evil and lends color to an inference that
> there is an alarming spread of the improper use of the
> drug, whereas the actual increase in such use may not
> have been inordinately large.[22]

That year the FBN strongly endorsed the new Uniform
State Narcotic Act and repeatedly stressed that the problem
could be brought under control if all the states adopted the
Act.[23] As late as January 1937, Commissioner Anslinger was
quoted as advising that the distribution of marihuana was an
"intrastate problem" and that "hope for its ultimate control
lies . . . in adoption by states of the Uniform Narcotic Act"
(*New York Times*, Jan. 3, 1937, section 3, p. 6). Study of the
annual reports reveal an increasing amount of space taken up
by marihuana-associated crime after 1935, but the FBN
continued to recommend the Uniform Act. There seem to be
several reasons why the FBN delayed advocacy of a federal
marihuana law.

The Commissioner recalls that marihuana caused few
problems except in the Southwest and the Western states.
There the growing alarm was directed at the "Mexicans"

whom the "sheriffs and local police departments claimed got loaded on the stuff and caused a lot of trouble, stabbings, assaults, and so on." These states were "the only ones then affected . . . we didn't see it here in the East at all at that time." To Anslinger, the danger of marihuana did not compare with that of heroin and, after the Act's passage in October 1937, he states that he warned his agents to keep their eyes on heroin. If an agent started to make a series of arrests for marihuana possession, he was told to get back to "the hard stuff" (H. J. Anslinger, oral communication, June 30, 1970).

In addition to questioning whether a federal law would significantly ameliorate the "marihuana problem," the Commissioner also doubted the possibility of a law which would be constitutional. When the idea of a transfer tax was first broached to him by the Treasury's General Counsel, Herman Oliphant, he thought the notion was "ridiculous." Even after the decision was made to recommend the transfer tax to Congress, Anslinger "couldn't believe it would go through." It was not that he did not abstractly favor a marihuana law, but he had doubts about its constitutionality and about whether it would have any substantial effect on the problem of marihuana use (H. J. Anslinger, oral communication, June 30, 1970).

Lastly, the FBN had "put sandbags against the door" whenever anyone suggested it take over control of barbiturates and amphetamines. Such controls would mean very difficult problems in adjudicating "proper uses" and legitimate exceptions. The FBN preferred heroin as a target; it had no legal uses whatever. The whole question of enforcement was enormously simplified by tracking down a totally prohibited drug. Such an attitude would be consistent with hesitating to take on marihuana which, unlike heroin, was not imported but rather grew, as the Commissioner ruefully pointed out in 1936, "like dandelions," and which had a few legitimate uses.[24] It is significant that when marihuana was finally controlled by the federal government, almost all uses were outlawed with the exception of its use in bird seed (and then only if sterilized). The regulations for its use by physicians were so complicated that possibly no general physician has legally prescribed it since 1937.

The pressure for a federal anti-marihuana law was,

Anslinger states, "political," traveling from local police forces in affected states to the governors, then to the Secretary of the Treasury, Henry Morgenthau, Jr., and from him to the General Counsel, and the Commissioner of Narcotics (H. J. Anslinger, oral communication, June 30, 1970). Apparently the decision to seek a federal law was made in 1935, since by January 1936 Anslinger was holding conferences on what course to take to accomplish that end. The FBN's search for grounds on which to base a federal law was almost unsuccessful. It first claimed that only the treaty-making power of the federal government could sustain an anti-marihuana statute. Such a treaty was then attempted, but with an appeal to other nations which had almost no chance of success. If the FBN did not actually want a federal marihuana law, it had performed faithfully the task it had been given and the effort was about to fall short, when, claims Anslinger, the Treasury's General Counsel ingeniously contrived the "transfer tax."

The pressure on the Treasury could well have been sufficient to induce such cleverness, as the following letter of 1936 (Anslinger papers, Box 6) from the editor of the Alamosa, Colo, *Daily Courier* suggests:

> Is there any assistance your Bureau can give us in handling this drug? Can you suggest campaigns? Can you enlarge your Department to deal with marihuana? Can you do anything to help us?
>
> I wish I could show you what a small marihuana cigarette can do to one of our degenerate Spanish speaking residents. That's why our problem is so great; the greatest percentage of our population is composed of Spanish speaking persons, most of whom are low mentally, because of social and racial conditions.
>
> While marihuana has figured in the greatest number of crimes in the past few years, officials fear it, not for what it had done, but for what it is capable of doing. They want to check it before an outbreak does occur.
>
> Through representatives of civic leaders and law officers of the San Luis Valley, I have been asked to write to you for help.

It was this kind of attitude which the Tax Act was

designed "to placate," according to Anslinger, although he felt that little besides a law on the books could be offered the fearful citizens of the Southwest and their importuning officials (H. J. Anslinger, oral communication, June 30, 1970).

With the goal of trying to figure out how the federal government could pass such a law, the Narcotics Commissioner traveled in January 1936 to New York. There he met with a group of distinguished experts—a representative of the Foreign Policy Association; Joseph Chamberlain, Professor of Law at Columbia; Herbert L. May, a member of the permanent Central Board of the League of Nations; and Stuart Fuller, Assistant Chief of the Division of Far Eastern Affairs of the State Department. They concluded, Anslinger reported to Assistant Secretary of the Treasury Stephen B. Gibbons in a confidential memorandum, "that under the taxing power and regulation on interstate commerce it would be almost hopeless to expect any kind of adequate control."[25]

The Commissioner's recommendation was to follow the example of the Migratory Bird Act which had been declared constitutional, although it entered into the police powers of the states, because it was enacted as a requirement of international treaties with Canada and Mexico (Mo. vs. Holland, 252 US 416). He suggested a treaty requiring the control of marijuana. Once the treaty was ratified by the Senate, a federal law could be enacted which would not meet the constitutional blocks which he felt sure an anti-marihuana law would face if based on federal tax or commerce powers. Otherwise, the various details which imperiled simple prohibition of marihuana were coming near solution:

> The State Department has tentatively agreed to this proposition, but before action is taken we shall have to dispose of certain phases of legitimate traffic; for instance, the drug trade still has a small medical need for marihuana, but has agreed to eliminate it entirely. The only place it is used extensively is by the veterinarian, and we can satisfy them by importing their medical needs.

The Marihuana Tax Act

We must also satisfy the canary bird seed trade, and
the Sherwin Williams Paint Company which uses hemp
seed oil for drying purposes. We are now working with
the Department of Commerce in finding substitutes for
the legitimate trade, and after that is accomplished, the
path will be cleared for the treaties and for federal
law.[25]

The Commissioner was permitted to try his idea in June of
the same year when he and Fuller represented the United
States at the Conference for the Suppression of Illicit Traffic
in Dangerous Drugs, held in Geneva. The United States
sought to incorporate a requirement for domestic cannabis
control in a treaty with twenty-six other nations. Perhaps to
have additional leverage, or perhaps to dramatize the opposition of other governments, the US delegation asked just
before the conference opened for permission to abstain if the
American proposals were turned down. Still recalling the
regrettable isolation which followed American departure
from a similar conference in 1925, the State Department
refused permission. So, although their views were outvoted,
the delegation stayed, but did not sign the Convention. It was
the only nation represented which did not do so.[12]

In the summer of 1936, therefore, it became obvious that
there would be no law to placate the police of the Southwest
unless some federal legislation under the traditional legal
powers was enacted. General Counsel Oliphant then suggested the marihuana transfer tax about which the Commissioner had strong doubts: (H. J. Anslinger, oral communication, June 30, 1970). The FBN loyally went along with the
plan, though, and did its best to present a very strong case to
Congress so as to ensure the greatest chance of passage. To
Anslinger, Congress did not seem very concerned and "the
only information they had was what we could give them in
our hearings" before the Appropriations Committee or when
the Tax Act was pending (H. J. Anslinger, oral communication, June 30, 1970).

The Treasury Department collected and considered scientific and medical opinion prior to the Tax Act hearings. But
the desire to present a solid front when the Department
appeared before the committees of Congress caused the
officials to ignore anything qualifying or minimizing the evils

of marihuana. As suggested above, the political pressure to put "something on the books" and the doubt that it could be done combined to make the marihuana hearings a classic example of bureaucratic overkill.

For a balanced interpretation of the hearings it is necessary to keep in mind that marihuana had been extravagantly condemned in the halls of Congress at least as early as 1910 and that in some areas of the nation it was at that time an object of horror to respectable and vocal citizens. The Bromberg study would have offered ample reason for concern, although it can be read as reassuring about the dangers of marihuana. After the Tax Act was passed, even Dr. Lawrence Kolb, Sr., certainly no booster of the FBN, warned that "Continued use of the drug causes insanity in many cases, but very unstable persons may have a short psychotic episode from only a few doses. . . . No matter by what means taken marihuana is a dangerous drug . . . much more harmful in certain respects than opium . . . Enough is known about the drug to brand it as a dangerous one that needs to be strictly controlled" (Federal Probation 2:22–25, 1938).

The Treasury presentation to Congress may, therefore, have been exaggerated, but it was not without foundation in the current thinking of medical research. The government's witnesses could also be fairly confident that the congressmen had no preconceived, favorable, or even informed opinions.

In the tradition of federal departments, everyone from the Treasury Department who appeared for the Tax Act gave it full support, while those who might have had more moderate views remained in the background. In particular, the Public Health Service was not represented, although the opinion of its Division of Mental Hygiene (now the National Institute of Mental Health) was available to the Treasury Department months prior to the hearings in April. Like other authorities, Dr. Walter L. Treadway was asked a series of questions about marihuana, probably in late 1936, when the Treasury was gathering expert opinion on the botanical, chemical, pharmacological, and behavior-modifying characteristics of cannabis. To the question "What are the proofs that the use of marihuana in any of its forms is habit forming or addictive, and what are the indications and positive proofs that such addiction develops socially undesirable characteristics in the users?" Dr. Treadway replied in full:

Cannabis Indica does not produce dependence as in opium addiction. In opium addiction there is a complete dependence and when it is withdrawn there is actual physical pain which is not the case with cannabis. Alcohol more nearly produces the same effect as cannabis in that there is an excitement or a general feeling of lifting of personality, followed by a delirious stage, and subsequent narcosis. There is no dependence or increased tolerance such as in opium addiction. As to the social or moral degradation associated with cannabis it probably belongs in the same category as alcohol. As with alcohol, it may be taken a relatively long time without social or emotional breakdown. Marihuana is habit forming although not addicting in the same sense as alcohol might be with some people, or sugar, or coffee. Marihuana produces a delirium with a frenzy which might result in violence; but this is also true of alcohol.[26]

Having received Dr. Treadway's opinion and that of other authorities, the Department held a conference in the Treasury Building on January 14, 1937. Attending were fourteen government officials and consultants, many of whom would testify a few months later before the Congressional committees deliberating on the Tax Act.[27] The purpose of the conference was to prepare a satisfactory legal definition of marihuana for the proposed legislation and to make some final arrangements for the presentation to Congress. Dr. Treadway was not present, although Dr. Carl Voegtlin, Chief of the Division of Pharmacology of the National Institute of Health, was there to assist, along with some chemists, pharmacologists, and Commissioner Anslinger. Two members of the Department's General Council's Office and the FBN's General Counsel were so present.

Fortunately, the conference was stenographically transcribed so that we can gain some appreciation of the attitudes surrounding the proposed legislation by the individuals who would present it to the House and Senate. Most of the conference was devoted to which part of the marihuana plant was pharmacologically active and what should be the name of the soon-to-be-taxed substance. Conversation was chiefly between the scientists and the Treasury lawyers and reveals that the Department did take into consideration scientific and medical opinion in the preparation of the marihuana legislation.

The upcoming hearing was on the minds of the participants. They knew that they would have to be prepared to rebut any suggested valid use or to include it through some exemption. The goal, however, was to have a prohibitive law to the fullest extent possible. Exceptions, particularly trade or medical exceptions, would make enforcement considerably more expensive and the Act's future cost concerned the conference. Such a desire prior to the Act and the lack of any increased appropriations for several years after the Act are consistent with Anslinger's claim that the Tax Act was no boon to his bureaucratic structure.[27]

Tennyson, the FBN's Counsel, emphasized to the group that every detail of the legislation would have to be worked out well ahead of the hearings, because "we have to support it and everything in it when we go before the Committee."[27] Perhaps a little defensively, the Commissioner wanted the group to know that the enterprise was not "a fishing expedition." Two hundred ninety-six seizures had been made of cannabis in 1936 alone. "The illicit traffic," he complained, "shows up in almost every state."[27]

After about an hour the scientific evidence on the plant and its active principle had been exhausted and the group reverted to the hearings. With regard to the effects of marihuana on the personality, S. G. Tipton of the Department's General Counsel's Office asked the Commissioner: "Have you lots of cases on this—horror stories—that's what we want."[27] The Commissioner did indeed have a collection. Then, in one of the most significant moments in the meeting, Anslinger asked the opinion of Dr. Voegtlin on whether marihuana actually produces insanity. The NIH pharmacology expert replied: "I think it is an established fact that prolonged use leads to insanity in certain cases, depending on the amount taken, of course. Many people take it and do not go insane, but many do."[27] To which the Secretary of the Treasury's Consulting Chemist, H. H. Wollner, responded with a characteristic comparison of American frankness to foreign vacillation: "At the League of Nations, they whitewashed the whole thing."[27]

The hearings before the House were held in late April and

early May.[28]   They were curious events. The Treasury's presentation to Congress has been adequately described many times, although no retelling has equalled reading the original transcript. As anticipated, the Representatives accepted whatever the Treasury Department asserted. The only witness to appear in opposition to the administration's proposal, AMA spokesman William C. Woodward, M.D., was barraged with hostile questions. One member of the Committee even questioned whether the veteran of many legislative battles dating back to before the Harrison Act actually represented the AMA. Nevertheless, he was able to get his message across: there was no need to burden the health profession with the bill's restrictions, the states could handle the problem without any additional assistance from the federal bureaucracy than was already available, and, finally, the evidence against marihuana was incomplete. He pointedly asked where the Public Health Service and Children's Bureau experts were, if it were true that the weed did have horrible physiologic effects and was wreaking havoc among America's school children. Dr. Woodward's arguments were ignored. One reason for his poor showing was that the AMA had aroused a lot of hostility by its successful defeat of President Roosevelt's plan to include health insurance in the Social Security Act. In a way reminiscent of the battle lines over the Harrison Act, the most "liberal" spokesmen were among the most eager to effect the protection of the public through the prohibition of cannabis.[29]

After the House and Senate hearings the bill was passed by Congress with no difficulty and came into effect on October 1, 1937. One of the regrettable aspects of the Marihuana Tax Act was that its role as a symbolic legislative gesture toward fearful groups made any qualification or moderation of the drug's intrinsic dangers a threat to the FBN. Anything less than prohibition would greatly diminish its value as a symbol as well as making enormously more difficult legal control with no additional appropriations. As regards enforcement, this task continued to be primarily the responsibility of local police aided by the occasional efforts of FBN agents. The arrest of those who violated the marihuana law was not difficult when compared to the task of stopping heroin smuggling, and, with no more agents, the FBN was able to put an impressive number of arrests before the public. After the Act's passage the educational campaign of the FBN stepped up, but other publicity campaigns, by lay organizations who claimed that the menace was still out of hand, were muted by FBN opposition. For example, the creators of the often reprinted marihuana poster warning children of the "Killer Drug Marihuana" were in fact put out of business by the FBN because their tactics were beginning to alarm the citizens of Chicago.[30] It may surprise some to learn that the FBN attacked such apostles of fear and had only contempt for their profit making. One reason for the FBN's action may have been its policy of designing educational literature in such a way that no youth would be tempted to try the substance.[31] Another reason may have been a reflection of the Commissioner's belief that the problem was under control in the vast majority of the nation's communities and any impression that it was out of control would only embarrass the Treasury Department.

On the other hand, the FBN resented later medical rebuttal of claims that marihuana was an extreme danger, as, for example, the La Guardia Report (1944).[32] Two responses from the FBN—closing down the Inter-State Narcotic Association for spreading disturbing scare stories and a strong and publically effective attack on the medical criticism of the FBN's position on marihuana—demonstrate both the effectiveness and the philosophy of the FBN. Two goals seem to have guided the FBN's actions: to show (1) that the FBN fought a great menace and (2) that the menace was under control.

Why the marihuana law was so eagerly desired by some and, when enacted, so effectively placating are fundamental questions. From the evidence examined, the FBN does not appear to have created the marihuana scare of the early 1930s nor can the law be simply ascribed to the Commissioner's determined will. Such scapegoating offers no more than it did in the era when marihuana was blamed for almost any vicious crime. When viewed from the narrow goal of placating fears about an "alien minority," the Act was serviceable for more than a quarter of a century. For the broader significance of the marihuana law and an understanding of the dynamics involved in prohibitive legislation, the Tax Act must be placed in its cultural and institutional context.

REFERENCES

1. *Pure Food and Drug Act,* 59th Cong., 1st Sess., ch 3915, § 8 (1901).

2. *Importation and Use of Opium,* hearings before the House Committee on Ways and Means, 61st Cong., 3rd Sess. (Jan 11, 1911).

3. Musto DF: The American antinarcotic movement: Clinical research and public policy. *Clin Res* 19:603, 1971.

4. *Importation and Use of Opium,* hearings before the House Committee on Ways and Means, 61st Cong., 3rd Sess. (Dec 14, 1910).

5. Letter from H. J. Finger to Dr. Hamilton Wright, July 2, 1911, in *Preliminary Inventories, No. 76,* Records of United States Participation in International Conferences, Commissions and Expositions, No. 39, "Correspondence of Wright with Delegate Henry J. Finger, 1911." Washington, DC, National Archives, 1955.

6. International opium convention. *Amer J Int Law* 6:177–192, 1912.

7. The Second Geneva Convention, reprinted in Terry CE, Pellens M: *The Opium Problem.* New York, Bureau of Social Hygiene, 1928, pp 945–961.

8. Letter from Dr. Oscar Dowling to Gov. John M. Parker, Aug 21, 1920, Records of the Public Health Service, File No. 2123. Washington, DC, National Archives.

9. Letter from Dr. Oscar Dowling to Surgeon-General Hugh S. Cumming, Aug 25, 1920, Records of the Public Health Service, File No. 2123. Washington, DC, National Archives.

10. Letter from Surgeon-General Hugh S. Cumming to Dr. Oscar Dowling, Sept 3, 1920, Records of the Public Health Service, File No. 2123. Washington, DC, National Archives.

11. Letter from Gov. John M. Parker to Commissioner John Kramer, Nov 26, 1920, Records of the Prohibition Unit, Bureau of Narcotics and Dangerous Drugs, Washington, DC.

12. Taylor AH: *American Diplomacy and the Narcotics Traffic, 1900–1939.* Durham, NC, Duke University Press, 1969, pp. 200–203.

13. Act of Jan 19, 1929, 70th Cong., Sess. 2, ch 82, 45 Stat. 1085.

14. Samora J.: *Los Mojados: The Wetback Story.* Notre Dame, Ind, University of Notre Dame, 1969, pp 38–46.

15. Fossier AE: The marihuana menace. *New Orleans Med Surg J* 84:247–251, 1931.

16. Hayes MH, Bowery LE: Marihuana. *J Criminal Law and Criminology* 23:1086-1098, 1933.

17. McLean RN: Tightening the Mexican border. *The Survey* 64:29, 1930.

18. Taylor PS: More bars against the Mexicans? *The Survey* 64:26, 1930.

19. Letter from the US Marshall of the Northern District of Oklahoma to Commissioner Anslinger, Dec 18, 1934. Papers of Harry J. Anslinger, Pennsylvania State University, Box 6.

20. Bromberg W: Marihuana intoxication. *Amer J Psychiat* 91:303-330, 1934.

21. Stanley E: Marihuana as a developer of criminals. *Amer J Public Sci* 2:252, 1931.

22. *Report by the Government of the United States of America for the Calendar Year ended December 31, 1931: On the Traffic in Opium and Other Dangerous Drugs.* Federal Bureau of Narcotics, 1932, p 51.

23. Uniform State Narcotic Act, reprinted in Eldridge WB: *Narcotics and the Law*, ed 2. Chicago, University of Chicago Press, 1967, pp 161-175.

24. Don't Be a "Mugglehead." Worcester, Mass, *Telegraph*, Oct 11, 1936. Papers of Harry J. Anslinger, Pennsylvania State University, Box 6.

25. Confidential memorandum from Harry J. Anslinger to Assistant Secretary of the Treasury Stephen B. Gibbons, Feb 1, 1936. Papers of Harry J. Anslinger, Pennsylvania State University, Box 12.

26. Marihuana questionnaire filled out by Dr. Walter L. Treadway, papers of Harry J. Anslinger, Pennsylvania State University, Box 6.

27. Transcript of the conference on *Cannabis sativa*, held Jan 14, 1937, 10:30 A.M., Room 81, Treasury Bldg Papers of Harry J. Anslinger, Pennsylvania State University, Box 6.

28. *Taxation of Marihuana,* hearings before the House Committee on Ways and Means, 75th Cong., 1st Sess. (April 27-30 and May 4, 1937).

29. Musto DF: The development of narcotic control in the United States, in Bell WJ Jr (ed): *Medicine and Society*, publication No. 4. Philadelphia, American Philosophical Library, 1971, pp 95-110.

30. "Inter-state Narcotic Association," FBN File 0145-18, Bureau of Narcotics and Dangerous Drugs.

31. *Report by the Government of the United States of America for the Calendar Year ended December 31, 1938: On the Traffic in Opium and Other Dangerous Drugs.* Federal Bureau of Narcotics, 1939, p 49.

32. Mayor's Committee on Marihuana: *The Marihuana Problem in the City of New York.* Lancaster, Pa, Jacques Cattell Press, 1944.

Appendix

Glossary, Conversion Tables, Biographical Notes

Glossary

Selected terms chosen to make *Marijuana: Medical Papers* more useful to the non-specialized reader.

agrypnia. Sleeplessness or insomnia.

angina pectoris. A disease marked by paroxysms of pain in the thorax, with suffocation and fainting. Due to a spasm of the coronary arteries. Occurs often with heart disease.

anodyne. A pain-killing agent, analgesic.

anorexia. Lack or loss of the appetite for food.

anti-diuretic effect. See *diuresis, diuretic effect.*

ataxia. Muscular incoördination.

bradycardia. An abnormal slowness of the heart, usually applied to a pulse-rate of 60 or less.

chorea. St. Vitus' dance, a convulsive nervous disease.

conjunctival suffusion. Bloodshot eyes.

corneal areflexia. A lack of the blinking reflex.

diuresis, diuretic effect. Increased excretion of urine.

dysmenorrhea. Painful and difficult menstruation.

dysphasia. An impairment of speech consisting of a failure to arrange words in their proper order.

dyspnea. Difficult or labored breathing.

eclampsia. A sudden attack of convulsions, usually of a puerperal cause.

enteralgia. Pain or neuralgia of the intestines.

febrile restlessness, febrile syndrome. The condition of feverish discomfort and restlessness.

gastrodynia. Pain in the stomach.

glottis spasm. Involuntary contraction of the vocal apparatus.

hyperemia. An excess of blood in any particular part of the body.

hyperesthesia. Excessive sensitiveness of the skin or of a special sense.

hypergeusia. An overly acute sense of taste.

hyperphagia. Overeating.

hyperreflexia. The exaggeration of reflexes.

hypoglycemia. A deficiency of sugar in the blood.

kymograph. An instrument for recording variations or undulations, arterial or otherwise.

laryngismus stridulus. A disease of children marked by a sudden spasm of the voice box, attended by a crowing inspiration and blueness of the skin.

macropsy. A condition in which things are seen larger than they really are.

menorrhagia. Abnormally profuse menstruation.

metritis. Inflammation of the uterus.

micropsy. A condition in which things are seen smaller than they really are.

myoclonic movement. A spasm of a muscle or muscles.

myodynia. Pain in muscle.

neuralgia. A pain in a nerve or nerves, or radiating along the course of a nerve.

neurasthenia. Nervous prostration; a nervous disorder characterized by abnormal fatiguability.

oedema of the eyelids. Watery eyes, tears, and swelling of the eyelids.

paresis. Slight or incomplete paralysis.

paresthesia. Abnormal sensations; a burning, prickling, etc.

peripheral neuritis. Inflammation of the nerve-endings or of terminal nerves.

peritonitis. Inflammation of the smooth, strong, colorless membrane lining the abdominal walls and containing the viscera.

phthisis. A progressive wasting away of the body or part of the body often with expectoration of opaque matter and sometimes blood.

placenta praevia. A placenta that comes between the intra-uterine cavity and the inner orifice of the cervical canal. It may lead to fatal hemorrhage.

praecordial discomfort. Discomfort in the region over the heart or stomach: the epigastrium and lower part of the thorax.

pruritis. Intense itching, a symptom of various skin diseases.

puerperal convulsions. Convulsions pertaining to childbirth.

pulmonary oedema. A condition in which the lungs fill with fluid.

rheumatism. A constitutional disease marked by inflammation of the connective tissue, especially the muscles and joints, attended by pain.

Roentgenogram. A photograph taken with Roentgen-rays (X-rays).

sacralgia. Pain in the sacrum, the five fused vertebrae wedged between the pelvic bones.

sciatica. A painful inflammation of the sciatic nerve, usually a neuritis attended with a partial paralysis of the leg and sometimes a wasting of the calf muscles.

sciatic nerve. A nerve running along the lower pelvis to the lower back and legs.

spinal sclerosis. A condition of the spinal cord characterized by a hardening from inflammation and overgrowth of tissue.

sudorific effect. Sweat-producing.

tachycardia. Excessive rapidity of the heart, a term usually applied to a pulse rate above 130 per minute.

thalamic structures. A mass of gray matter at the base of the brain.

tic douloureux. A spasmodic facial neuralgia.

torticollis. A contraction of muscles resulting in a twisted neck and abnormal position of the head.

trismus. Lock-jaw, a condition accompanying tetanus.

urticaria. Nettle-rash or hives; smooth, slightly elevated patches, usually whiter than surrounding skin and attended by severe itching.

uterine leucorrhea. A thick whitish discharge from the uterus and vagina. Symptomatic of vaginal and uterine congestion.

vasodilation. Dilation of blood vessels.

Conversion Tables

Apothecaries' Weight and Metric Equivalents

	Gramme			Grammes			Grammes
$1/100$ grain	= 0.0006	2 grains	= 0.13		$1\frac{1}{2}$ drachms	=	5.85
$1/64$ "	= 0.001	3 "	= 0.2		$1\frac{3}{4}$ "	=	6.81
$1/50$ "	= 0.0013	4 "	= 0.26		2 "	=	7.78
$1/40$ "	= 0.0016	5 "	= 0.32		$2\frac{1}{2}$ "	=	9.72
$1/32$ "	= 0.002	6 "	= 0.39		3 "	=	11.65
$1/20$ "	= 0.003	8 "	= 0.52		4 "	=	15.55
$1/16$ "	= 0.004	10 "	= 0.65		5 "	=	19.43
$1/12$ "	= 0.005	12 "	= 0.78		6 "	=	23.3
$1/10$ "	= 0.006	15 "	= 0.97		1 oz. (480 grs.)	=	31.1
$1/8$ "	= 0.008	15.4 "	= 1.		2 ounces	=	62.2
$1/6$ "	= 0.011	20 "	= 1.3		3 "	=	93.3
$1/5$ "	= 0.012	24 "	= 1.55		4 "	=	124.4
$1/4$ "	= 0.015	30 "	= 1.94		6 "	=	186.6
$1/3$ "	= 0.022	40 "	= 2.6		8 "	=	248.8
$1/2$ "	= 0.032	45 "	= 2.92		10 "	=	311.
$3/4$ "	= 0.048	50 "	= 3.23		12 "	=	373.2
1. "	= 0.065	60 grains or 1 drachm	= 3.89				

Apothecaries' Measure and Metric Equivalents

1 minim	= 0.06 Cc.	60	minims or 1 fluidrachm		=	3.70 Cc.	
2 minims	= 0.12 "	$1\frac{1}{4}$	fluidrachms	- -	=	4.65 "	
3 "	= 0.18 "	$1\frac{1}{2}$	"	- -	=	5.60 "	
4 "	= 0.24 "	$1\frac{3}{4}$	"	- -	=	6.50 "	
5 "	= 0.30 "	2	"	- -	=	7.50 "	
6 "	= 0.36 "	3	"		=	11.25 "	
7 "	= 0.42 "	4	"	-	=	15.00 "	
8 "	= 0.50 "	8	fluidrachms or 1 fluidounce	=	30.00 "	
9 "	= 0.55 "			(more exactly, 29.57)		
10 "	= 0.60 "	2	fluidounces	- -	=	59.15 "	
15 "	= 0.92 "	3	"		=	88.72 "	
20 "	= 1.25 "	4	"	- -	=	118.29 "	
25 "	= 1.54 "	8	"	-	=	236.59 "	
30 "	= 1.90 "	16	fluidounces or (1 pint)	=	473.18 "	
40 "	= 2.50 "	32	fluidounces	- -	=	946.36 "	
45 "	= 2.80 "	128	fluidounces or 1 gallon	=	3785.43 "	
50 "	= 3.10 "						

Avoirdupois Weight and Metric Equivalents

1 AV. OZ. = 437.5 GRAINS

$1/8$ oz.	=	3.54 Gms.	7 ozs.	= 198.45 Gms.	1 ℔.	=	453.60 Gms.
$1/4$ oz.	=	7.09 "	8 ozs.	= 226.80 "	2 ℔s.	=	907.18 "
$1/2$ oz.	=	14.17 "	9 ozs.	= 255.15 "	2.2 ℔s.	=	1000.00 "
1 oz.	=	28.35 "	10 ozs.	= 283.50 "	3 ℔s.	=	1360.78 "
2 ozs.	=	56.70 "	11 ozs.	= 311.84 "	4 ℔s.	=	1814.37 "
3 ozs.	=	85.05 "	12 ozs.	= 340.20 "	5 ℔s.	=	2267.96 "
4 ozs.	=	113.40 "	13 ozs.	= 368.54 "	6 ℔s.	=	2721.55 "
5 ozs.	=	141.75 "	14 ozs.	= 396.90 "	8 ℔s.	=	3628.74 "
6 ozs.	=	170.10 "	15 ozs.	= 425.25 "	10 ℔s.	=	4535.92 "

Metric Weight and Apothecaries' Equivalents

Grammes		Grains	Grammes		Grains	Grammes		Grains	Grammes		Grains
0.001	=	$1/64$	0.04	=	$2/3$	0.6	=	9	10.	=	154.3
0.0015	=	$1/40$	0.05	=	$3/4$	0.65	=	10	15.	=	231.3
0.002	=	$1/32$	0.065	=	1.	0.7	=	10.8	20.	=	308.6
0.003	=	$1/20$	0.08	=	$1 1/4$	0.8	=	12	25.	=	385.8
0.004	=	$1/16$	0.1	=	$1 1/2$	1.0	=	15.432	30.	=	463
0.005	=	$1/12$	0.15	=	$2 1/4$	1.5	=	23	40.	=	617.3
0.006	=	$1/10$	0.2	=	3	2.	=	30.8	50.	=	771.6
0.008	=	$1/8$	0.25	=	4	4.	=	61.5	60.	=	926
0.01	=	$1/6$	0.3	=	$4 1/2$	5.	=	77			
0.015	=	$1/4$	0.4	=	6	6.	=	92.5			
0.03	=	$1/2$	0.5	=	$7 1/2$	8.	=	123.4			

Metric Weight and Avoirdupois Equivalents

Grammes	Grammes	Grammes
25. = 385.8 grs.	60. = 2 oz. + 50 grs.	300. = 10 oz. + 255 grs.
(approx. $7/8$ oz.)	70. = 2 oz. + 205 grs.	400. = 14 oz. + 48 grs.
28.35 = 1 oz. = 437.5 grs.	75. = 2 oz. + 282 grs.	500. = 17 oz. + 279 grs.
30. = 1 oz. + 25 grs.	80. = 2 oz. + 360 grs.	(approx. 1 ℔., 1 $5/8$ oz.)
32. = 1 oz. + 56 grs.	90. = 3 oz. + 76 grs.	600. = 21 oz. + 72 grs.
33. = 1 oz. + 72 grs.	100. = 3 oz. + 231 grs.	700. = 24 oz. + 303 grs.
34. = 1 oz. + 87 grs.	(approx. 3 $1/2$ oz.)	750. = 26 oz. + 198 grs.
35. = 1 oz. + 103 grs.	120. = 4 oz. + 102 grs.	800. = 28 oz. + 96 grs.
36. = 1 oz. + 118 grs.	125. = 4 oz. + 179 grs.	900. = 31 oz. + 326 grs.
40. = 1 oz. + 180 grs.	150. = 5 oz. + 127 grs.	1000. = 35 oz. + 120 grs.
45. = 1 oz. + 218 grs.	200. = 7 oz. + 24 grs.	(approx. 2 $1/5$ ℔s.)
50. = 1 oz. + 334 grs.	250. = 8 oz. + 358 grs.	

Metric Measure and Equivalents in Apothecaries' Measure

Cc.	Cc.	Cc.
0.06 = 1 minim	6 = 1.62 fluidrachms	120 = 4 fluidounces
0.1 = 1.5 minims	8 = 2.16 "	150 = 5 "
0.2 = 3 "	10 = 2.71 "	200 = 6.75 "
0.3 = 5 "	15 = 4 "	300 = 10.14 "
0.4 = 6 "	20 = 5.42 "	400 = 13.53 "
0.5 = 8 "	25 = 6.75 "	473 = 16.00 (1 pt.) "
0.6 = 10 "	30 = 1 fluidounce	500 = 16.90 "
0.7 = 11 "	40 = 1.3 fluidounces	600 = 20.30 "
0.8 = 12 "	45 = 1.5 "	700 = 23.67 "
0.9 = 14 "	50 = 1.7 "	750 = 25.36 "
1 = 16.2 "	60 = 2 "	800 = 27. "
2 = 32.4 "	70 = 2.3 "	900 = 30.43 "
3 = 48.6 "	75 = 2.53 "	1000 = 33.81 "
4 = 64.8 "	90 = 3. "	(= 1 liter)
5 = 1.35 fluidrachms	100 = 3.38 "	

Biographical Notes

Roger Adams completed his Harvard doctorate in chemistry in 1912. From 1922 to 1932 he was editor of the *Journal of the American Chemical Society* and contributed nineteen essays on cannabis chemistry from his research at Noyes Chemical Laboratory, University of Illinois, during the 1940s. The Harvey Lecture reprinted in this volume is a report on his cannabis research up to 1924.

Samuel Allentuck, M.D., is a member of the American Board of Psychiatry and Neurology. He was director of the clinical experiments at the Welfare Island Hospital under Mayor La Guardia's Commission on Marihuana. He is a psychiatrist in private practice in New York City.

Frances Rix Ames received her M.D. from the University of Capetown in 1942 and her M.Med. in 1954. She also holds a doctorate of psychiatric medicine and is on the staff of the department of neurology at the Groote Schuur Hospital.

John Bell was elected a fellow and councilor for the New Hampshire Medical Society in 1846. He published numerous articles on various botanical subjects and published a paper describing the effects of consanguinity upon the physical and mental makeup of offspring in 1859.

Edward Birch, M.D., entered the India Medical Service in 1866 and spent nearly the whole of his service in Bengal. He was civil surgeon of Hazaribagh, later superintendent of the Presidency General Hospital, and later still principal of the Medical College, Calcutta. In 1902 he completed his fourth edition of *Birch's Management of Children in India.*

Alfred Crancer, Jr. received a master's degree from American University in 1963 in mathematics and statistics. He was formerly director of research for the State of Washington Motor Vehicle Department and currently serves as evaluation coordinator for the U.S. Department of Transportation Office of Alcohol Countermeasures. He has published many other papers on the applications of driving simulator technics in the assessment of effects of various drugs on driving ability.

John Preston Davis became a physician in 1934 at the University of Pennsylvania School of Medicine. He is a member of the American Board of Internal Medicine and a professor at Bowman Gray School of Medicine of Wake Forest College, Winston-Salem, North Carolina.

James Foulis studied under Lister at both Glasgow and Edinburgh schools of medicine. He received his M.D. from Edinburgh University in 1875. He published several papers on obstetrics and received numerous awards for his medical scholarship.

Herbert C. Hamilton, M.S., was a full-time chemical engineer for the Parke-Davis company. He published several other papers on pharmaceutical effects of cannabis in pharmaceutical journals. He was a member of the American Pharmaceutical Association and retired from the company in 1934.

Hobart Amory Hare received his M.D. from the University of Pennsylvania in 1884, became professor of materia medica at Jefferson Medical School, wrote numerous prize-winning medical research articles, and edited numerous medical and scientific publications, including *Therapeutic Gazette.* He was a president of the Philadelphia College of Physicians and a member of many medical specialty societies.

Walter Siegfried Loewe, M.D., Ph.D., was educated at the universities of Freiburg, Berlin, Munich, and Strasbourg, and became an M.D. in 1908. A professor of pharmacology in several German universities, Loewe left Germany in 1934 to join the medical staff at Mt. Sinai Hospital. As a research fellow for ten years, beginning in 1936, at Cornell Medical College, he conducted his pharmacological experiments on marijuana. In 1946 Dr. Loewe became Research Professor of Pharmacology, College of Medicine, University of Utah.

Charles Robertsham Marshall obtained an M.A. at Cambridge and an Ll.B. at St. Andrews College before receiving an M.D. from Victoria College in 1899. He was professor of materia medica at the University of Aberdeen and author of a textbook on materia medica.

Jansen Beemer Mattison was graduated M.D. from Bellevue Hospital Medical College in 1867. A member of the Brooklyn Neurological Society and the American Association for the Cure of Inebriety, he devoted himself to the study and treatment of narcotic inebriety and authored more than seventy papers on various phases of this disease.

Tod Hiro Mikuriya, a psychiatrist in private practice, was formerly in charge of marijuana research at the National Institute of Mental Health. He was a consultant to the National Commission on Marihuana and Drug Abuse. Dr. Mikuriya has authored a number of essays on a spectrum of marijuana topics, including "Marijuana in Morocco," "Marijuana in Medicine, Past, Present, Future," and "Historical Aspects of Cannabis Sativa in Western Medicine."

David Franklin Musto acquired his M.D. at the University of Washington School of Medicine in Seattle in 1963. His medical specialties include psychiatry and internal medicine. Dr. Musto, as assistant professor of history and psychiatry at Yale, has conducted research in association with the Child Study Center there. He is a consultant to the National Commission on Marihuana and Drug Abuse and has recently published a book on the history of drugs and the law.

John Christopher O'Day, M.D., graduated from National Normal University College of Medicine in 1896 and from Rush Medical College in 1900. He was a member of the American College of Surgeons.

Sir William Brooke O'Shaughnessy, upon graduating as M.D. from Edinburgh University, entered the East India Company's service as a surgeon in Bengal and Agra and as professor of chemistry in Calcutta. He devoted much of his interest to the electric telegraph and in 1854, as director-general of telegraphs in India, he oversaw the laying down of four thousand miles of lines between major Indian cities. A message over these lines saved a garrison during the Sepoy Rebellion, for which he was knighted in 1856.

Joseph Price Remington, Ph.M., F.C.S., graduated in 1866 from Philadelphia College of Pharmacy, where he then became professor of theory and practice of pharmacy. He became the leading figure of his time in American pharmacy as a promoter and director of research, vice-chairman of the U.S. Pharmacopoeia (1880–1891), and chairman of the council of the American Pharmaceutical Association.

Sir John Russell Reynolds took up a practice in London upon acquiring an M.D. in 1852. He became professor of Medicine at University College and specialized in the study of nervous diseases, electrotherapy, and scientific evaluations of the legal tests for insanity. He was physician to the queen's household and twice president of the Royal College of Physicians.

Alexander Theodore Shulgin completed his college education at the University of California with a doctorate in biochemistry in 1954. As a research chemist for Dow Chemical Company and an expert in phenethylamine chemistry, Dr. Shulgin's work in myristicin chemistry led to the first synthesis of DOM (STP) and MMDA.

Robert P. Walton was born in Guthrie, Kentucky, received a Ph.D. from Columbia University in 1929, and became an M.D. at the University of Chicago in 1941. In 1939 he authored a comprehensive report, *Marihuana, America's New Drug Problem*, from which this volume has reprinted two chapters. In 1942, Dr. Walton became professor of pharmacology and therapeutics at the Medical College of South Carolina, a post he held until his death.

Andrew T. Weil concluded his Harvard education with an M.D. in 1963. He has contributed several essays dealing with clinical research on marijuana and β-phenethylamines. He is the author of *The Natural Mind*, a book on altered states of consciousness, and recently conducted a botanical and anthropological expedition in Brazil's Orinoco River basin.

Author Index

Aaron, 404
Adams, Roger, 218, 292, n. 375, 376, 378, 379, 402, 403
Ali, Syed Keramut, 4, 10
Allentuck, Samuel, xx, 177, 218, 345, 361, 369, 371
Ames, 177
Amoroso, Peter F., 196
Andrews, Dr. Robert, 129
Anslinger, Harold J., 417, 427, 428, 429, 430, 431, 432, 434, 435
Anstil, 153, 154
Atlee, Dr., 98, 133
Aubert-Roche, 83, 160
Ainslee, Dr., 15
Audie, 162
Austin, Dr., 127

Bain, Dr., 4
Baker-Bates, Dr., 100
Baker, B. R., 348
Banks, Sir Joseph, 118
Barker, xix
Bartholow, 151
Bastedo, 163
Bastian, 153
Bates, J. W., 252
Batho, 164
Batterman, Dr. Robert C, 200
Baudelaire, 109
Baxter-Tyrie, 99
Bayer, V., 107
Beane, 93
Beddoe, 154
Becchner, 266
Beitar, Ibn, 11, 16
Bell, Dr. John, 31, 93, 120
Benedict, 99
Beringer, K., 107, 247, 248
Beron, 120
Berthier, 163
Bicknell, 99
Billah, Khalif Mostansir, 11
Binet-Sangle, 90
Birch, xiv, 164
Blatt, A. H. 347, n. 375
Boner, Dr., 136, 137
Bourhill, C. U. G., 220, 221
Bowman, 218
Bragman, 163
Braun, 411
Breyer-Brankwijk, 221
Bromberg, Walter, M.D., 111, 112, 218, 427
Brown, 94, 164
Buchwald, 96
Buckingham, Dr. C. E., 125, 126

Burgi, 384
Burr, 90, 248

Cabot, Dr., 125
Cahn, R. S., 348, 349, 377
Cain, C. K., 348
Campbell, Dr., 5, 93
Caswell, George, 51
Chamberlain, Joseph, 431
Chevalier, 14
Chopra, I. C., 253
Chopra, N. R., 253
Christison, Dr., 123, 165
Churchill, Dr., 123
Circe, 64
Clark, J. H., 348
Clark, Stafford, 218, 249
Clarke, Dr., 84, 126
Claussen, 409
Clendinning, 163
Cohen, 162
Cornbleet, 163
Crancer, A., 177, 287
Crump, xvii
Cunningham, n. xxiii

DaCosta, 4, 10, 12
Dalton, Dr. John C. Jr., 125
Dante, 62
David (King of Israel), 42
de Lens, 14
De Quincey, Thomas, 31, 58
De Sacy, 10, 15
Dhur, Dinonath, 22, 29
Dioscorides, xiv, 11
Dixon, W. E., 163, 336
Dlugosch, 409
Dohme, A. R. L., 338
Domino, xxii
Donahoo, Dr. H. J., M.D., 126
Donovan, 84, 119, 123, 154
Dontas, 109
Dowling, Oscar, 423
Downer, 99
Dozier, Horace, 161
Dresbach, Dr. E., 124, 125
Dreury, 111
Duncan, Dr., 18, 87, 123
Dunglison, Dr., 119
Durand-Fardel, 146
Dutcher, Dr. A. P., 133

Easterfield, Dr., 107, 217, 301, 303, 309, 318, 340, 347
Eckhardt, G., 356
Edes, 164
Egerton, Dr., 24

Eichhorn, 163
Elijah, Khizer (Mohamedan Saint), 215
Eschenmoser, 412
Esenbeck, Ness V., 14
Esquirol, 39, 47, 48, 49
Ewens, 357

Famulener, 340
Fantus, 162, 163
Farlow, 162
Fee, 14
Finger, Henry J., 422
Fischlowity, 97
Florshinger, 163
Foulīs, Dr. J., 31, 62
Fraenkel, J., 102, 109, 113, 340, 357, 358
Freusberg, 109
Fronmueller, Dr., xv, 119, 120, 154, 163
Fuller, 154
Fuller, Stuart, 431, 432

Galen, xiv, 14
Gaoni, 407, 410, 412
Gautier, 109
Gayer, H., 104, 106, 357, 358, 386
Geiser, 97
Gibbons, Stephen B., 431
Gillman, A., 216, 259, 389
Githens, M.D., 162
Gitzelter, Dr. Louis, 207
Glickman, 252
Goethe, C. M., 426
Goodeve, Dr., 4, 23
Goodman, L. S., 167, 216, 259, 387, 289
Goopto, Modoosudun, 4, 9
Goosen, C. C., 252
Green, Richard, 153
Gregor, Dr., 124
Grigor, 165

Hackell, 408
Haefliger, 411
Haider, Sheikh, 10, 11
Hall, Marshall, 146
H a m a k e r ,
Hamburg, 93
Hamilton, H. C., 31, 69, 70, 80, 334
Hardman, Dr. Harold F., xxii
Hare, Dr. H. A., xvii, 151, 154, 156, 162,
    163, 291
Harris, xxii
Hassan, 10
Henry, 14
Herodotus, xiv, 118
Hewitt, Graily, 154
Hiller, 163
Hippocrates, 11
Homer, 118
Hooper, 336, 339
Houghton, 69, 80
Hoa-tho, xiv
Hunt, Madison, 348

Indee, 120

Isbell, 257
Iwanow, 108

Jaffe, 259
Jahns, 340
Jelinek, Charles F., 348
Joel, 102, 109
Jones, xxii
Judee, 93
Julien, M., 118

Kant, 104, 106
Kelly, 94
Kendricks, Dr. O. C., 130
Kincaid, Dr. W. P., 135, 140
Kionka, 312, 313
Klug, 69
Kobert, 340
Kobylanski, 165
Kolb, Dr. Lawrence Sr., 433
Korte, 409
Kramer, John F., 423
Krapf, 104
Kubie, Dr. L., 385
Kuykendall, 86

La Guardia, Mayor, xx, 361
Lamarck, 333
Lambert, Dr. Alexander, 420, 421
Lange, 93
Lanslerer, 120
Laplin, Leif, 309
Lenard, 408
Lescohier, Dr. A. W., 31
Levine, J., 355, n. 376
Lewin, L., 214
Lewis, 163
Liataud, 357
Lindemann, 165
Lindley, 4, 5
Linnaeus, 118
Lloyd, B., 249
Loewe, J., 167, 217, 249, 292, 345, 355, 357,
    358, 359, 363, 378

MacKenzie, 153, 154, 162
Mahneman, 3
Makrizi, Takim Eddin, 10, 11, 12 15
Malamud, 165
Mantz, H. W., 357
Marshall, Dr. C. R., 89, 291
Marx, 106
Matchett, Dr. J. R., 345, 347, 355, n. 376
Matsui, 409
Mattison, xvi
May, Herbert L., 431
McCann, 4, 6
McCrae, 162
McConnell, N. F., 154, 163
McFarland, Dr. J. A., 125
McKinnon, Dr., 6
McMeens, Dr. R. R., 135
McPhee, 348

Mechoulam, 407, 410, 412
Meggendorfer, 106
Mendel, 157
Mendelssohn, Jack H., 169
Merat, 14
Mercer, 162
Merek, 156
Meyer-Gross, 247
Mikuriya, Tod H., M.D., 67
Milks, 163
Miller, 123, 163
Mills, George, 18
Mitter, Nobinchunder, 4, 18
Mooney, Dr. M. D., 130
Moore, 312
Moreau, Dr. J. J. (de Tours), 41, 42, 43,
    44, 83, 109, 160, 164, 247
Morgenthau, Henry Hr., 430
Morton, n. xxiv
Munch, J. C., 357
Musto, Dr. David, 417

Napoleon, 15, 216
Neil, 207
Nicholson, Dr., 28
Nickerson, 388

O'Brien, 4, 25, 26
O'Day, Dr. J. C., 31, 52
Ohloff, 412
Oliphant, Herman, 429, 432
O'Shaughnessy, Dr. W. B., xiii, xv, xxii,
    1, 4, 26, 83, 119, 122, 160, 301, 306
Osler, xviii, 162
Osmond, 218
Owen, 93
Oxley, 154

Parker, 218
Parker, John M., 423
Pars, 404
Pease, D. C., 348
Pereira, 118, 334
Perkins, R. A., 31
Personne, M. J., 303
Petrzilka, 411
Phillips, 154
Plaut, Albert, 420
Pliny, 11
Polli, 93
Potter, Dr., 151, 154
Poulsson, 163
Prentiss, Dr., 96
Prichard, 40
Prior, 156
Pusinelli, Dr., 96

Ragsky, 93
Ratier, 14
Ray, 49
Rech, 120, 164
Reich, 84
Renz, 93
Reynolds, Russell, xvii, xviii, 153

Rhazes, Abdul Mirza, 4, 6, 10, 13
Rheede, 14
Richard, 14
Richet, 93
Richter, 96
Ringer, 152, 154
Robertson, 301
Robinson, 90
Rockwood, 312
Rolls, E. J., 218, 249
Roosebelt, 436
Roques, 14
Rosetti, 62
Roux, I., 303, 340
Rouyer, M., 15
Royle, Dr., 118
Rumphius, 13, 14
Ruppaner, xix
Rusby, Dr. H. H., 69, 70

Sakinofsky, S., 252
Sapeika, Prof. N., 252
Saul (biblical personage), 42
Saunders, Dr. Stewart, 237, 252
Savignac, 165
Sawtelle, Dr., 98
Schieffelin, Dr. Wm. J., 421
Schlesinger, 339
Schmidt, 101
Schneider, 92
Schroff, 109, 120
See, Germain, 161
Sequin, Dr. E. C., 152
Seifert, Dr., 96
Shen-nung, xiv
Shirazi, Djafar Hassan, 10
Shoemaker, 163
Shulgin, 292
Shvo, 407
Siddons, 21
Sieper, 408
Sikemeier, 411
Silver, Dr., 18
Sim, Dr. Van M., xxii
Simpson, Dr., 118, 123
Sinkler, Dr. Wharton, 153
Skliar, 108
Smit, Dr. Ryno J., 252
Smith, 266
Smith (brothers), 119, 301, 337
Smith, C. M., 348
Smith, Southwood, 39
Smythies, 218
Solis-Cohen, 162
Soubeiran, 14
Speigel, E. A., 250
Spivey, 107, 217, 301, 318, 340, 347
Squire, Peter, 145
Stevens, 162
Sticker, Dr., 95
Stille, 151, 152
Stockings, 218
Straub, Prof., 104, 105, 164
Strauss, Dr. Hans, 208

Stringaris, 108
Suckling, Dr., xvi, 153, 154, 157
Swinburne, 62
Syce, Chundov, 25

Tamarin, 169
Taylor, 407
Taylor, Bayard, 87, 120, 133
Tennyson, 435
Tennyson, Lord Alfred, 62
Thomas, Dr., 86
Tipton, S. G., 435
Todd, 400, 402
Toman, 387
Tamert, John S., M.D., 169
Towns, Charles B., 421
Treadway, Dr. Walter L., 433, 434
True, 69
Tschirch, 335
Tyrell, 154

Valenti, 303
Van Slyke, 207
Vedder, Dr., 252
Vedder, Senator, 219
Vidyadanka, Kamalakantha, 4, 9
Vignola, 303
Virgil, 62
Voegtlin, Dr. Carl, 434, 435
Vogelsgesang, 156
Von Mering, 89

Von Schrenck, 166
Von Schroff, 93

Wallich, Dr., 14
Walton, R. P., M.D., Ph.d., xviii, 31, 115,
    217, 218, 248, 292, 357, 360
Watt, Prof. J. M., 221, 252
Wearn, R. B., 348
Weil, A. T., 177, 288
Wellner, Dr. H. J., 345
West, Charles A., 420
West, Dr., 124, 154
Wheeler, L. M., Ph.d., 68
Wiltshire, 87
Wiley, Dr. Harvey Washington, 421
Wilker, A., 249
Williams, Dr. C. J. B., 93, 145, 257
Willis, Dr. J. P., 124, 129, 164
Windscheid, Dr., 96
Wolff, 120
Wolff, Hans, 348
Wollner, H. J., 216, 355, n. 376, 378, 435
Wood, Prof. H. C. Jr., 53, 69, 85, 107, 118,
    119, 123, 151, 152, 155, 162, 217, 301,
    303, 317, 334, 335, 340, 347, n. 375
Woodward, William C., M.D., 436
Wright, Dr. Hamilton, 419, 422
Wrigley, 218

Zis, 109

Subject Index

abdomen, sensation of warmth in, 34, 35, 232
abdomen, sensation of oppression in, 38
abdominal cramps, 241
abnormal electrocardiograms, 200 see also electrocardiograms
acetanilide, xviii, 160, 421
acetate of lead, 25
acetone, 217
acetylcannabinol, 317
addiction, xix, 108, 115, 152, 161, 393
addiction-maintenance, 422, 423
addiction treatment, 241
addicts, 243, 245, 248 see also addiction, habituation, habitues
adrenaline, 225
Advisory Committee of the Traffic in Opium and Other Dangerous Drugs (League of Nations), 424
agrypnia, 155
albino mice, 357
albumen, 203, 335, 339
alcohol, 5, 119, 126, 134, 171, 172, 391, 338, 340
alcohol (liquor) compared to marijuana, xxii, xxiii, 16, 29, 33, 38, 40, 153, 170, 173, 176, 177, 221, 241, 244, 261, 286, 287, 289, 295, 346, 364, 366, 421, 423, 434
alcoholic dependence, alcoholism, xx, 115, 169, 175, 176, 311, 341, 369, see also episodic drinking
alcoholic, 169, 175
alcoholic delirium, xxviii, 146, see also delirium tremens
alimentary canal, 38, 107, 312, see also gastrointestinal tract
alpha rhythm, 241, 249
American hemp, 375, see also marijuana
American marijuana, 255, see also marijuana
American Medical Association, 160, 177, 417, 420, 436
American Psychiatric Association, 427
amine oxidase, 249
amphetamines, 429
amputation, 25, 139
Amytal, 165
anaemia, 153
analgesia, xiii, 115, 161, 390, 391
analgesic drugs, 115, 159, 216
analgesic effect of marijuana, xviii, 152, 162, 291, 292, 317, 343, 388, 393
analgesic-hypnotic effect, xviii, xxiv
analgesic-soporific drugs, 151
anasarca, 13
anascha, 101, 102, 109, 215
"anaschisten", 108

anesthesia, 91, 95, 98, 104, 152, 160, 357 see also semi-anesthesia
anesthetic effect of marijuana, 152, 299
angina pectoris, 62
anodyne, xvi, 123, 128, 151, 152, 153, 154, 155, 157, 163
anorexia, 142
Antabuse, 170, 174
antagonist of spastic conditions, antispasmodic, 216
anthrax, 219
anti-asthmatic, xxiv
antibiotic properties, xiii, xxiv, see also bacteriological properties
anticonvulsant action, xiii, 29, 292, 387, 390
antidepressant-tranquilizer, xxiv
antidiuretic effect (lack of), 205
antielectroshock effect, 387, 388, 390, 391
antiepileptic-antispasmodic activity, xxiv, 249, 390, 391, 393
anti-marijuana laws, 429
anti-petit mal activity, 387, see also epilepsy therapy; petit mal
antipyrine, xvi, 160, 421
anti-tussive effect, xxiv
anxiety, 152, 179, 182, 183, 190, 191, 196, 197, 226, 230, 232, 247, 295, 365
aphrodisia, aphrodisiac effect, 8, 20, 29, 65, 86, 87, 100, 104, 122, 243, 365
appetite, appetite stimulation, xiii, xviii, xxiv, 8, 13, 122, 134, 245, see also desire for food
Arabic authors, xii, 9, 10
Arab poet, 11
areflexia, 387
aromatics, 398
arsenic, 147
arterial pressure, 296, 297, 298, 363, see also blood pressure, venous pressure
assay, 94, 340, 341, 342, 359, 376, 404, see also bioassay
association, difficult with marijuana, 104
asthma, xvii, 14, 127, 128, 148, 154
Astrachan Psychiatric Clinic, 108
ataraxia, xiii
ataxia, 90, 167, 179, 180, 184, 196, 217, 234, 305, 306, 314, 341, 342, 356, 360, 365, 371, 376, 380, 384, 385, 386, 389, 390, 391, 392, 403, see also incoordination, muscular
ataxia-active THC, 387
ataxia analysis, 403
ataxic incoordination, 390
auditory hallucinations, 221, see also hallucinations
autistic personality, 363
autonomic changes, 250

autonomic disturbance, xiii
autonomic imbalance, 248

bacteriological properties, xxi, see also
    antibiotic properties
"Balsamum Cannabis Indica'" 96
barbitals, xviii, 160, 216
barbiturates, 357, 364, 384, 388, 392, 429
barium test, 206
basal metabolic rate, 208, 209, 210, 363
basal metabolism test, 190, 197
"beginner's habituation", xvii
Bellevue Hospital, 111, 193
beta (wave) activity, 235
bhang, bangh subjee, bang, 6, 7, 13, 15,
    143, 215, 219, 335
bile, flow of, xvii, 13, 14
bioassay of marijuana, xiii, 358, 359, 385,
    389, 392 see also assay
biosynthesis, biosynthetic, 399, 405
bladder, 230
blood, 127, 383
blood cells, 204
blood chemistries, 363, 365
blood composition, 197
blood counts, 200
blood glucose level, 265
blood pressure, 75, 103, 179, 180, 198, 210,
    233, 256, 259, 314, 315, 363, 364
blood studies, 202
blood sugar (level), 202, 203, 205, 210, 223,
    236, 238, 241, 252, 259
blood tests, 175
blood urea, 202
blood vessels, 315
botanical description of marijuana, 4, 5,
    118, 256, 333, 334, 335, 338
bowels, 27, 129
bowels, disordered, 142
Brahmins, 9, see also Hindus, Hindu
    Tantra
brain, xv, 37, 59, 64, 65, 85, 120, 121, 134,
    163, 206
brain disease, 265, 266
brain metabolism, 206
brain-softening, 146
brain stem, effect of marijuana on, 250
brain tissue, 206
brain tumor, 147
brain waves, see alpha (wave) activity,
    alpha rhythm, beta (wave) activity
Bright's disease, 154
British East India Co., 1
British Medical Journal, 153
British Pharmacopoeia, 338
Bromberg study, 433
bromine, 147
bromsulfalein, 204, 210
bronchitis, 133, 134
bronchopneumonia, 164
buccal mucus, 306
Bulletin de Pharmacie, 15
butyl-bromoallyl barbituric acid, 357

caffeine, 265, 421, see also coffee
calabash, 215
calcium, 200, 202
California Board of Pharmacy, 422
calmative (drug) effect, 108, 111, 123, 135
Cambridge, 217, 301
Cambridge Philosophical Society, 303
camphor, 14, 34, 122, 129
canamo, 333, see also marijuana
"cancer cures", 219
cannabene, 303, 339
cannabichromene, 406
cannabicyclol, 406
cannabidiol, 349, 350, 351, 352, 355, 358,
    361, 364, 376, 389, 389, 386, 392, 402,
    405, 413
cannabidiol diacetate, 355
cannabidiolic acid, xxi, 40
cannabidiol molecule, 350
cannabigerol, 405, 413
cannabin, 119, 304, 339, 340
cannabindon, 340
cannabinoid group, 398, 399, 400, 404, 405,
    407, 411
cannabinol(s), 89, 90, 106, 188, 216, 217,
    249, 303, 304, 306, 307, 310, 311, 313,
    314, 315, 317, 340, 344, 347, 349, 352,
    376, 378, 380, 383, 385, 387, 388, 390,
    391, 392, 393, 398, 399, 405, 411
cannabinol molecule, 348
cannabinol phosphate, 314, 317
cannabinol therapy, 167, 388
cannabinon, 95, 96, 307, 309
cannabinone, 156
cannabis, xiii, xiv, xv, xvi, xvii, xix, xx,
    xxi, xxiii, 79, 93, 128, 143, 151, 153,
    159, 160, 161, 165, 170, 172, 175, 176,
    213, 214, 216, 217, 218, 221, 223, 232,
    235, 236, 237, 239, 242, 247, 251, 255,
    256, 253, 292, 312, 314, 316, 334, 338,
    343, 357, 358, 375, 385, 386, 392, 398,
    402, 419, 420, 422, 423, 424, 425, 427,
    432, 433, see also marijuana
"cannabis activity", 376, 383, 386
cannabis addiction, xix, 214, see also
    addiction, habituation
Cannabis americana, xiv, 67, 70, 73, 75, 78,
    79, 101, 102, 334, see also marijuana
cannabis analgesia, 291, see also analgesia
cannabis euphoria, 172, see also euphoria
cannabis fluid extracts, 361
cannabis habit, 214, see also addiction,
    cannabis addiction, habituation
Cannabis indica, xiv, xviii, 4, 33, 40, 50,
    51, 58, 67, 69, 70, 78, 84, 90, 92, 96, 97,
    98, 100, 102, 117, 118, 125, 126, 127,
    128, 130, 132, 135, 139, 142, 145, 146,
    151, 157, 293, 294, 295, 299, 304, 306,
    310, 314, 333, 334, 339, 340, 422, 434,
    see also marijuana
cannabis intoxication, 218, 249, 250, see
    also intoxication
cannabis market, 424
cannabis pharmacology, 250

cannabis products, 115, 291
cannabis psychoses, 106
cannabis resin, 313, *see also* resin
Cannabis sativa, xiv, 4, 69, 80, 81, 118, 213, 219, 221, 222, 224, 251, 255, 333, 334, 345, 379, 399, 404, 405, 406, 413, 416, *see also* marijuana
cannabis smokers, 221
cannabis users, 425
carbohydrates, 398
carbon-dioxide, 309
carbon-dioxide concentration, 207
carcinoma, pain of, 239
cardiac depression, 298
cardiac disease, 154
cardiac palpitation, 186
carotid artery, 206
castor oil, 25, 28
casts, 203
cats, 304, 315, 320, 329, 344, 357, 387
cauterization, 118
cell count, 202, 210
central nervous mechanism, 389
central nervous stimulant action, 385, 386
central nervous system, 211, 217
cerebral cells, 315
cerebral depression (in the frog), 298
cerebral disease, 218, *see also* brain cerebral disturbance, 249
cerebral excitation, 210, *see also* excitement
cerebral hyperaemia, 250
cerebral palsy, 167
cerebral system, 16
cerebral tissue, 249
cerebrum, 299
Chanvre de l'Inde, 333, *see also* marijuana
charas, churrus, 5, 6, 12, 16, 89, 119, 291, 301, 303, 307, 336, 337, 339, 340, 346, 398, *see also* marijuana
charas tetrahydrocannabinol, 376, 384, *see also* tetrahydrocannabinol
Chemical Abstracts convention, 399
chest, tightness of, 186
childbirth (labor), xxiv, 124, 164, 165, 219
Children's Bureau, 436
chloral hydrate, xviii, 142, 143, 153, 154, 156, 160, 216, 419
chloral hydrate, chronic poisoning by, 164
chloroform, 123, 126, 127, 136, 137, 139, 142
chlorophyll, 5, 339, 413
chlorpromazine, n. 241, 266
chocolate powder, 105
cholera, 1, 23, 30, 123
choline, 339
chordee, 154
chorea, 83, 124, 140, 148, 154, 161
choreiform restlessness, 107
chromatographic analysis, 405
chronic users, effect of cannabis, 109
cicuta, 127
cigarettes, *see* smoking
Cincinnati Lancet and Observer, 133

circulation, 197
clap, 154, *see also* gonorrhea
claustrophobia, 190
clinical studies, xxii
clonic spasms, 95, 147
coadjutor muscles, 19
cocaine, 152, 154, 165, 419, 420
coca leaves, 423
codeine, 152
coffee, 33, 99, 100, 121, 132, 148, 434, *see also* caffeine
Collodium Sidicylici Composita, 344
colocynth, 142
coma, 147, 217
comatose state, 182
Commission on Law Enforcement and the Administration of Justice, 257
Committee on Cannabis Indica (of the Ohio State Medical Society), x
comp. tinct. opii., 128, 137
concentrate (of cannabis), 189
concentration, difficulty in (due to marijuana), 196, 257
Confessions of an English Opium Eater, 34, 58
confusion, *see* mental confusion
congestion, 29, *see also* chest, tightness of
conjunctival blood vessels, 364
conjunctival suffusion, 7, 233, 239, 247, 250
conjunctival vascular state, 265
constipation, 86, 315
Continuous Performance Test (CPT), 265, 266
convulsions, 27, 147, 218, 248
convulsive disorder, 4, 26, 194
convulsive movements, 120
copavia, 154
cornea, 358
corneal anesthesia, 104, 357
corneal areflexia, 386, 390, 391, 392, 402
"corneal units", 106
Cornell Medical College, 345
cortex, 250, *see also* brain
cortical effects, 161
cough, 103, 110, 133, 161, 294
cough reflex, xvii
Count of Monte Cristo, 420
criminal acts, 346
Crusades, 118
crystalline paraffin, 303, 340
curative powers, 124
cutaneous eruptions, 161
cyanosis, 84
cyclothymic personality, 133, 363, 369
cystitis, 97

dagga, 213, 219, 220, 221, 222, 224, 245
"dagga insanity", 221
"dagga lunacy", 221
Daily Courier, 430
Dannemora, 195
Datura stramonium, *see* stramonium, datura

dawamese, 83
deafness, 97
Defense Department, xiii, xxii
delirium, 20, 85, 94, 124, 147, 148, 153, 343, 434
"delirium form", 146
delirium tremens, 29, 124, 140, 161, see also alcoholic delirium
Delphic Oracles, 23
delusion(s), 38, 45, 49, 99, 108, 143, 232
dementia, 47
dentists, 299
Department of Agriculture, 421
Department of Treasury, see Treasury Department
depersonalization, 218
depression, xx, 57, 84, 89, 108, 169, 179, 190, 193, 218, 232, 241, 304, 316, 317, 339, 343, 359, 367, 369
depressive states, 384
desire for food, 242, 366, 369, see also hunger, incceased appetite
desire for sweets, 18, 205, see also hypoglycemia, sweet candies
detoxification, 189, 391
dextrose, 291
diarrhea, 12, 14, 15, 23 370
dibenzopyran derivative, 216
Dictionnaire des Sciences Medicales, 15
digestive tract, 120, see also alimentary canal, gastrointestinal tract
digitalis, 148, 152
Digit-Symbol Substitution Test (DSST), 265
dihydrocannabinols, 380
Dilantin, (diphenylhydantoin), xx, 167
diphenyl-hydantoin, 387, 392, 393, see also hydantoids
disorientation, 113
Dispensary of the U.S.A., 291
dissociation, 366
dissociational ideas, 247
disulfiram, 170
diuresis, 108, 239, 245, 249
diuretic (drug), 126, 143, 251
diuretic effect, 11, 12, 34, 205, 237
dizziness, 93, 100, 101, 162, 179, 180, 185, 189, 192, 196
dog(s), 52, 67, 68, 70, 80, 98, 217, 296, 298, 299, 304, 306, 314, 315, 316, 317, 319, 321, 322, 323, 324, 325, 326, 327, 328, 341, 342, 343, 344, 357, 358, 359, 360, 371, 376, 384, 385, 386, 389, 390, 392
dog-ataxia tests, 355, 359, 363, 403
"dope farm", 31
"double-blind" experimentation, xxiii, 218, 257, 263
Doveri, 128
Dover's powder, 17, 131
"down", 88, 211
dreams, 65, 73, 164, 296
drowsiness, 71, 79, 100, 163, 180, 181, 187, 191, 194, 343, 365
drug addicts, 195, see also addicts

dryness of lips, mouth, and throat, 34, 35, 84, 85, 89, 91, 92, 93, 97, 100, 101, 103, 106, 108, 110, 179, 183, 185, 186, 189, 196, 225, 240, 242, 245, 248, 306, 364, 467, 470
dysentery, 219
dysmennorrhea, xvii, 124, 148, 154, 164
dysphasia, 226
dysphoria, 369
dyspnea, 192, 225, 232, see also inspiratory dyspnea

ears, ringing in, 184
eclampsia, 147
ecstasy, 87, 107
ecstatic rapture, 103
eczema, itching of, 152
ego, 175
elation, 108, 190, 197
electrocardiogram(s), 200, 207, 210, 223, 227, 249, 363
electrocardiograms, abnormal, 200
electrocardiographic records, 198, 207, 223, 227, 238, 252
electro-convulsive therapy, 220, 232
electroencephalogram (EEG), 227, 232, 235, 241, 388
electroencephalographic changes, 214, 365
electroshock, 387, 388, 390, 391, see also anti-electroshock
Eli Lilly Company, 67, 291
Elmira Reformatory, 194
emetics, 18, 100
enema, 14, 21, 25
engram, 111
enteralgia, 147
epilepsy, 136, 137, 138, 139, 147, 148, 153, 167, 192
epilepsy therapy, 39$
epileptic attacks, 194
epileptic children, 115, 167
epileptics, 194, 197
epileptic-sedative action, 386
epileptiform convulsions, 147
episodic drinking, 167, see also alcoholic dependence
erection of the penis, 98
ergot of rye, 123, 124, 165, 309
erotic ideas, 196
eroticism, 182
erotic sensations, 90
esrar, 214, see also marijuana
ether, 5, 119, 126, 198, 301, 340
euphoria, 83, 90, 91, 103, 107, 108, 111, 164, 169, 172, 175, 179, 180, 181, 183, 191, 196, 198, 198, 231, 240, 245, 246, 251, 257, 365, 369, see also well-being, sense of
euphoric effects, 186, 189
euthanasia, 154, 29615
excitement, 56, 57, 59, 96, 113
exhibitionism, 183
expectoration, 128, 131, 133
expiratory dyspnea, 232, see also dyspnea

extract of cannabis, 343
extract of hemp, 122
Extractum Cannabis Indicae (ethereum), 122, 134, 303, 311, 344
eyes, 184, 230, 299, 306
eyes, burning of, 184, *see also* inflammation of eye membrane
eyes, dilated, *see* pupils

fakirs, 10
fantasia, 37, 40, 45, *see also* phantasies
fatigue, xix, 104, 106, 152, 161, 189, 192, 220, 336, 365
fear of death, 57, 58, 88, 91, 95, 179, 182, 185
febrile syndrome, 107
febrile restlessness, 39
Federal Bureau of Narcotics, xxi, 260, 261, 263, 417, 425, 427, 428, 429, 430, 433, 434, 435, 436, 437
Federal Bureau of Narcotics and Dangerous Drugs, xxiii
Federal Food, Drug and Cosmetic Act, 414
Federal Government, 417
First Hague Conference, 422
fluid extractum cannabis, 87, 344
Flushing Parental School, 191
Food and Drug Administration, xxiii
Food and Drug Control Laboratory (Washington), 67
formaldehyde, 352
frog, 298
"functional disturbances", 107

ganjah, gunjah, 5, 6, 7, 15, 16, 19, 30, 143, 215, 335, 336, 337, 346
gastric motility, 206, 210, 364
gastric secretion, 206
gastric ulcer, 154
gastrodynia, 126, 147, 154
gastrointestinal absorption, 258
gastrointestinal function, 197
gastrointestinal tract, xvii, *see also* alimentary tract, digestive tract
gelsemium, 293, 294
"general paralysis", 146
geneva Opium Conference, 424
genitalia, 230, *see also* erection of the penis, penis
genito-urinary disorders, 154
ghee, 7, 15
glacial acetic acid, 313
glottis spasm, 136
gonorrhea, xvi, 9, 12, 13, 14, 130
grand mal epilepsy, 167, 386, *see also* epilepsy
Groote Schuur Hospital, 213
guilt, 169
gunja sativa, gunja agrestis, 14, *see also* marijuana

habituated person, 7, *see also* addicts, habitues
habituation, 214, 389, 393, *see also* addiction

habitues, 154, 156, *see also* addicts, cannabis addicts
haemorrhoids, 13, 15
Hague Convention, 422, *see also* First Hague Conference
Hague Opium Convention, 424
hallucinations, 4, 7, 49, 84, 85, 88, 90, 91, 98, 100, 108, 110, 111, 112, 113, 133, 189, 218, 228, 249, 316, 339, 423
harmful effects of marijuana, 183, 189, *see also* toxic effects, toxicity
Harrison Narcotic Act, 419, 423, 425, 427, 436
hash, hasheesh, haschisch, hashish, 3, 31, 33, 34, 35, 38, 40, 42, 43, 44, 45, 55, 58, 83, 84, 85, 87, 89, 90, 93, 101, 102, 104, 106, 107, 109, 111, 113, 114, 121, 122, 133, 155, 166, 213, 215, 255, 258, 336, 339, 346, 375, 388, 398, 420
hashish delirium, 165, *see also* delirium
hashish-eaters, 103, 215
hashish, effects of, 84
hashish euphoria, 164
hashish experiments, 108
hashish, habit, 159, *see also* cannabis addiction, habituation
hashish resin, 378, *see also* resin
hay asthma, 154, *see also* asthma
hay fever, 154
headache, 20, 23, 73, 88, 98, 129, 152, 153, 156, 157, 192, 225, 232, 233, 239, 337, 368
heart, 142, 197, 210
heart beats, 72, 306, *see also* pulse
heart disease, 200, 316
heart rate, 259, 265, 384
Heidelberg Psychiatric Clinic, 106
hematological surveys, 362, 365
hematology, 200
hemoglobin, 108, 200, 211
hemorrhage, 129, 218
hemp extracts, 357, 371
hepatic derangement, 128, *see also* liver
"Herba Cannabis Indica", 105, 333, *see also* marijuana
hernia, 14
heroin, 193, 346, 429; heroin addict, 190, 194
heroin addiction, 197
heroin smuggling, 436
hexahydrocannabinols, 380
"high", 177, 181, 186, 189, 192, 206, 210, 244, 262, 267, 286, 289, 365, 369
Hindoo Medical Works, 9
Hindus, 26, 118, 215
Hindu Tantra, 9
homosexuals, 427
homosexual tendencies, 113
honopay, 214, *see also* marijuana
hookah, 7, 24
Hortus Malabaricus, 14
hunger, xvi, 29, 77, 86, 104, 184, 186, 205, 210, 233, 256, 259, 365, 366, 368, *see also* appétite, increased; desire for food

hydantoids, 388, *see also* Dilantin, diphenyl-hydantoin
hydrochloric acid, 317
Hydrogen-ion concentration, 108
hydrogentecannabinol, 217
hydrophobia, 1, 4, 20, 30, 161, *see also* rabies
hyoscyamus, 127, 131
hyperemia of the brain, xx, *see also* cerebral hyperemia
hyperemic conjunctivae, 97, 109, *see also* conjunctival hyperemia, conjunctival suffusion
hyperesthesia, 97
hypergeusia, 366
hyperkinetic states, 248
hyperphagia, 256, 259
hyperreflexia, 365
hypnotic drugs, xvii, 134, 313, 357, 386
hypnotic (drug) effect, xvi, 123, 135, 151, 153, 156, 157, 163, 292, 317, 343, 386, 392
hypnotics (synthetic), xviii, 159, 386
hypnotism, 166
hypochondria, 48
hypodermic injection, 298, 369
hypodermic syringe, xix, 152
hypoglycemia (due to overdose of marijuana), xx, 108, 259
hypokinetic states, 248
hysteria, 124, 128, 130, 136, 139, 156, 248, 258
hysterical attacks, 190
"hysteric pains", 147

identity, loss of, 99
idiopathic epilepsy, 192, *see also* epilepsy
illusions, 47, 49, 84, 89, 105, 110, 112, 121, 246, *see also* hallucinations
impotence (alleged), 8, 102
inability to urinate, 232
incoordination (muscular), 77, 90, 189, 193, 341, 342, 343, 357, 390, *see also* ataxia
increased appetite, *see* appetite; desire for food; hunger
Indian Cannabis, 339, *see also* marijuana
Indischer hanf, 333, *see also* marijuana
Indian hemp, xiv, 33, 55, 118, 145, 148, 149, 151, 152, 157, 301, 306, 310, 311, 315, 316, 333, 339, 425, 248, *see also* marijuana
Indian hemp resin, 376, *see also* resin
infantile convulsions, 125
inflammation, 29, 130, 335
inflammation of eye membrane, 64, 299, *see also* eyes, burning of
influenza, 57, 312
ingestion, 206, *see also* mouth; oral administration
inhibitions, loss of, 189, 256, 257, 427
insane, insanity, 39, 41, 42, 84, 126, 130, 131, 184, 417, 435
insolubility of marijuana, xiii, xvi, 258, 314

insomnia, 142, 143
inspiratory dyspnea, 101, *see also* dyspnea
Internal Revenue Service, 31
Inter-State Narcotics Association, 437
intestinal hemorrhage, 389
intestinal motility, 365
intestinal tract, 93, 189
intestine, 312, 313
intoxication, 7, 12, 17, 21, 24, 64, 69, 75, 78, 80, 81, 99, 100, 103, 108, 111, 1113, 155, 169, 180, 197, 218, 221, 249, 250, 251, 258, 259, 267, 337, 363, 364, 365, 366, 367, 369, 423
intoxication, acute, 221, *see also* overdose
"intra-individual potency comparison", 376
intra muscular injection, 364, *see also* hypodermic injection
intravenous dextrose, 241
intravenous doses, 359, 386, 390
intravenous electrolyte therapy, xv, 1
intravenous injection, 357, 383
iodine, 147
ipecacuanha wine (vin. ipecac.), 58, 63, 128, 138
iron, 147
itching of eczema, 152

Jesus, marijuana offered to, *see* Savior, marijuana offered to
Journal of the A.M.A., 165, 177
Journal de Pharmacie, 15
jugular vein, 206, 296, 298

kidney(s), 93, 197
kidney function, 204, 210, 365
kif, 214, *see also* marijuana
klip-dagga, 219, 221, *see also* dagga; marijuana
konaba, kanaba, 214, *see also* marijuana
kymograph, 205

labor, xxii, 124, 164, 165, 219, *see also* childbirth
La Guardia Committee Report, 256, 383, 388, 437
Lancet, 18, 145
Lands of the Saracen, 120
largactil, 241
laryngismus stridulus, 133, 136
laudanum, 132, 142
"laughing jag", 187
laughter, 41, 60, 74, 75, 76, 77, 78, 79, 84, 89, 90, 96, 105, 106, 121, 179, 181, 188, 190, 197, 232, 244, 246, 312
League of Nations, 424
Leonotis leonotis, 219; L. leonurus, 219, 221
lethal dose (L.D.), 317, 385, 389
lethal effect, lethal action, 386, 388, 390, 393
libido, 108
licorice root, powdered, 224
lips (dry), 85, 367, *see also* dryness of lips, mouth, and throat

liver, 129, 175, 197
liver damage, 13, 204, *see also* hepatic derangement
liver function, 365
lock-jaw, 23, *see also* tetanus
Louisiana Board of Health, 423
"LSD-like" effects, 258
lumbago, 147
lung diseases, 124
lungs, 13, 294, 384
lycergic acid, 213
mocoha, 214
macropsy, 108
"macroscopic centrale", 90
madness, 8, 12, 160, 155, *see also* insanity, mental illness
majoon, 6, 7, 8, 13, 15, 16
malaria, 219
malarial cachexia, 97
mania, 39, 44, 47, 124, 135, 153, 190
mania-a-potu, 136
manic, manics, 164, 240, 241, 250
manic depressive, 106, 113
Massachusetts Bureau of Drug Abuse and Drug Control, 260
mass media, 260
masturbation, 244
marijuana, xiii, xiv, xix, xxi, xxii, xxiii, 1, 101, 102, 112, 113, 115, 167, 170, 174, 177, 179, 190, 191, 193, 196, 200, 203, 204, 205, 206, 207, 208, 209, 210, 213, 215, 255, 256, 257, 258, 260, 261, 262, 263, 267, 268, 287, 289, 293, 345, 346, 347, 352, 357, 358, 361, 363, 365, 366, 367, 375, 398, 405, 412, 413, 415, 416, 423, 424, 425, 426, 427, 428, 429, 431, 433, 436, 437, *see also* American hemp, American marijuana, *anascha, bhang,* cannabis, cannabis americana, cannabis indica, cannabis sativa, *canamo,* charas, *chanvre de l'Inde, dagga, esrar,* ganga, hashish, Indian hemp, *Indischer hanf, kif, konaba, klip dagga, macoha, mbanzhe,* momea, qunubu, "rup," "tea," "weed"
marijuana activity, 354, 357, 369, 371
"marijuana bill", 346
marijuana cigarettes, 120, 179, 180, 181, 184, 185, 191, 192, 194, 258, 263, 364
marijuana concentrate, 192, 194, *see also* marijuana preparations
marijuana habit, 159
marijuana homologues, 292
marijuana ingestion, 197, *see also* ingestion, oral administration
marijuana intoxication, 197, 207, 255, 259, *see also* intoxication
marijuana laws, legislation, 417, 435
marijuana overdose, 364, *see also* low toxicity, toxicity, hypoglycemia from O.D.
marijuana pills, *see* pills, marijuana
marijuana psychosis, 191, *see also* psychosis

"marijuana reaction", 267
marijuana smokers, 287
marijuana-smoking prisoners, 389
marijuana study, xxii, 192, 194
marijuana symptoms, 198
Marijuana Tax Act, xix, 436
Materia Medica, 14, 30, 43
Matteawan State Hospital, 193, 194, 195
mbanzhe, mbangi, matakwane, 215, *see also* marijuana
Medical Record, 152
Medical and Surgical Journal, 124, 125, 129
melancholia, 43, 153, 218
melancholics, 164
menorrhagia, 124, 164
menstruation, 124
mental confusion, 88, 101, 106, 162, 190, 191, 197
mental depression, 65, 343, 369, *see also* depression
mental derangement, 11
mental deterioration (alleged), 221, 346
mental disease, 40
mental disturbance, 36, 45
mental illness, xx, 31, *see also* insanity, madness
mental pain, 154, *see also* psychic pain
mental retardation, 167
mercury, 147
Mesantoin, 167
mescal button, 315
mescaline, 213
metabolic rate, 207, 209, 365
metabolic rate of the brain, 206
metacarpal bones, 25
metritis, 154
mice, 358, 385
micropsy, 108
migraine, xviii, xxiv, 97, 147, 152, 153, 154, 156, 162, 163, 294, 343
Miller-Abbott balloon, 206
"model psychoses", 213, 251
mode of action (of marijuana), xi
modus operandi (of marijuana), 34, 133
Mohamedanism, 33
Mohamedans, 7, 14
Mohamedan sects, 215
momea, momeea, mimea, 6, 337
mono-terpene, 303, 398
moral deterioration, 196
morals (lack of), 346
morphia, xvi, 61, 126, 152, 154, 156, 157, 163
morphine, 60, 84, 126, 140, 152, 165, 193, 266, 316, 346, 385-388
morphine derivatives, 160, *see also* addiction, analgesic drugs, heroin
Moslem fanatics, 215
motor ataxia, 376, *see also* ataxia, incoordination
motor-spinal tract palsy, 299
"mouse sleep prolongation test", 357
mouth, 232, 245, 313, *see also* dryness of

lips, mouth, and throat; ingestion; oral administration
mucus, 25, 95, 294
mucus membranes, 185, 335, 364
mucus secretion, 35, 134
"muggles", xix, *see also* marijuana
Munich Psychiatric Clinic, 104, 106
muscae volitantes, 147
muscle spasms, xviii, 246
muscular contractions, 232
muscular weakness, 193, 306
myoclonic movements, 107
myodynia, 147

narcoanalysis, 384
narcocatharsis, 384
narcosuggestion, 384
narcotic addicts, 370, *see also* addiction, addicts, habituation
Narcotics Division of United Nations Publication, 218
narcotic effect, 213, 247, 248
narcotics, 393, 423, 424
National Academy of Sciences, 365
National Formulary and Pharmacopeia, xiv
National Institute of Health, 417, 433, 434, 435
National Institute of Mental Health, xxii, xxiii
National Wholesale Druggists' Assoc. (NWDA), 420
nausea, xviii, 7, 70, 71, 74, 76, 78, 90, 93, 108, 110, 128, 179, 184, 186, 205, 210, 233, 295, 370
nerve centers, 343
nerve-trunks, 299
"nervous headache", 162
nervousness, 59, 73, 124, 191
nervous system, 38, 120, *see also* central nervous system
neuralgia, xvii, xxiv, 86, 87, 97, 98, 123, 146, 147, 153, 154, 161, 294, 311, 312
neuralgic paroxysms, 153
neurological tests, 256
neurasthenia, 343
neuronal enzyme systems, 249
neuroses, 195
neurotic depression, 218, *see also* depression
New York Times, 428
nicotine, 264
nitro-cannabinolactone, 217
nitrogen 404
nitrogenous compounds, 360
nux-vomica, 8, 15, 148

ocular muscles, 316
oedema of the eyelids, 233
Office of the Attorney General of Mass., 260
Ohio State Medical Society, xv, 117, 135
olfactory sense, depression of, 305
opiate addiction, xx, xxiiv, 152, *see also* addiction, addicts, habituation, heroin,

heroin addiction
opiates, xvii, xix, 27, 115, 160, 419, 423
opisthotonos, 99
opium, xv, 14, 16, 25, 33, 34, 38, 40, 55, 124, 125, 133, 134, 135, 142, 143, 154, 157, 161, 162, 163, 216, 295, 314, 343, 417, 420, 422
opium addiction, 434, *see* ~lso addicts, addiction, opiate addiction, habituation
opium addicts, 425
opium, chronic poisoning by, 164
opium derivatives, 365, 369
optical activity of marijuana derivates, 349, 354, 357-361, 402, 411
oral administration of marijuana, 121, 180, *see also* ingestion; mouth
oral tremors, 364, *see also* tremors
organic solvents, 347, *see also* alcohol; ether; petroleum ether; etc.
overdose of marijuana, 91, 120, 211, *see also* hypoglycemia due to overdose of marijuana, sweet candies (antidote)
oxazolidinediones, 386
oxidation, 309, 310, 344
oxycannabin, 317
oxygen concentration, 208
oxytocic, xiv, 165

pain relief from marijuana, xv, xvii, 16, 20, 97, 118, 122, 126, 294, 295, 305
pallor, 110, 190, 233
palsy, 124, 167, *see also* cerebral palsy; motor-spinal tract palsy; spinal palsy
parahexyl, 384, 389, *see also* synhexyl, pyrahexyl
paraldehyde, xviii, 160, 216
paralysis, 84, 95, 146
paralysis agitans, 148
paranoid behavior, 167
paranoid episode, 388
paranoid trends, 190
paresis, 153
paresthesia, 91, 100, 106, 110, 111, 232, 239, 245, 312
Parke, Davis and Co., 31, 67, 291
patellar reflexes (increased), 97, 119
pathological conditions, 135
peak effect, 383
penis, 98, 230
"peripheral neuritis", 240
peritonitis (chronic), 48
Pernoston, 357, 386
Persian authors, 9, 10
perspiration, 370
petit mal, 148, 192, 387, *see also* epilepsy
petroleum ether, 301, *see also* organic solvents
phantasies, 34, 39, *see also* fantasia Pharmacological Assoc.
pharmacology, 118
pharmaceutical industry, 417
pharmacological studies, 256, 291, 317, 357
pharmacopoeia, xiii, 148, 421, *see also*

American Pharmacopoeia, British Pharmacopoeia
pharynx, 19
Phenacetin, 421
phenobarbital, 167, 192
phenol-aldehyde, 340
phenolsulfonphthalein, 210
phenolsulfonphthalein test, 204
phosphate of zinc, see zinc phosphate
phosphorus, 200, 202, 210
phthistical patient, 94
phthisis, 124, 154, 294, 295
physical dependence, xiii, xvii, see also addicts, addiction, habituation, tolerance
physical deterioration, 196
physical effects of marijuana, 364
physical examination, 363
physical symptoms, 183
physiological action of marijuana, 117, 294, 345
physiological tests, 340
pills, marijuana, 20, 99, 224, 311, 363
pipe, 7, 12, 110, 219, 220
pitch, 307
placebo, 259, 263, 264, 268, 363
placenta praevia, 129
pleasurable sensations, effects, 41, 70, 73, 74, 78, 84, 89, 186, 295, 307
pneumonic inflammation, 130, 133, see also bronchopneumonia
podophyllin, 129
poisoning, 164, 191
poppy seeds, 15, see also opium
praecordial discomfort, 232
pregnancy, 390, see also childbirth; labor
preparation of the drug, 342
Pretoria Mental Asylum, 221
prison psychosis, 197, see also psychosis
prophylactic use of marijuana, xxiv, 293
pruritis, 161, 163
pseudo-cannabinol, 340
pseudo hallucinations, 119
"psychedelic" environments, 260
"psychedelic revolution", xix, xxi
psychiatric analysis, 113, 165
psychiatric clinics, 102, see also Astrachan pyschiatric clinic; Heidelberg psychiatric clinic, Munich psychiatric clinic, Utrecht psychiatric clinic
psychiatric effects, 365
psychiatric episodes, 385
psychiatric examination, 363
psychiatric studies, xx, 102, 292
psychiatrist, 195, 261
psychiatry, xx
psychic action of marijuana, 371, 384-391
psychic anodyne, use of marijuana as, 153
psychic changes caused by marijuana, 346
psychic defenses weakened by alcohol, 169
psychic disturbances caused by marijuana, 167, see also mental disturbances
psychic effects caused by marijuana, x
psychic pain soothed by marijuana, 169

psychic phenomena caused by marijuana, 110
"psychic relaxation" with marijuana, 384
psychic side effects from marijaana, 388, 389, 391
psycho-active drugs, xiv, 259, 261
psychological tests, 256, 259, 265, 267, 384
psychological treatments, 170
psycho-motor performance, 177
psychoneurosis, 369, see also neurosis
psychoneurotics, 166
psychopathic personality, 195
psychopathological phenomena, 106
psychoses, 113, 195, 213, 250
psychosis, 111, 113, 193, 194, 195, 197, 221, 222, 261
psychosis delirium, 192
psychotherapy, 218, 251
psychotic, 232
psychotic changes, 364
psychotic episodes, 179, 182, 185, 186, 189, 191, 196, 210, 433
psychotic personality, 197
psychotic states, 112, 197
psychotic symptoms from marijuana overdose, 364
psychotomimetic effects of marijuana, 157
psychotropic materials, 398
Public Health Service, 424, 425, 436
puerperal convulsions, 124, 161
puerperal mania, 135
pulmonary affections, 134, see also lungs
pulmonary oedema, 218, 389
pulse rate, 24, 58, 72, 75, 83, 86, 87, 92, 95, 97, 99, 100, 104, 107, 110, 127, 131, 136, 179, 180, 190, 198, 210, 223, 225, 239, 241, 256, 289, 296, 297, 305, 306, 363, 364
Pulv. Trag. Cr., 224
pupils, 58, 89, 91, 95, 96, 97, 99, 100, 132, 139, 179, 180, 184, 196, 248, 259, 265, 305, 306, 363, 394
Pure Food and Drug Act, 419, 422, 425
pursuit rotor, 265, 266
pyrahexyl, 249, 403, see also synhexyl, parahexyl

quinine, 147
qunubu, qunnabu, 214, see marijuana

rabbit corneal areflexia, 104, 402
rabbits, 104, 304, 306, 315, 316, 320, 329, 357, 358, 386
rabies, 1, see also hydrophobia
Randall's Island, 191
rats, 387
reaction formation, reduction of, 169
"recreational" smoking, xiii, xix
red oil, 291, 340, 345, 347, 349, 355, 358, 371, 376, 402, 403, 404, 405
"reefers", 113, 184, 186, 188
reflexes, augmentation of, 97, 111, 119
rehabilitation, 176, 370
rehabilitative value of marijuana, 175

renal disease, 154
repression, reduction of, 169
resin, xiv, 5, 17, 20, 25, 26, 28, 29, 30, 89, 119, 161, 255, 256, 303, 304, 307, 313, 335, 336, 337, 339, 340, 345, 347, 357, 378, 398, 399, 400, 408, 412, 413, *see also* Indian hemp resin
resina Cannabis Indicae, 303
resinous body (cannabinol), 303
resinous extract, 30, 224, 339, 413, 415
resinous exudate, 102, 119, 214, 336, *see also* resin
respiration, 73, 92, 98, 131, 136, 298, 306, 315, 384
respiration movements, 110, 365
respiratory center, 161, 164
respiratory mechanism, depression of, 165
respiratory mucus membrane, 185
respiratory rate, 90, 91, 259, 265
respiratory symptoms, 191
restlessness, 56, 124, 179, 183, 189, 192, 196, 295, 343, 370
retention of the urine, 154, *see also* inability to urinate
retina, 49
rheumatic heart disease, 202
rheumatic neuralgia, 161
rheumatism, 1 17, 19, 29, 48, 94, 125, 154, 161
riamba (calabash), 215
Riker's Island, 192, 194
Roentgenograms, 206
Rorschach test, 113
rum, 152
Rumphius Herbarium Amboinense, 13
"rup", 336

saccharin, 298
sacralgia, 147
safety of marijuana, xx, 267
salivation, 89, 110, 305, 316
Sanborn equipment, apparatus, 190, 207
sanity, 316
SAR (Structure Activity Relationship), 292, 315, 380, 381, 383, 391
Savior, marijuana offered to, 118
schizophrenia, 106, 194, 213, 227, 231, 232, 250
schizophrenics, 113, 166, 196
sciatic, 298
sciatica, 147
Science (magazine), 177
Second Geneva Convention, 422
secretions, 34, 35, 38, 157, 343, *see also* gastric secretion, mucus secretion, salivation
sedative effects, xvii, 12, 16, 143, 163, 313
sedative hypnotic, 291
sedatives, 115
seeds of marijuana, 4, 11, 14, 118, 255, 335, 345, 379, 398, 413, 432
self-rating bi-polar mood scale, 265, 266
semi-anesthesia, 164, *see also* anesthesia
seminal secretion, restraint of, 12

semi-synthetic THC, 378, 379
senile insomnia, xvii, 146, 153
sensory nerve trunks, 298
seonotic lenurus, 221
sesqui-terpene, 303, 304, 340, 398
sex cycles in dogs, 390
sex offenders, 195
sex perversion, 195, 196
sexual excitation, stimulation, due to marijuana, 9, 83, 86, 111, 112, 113, 180, 182, 425, 427
sidhee, 6, 7, 13, 15, *see also* bhang, marijuana
sinus bradycardia, 200, 210
sinus tachycardia, 200, 210, 233, 248
skin reflexes, heightened, 97
sleep, 28, 64, 70, 75, 79, 89, 92, 96, 97, 98, 120, 123, 124, 125, 132, 135, 165, 187, 242, 256, 294, 298, 315, 317, 341, 343, *see also* drowsiness
sleep deprivation, 265
sleepiness, 163, 304, 306
"sleep producers", 317
sleep prolongation, 386
smokers, 112, 184, 259
smokers of ganjah, 13
smoking, 7, 12, 100, 108, 109, 111, 188, 191, 221, 242, 244, 245, 255, 257; calabash, 215; cigarettes, 101, 102, 11,1, 113, 179, 180, 184, 185, 186, 189, 191, 192, 194, 197, 228, 241, 242, 258, 261, 364; dagga, 220, 221, 222, 241, 242; hashish, 110, 111, 215, 336; hookah, 206, 346, 388; narghile, 111; pipe, 7, 12, 111, 219, 220; *see also* "recreational" smoking
Social Security Act, 417
sodium bromide, 163, *see also* bromide
Solanaceae, 38
somatic changes, 346
soothing effects of marijuana, 163
soporific action of marijuana, 155, 163, 386
space perception, alteration of, 246
spasms, muscular, 24, 28, 94, 136, 137, 232, *see also* convulsive disorders; clonic spasms
spasmodic dysmenorrhea, *see dysmenorrhea*
spasmodic pain, 162
spasm of the glottis, 136
spasm, vesicle, 154
spectroscopic analysis, 258, 406
spinal cord, 163, 299
spinal palsy, 298
spinal sclerosis, 148
standardization of marijuana preparations, 94, 258, 340
State Department, 417, 424, 431, 432
stimulant effects of marijuana, 12
stomach, 7, 14, 20, 73, 78, 88, 95, 98, 121, 134, 157, 196, 206, 217, 313, 366
stomach tube, 358
stramonium, datura, 15, 127
stramonium seeds, datura, 8

Structure and Activity Relationship, *see* SAR
strychnine, 99
strychnine poisoning, 161
subconscious, 165
subjective symptoms of marijuana, use, 183
submur-hydrarg, 128
sudorific effect of marijuana, 34
sugar, 15, 434, *see also* blood glucose level
suicidal impulses, 247, 251
sulfanol, xvi, 155, 160
sulphuric acid, 309, 313
superego, 175
Supreme Court, 422
surgery, 118
surgery, brain, xxii
sweet candies (antidote for overdose), 211, 364
sweets increasing effects of marijuana intoxication, 12, *see also* desire for sweets
synhexyl, 218, *see also* parahexyl, pyrahexyl
synthetic anodynes and hypnotics, 159
synthetic drugs and agents, 115, 159, 392
synthetic cannabinol, 387
synthetic THC, 379, 380, 381, 414, 415
syphilitic infection, 195
syrup rhei, 123
syrup aurantii, 123

tachycardia, 107, 232, 238, 242, 245, 248, *see also* sinus tachycardia
"tahgalim", 336
talkativeness, 56, 96, 111, 137, 181, 183, 185, 190, 196, 198, 244, 245
tannate of cannabin, 156
Tax Act, 430, 432, 433, 434, 435, 437
tax stamps, xxi
"tea", xix, 148, 186
tea pad parties, 186, 189
"tea pads", 185, 186, 346
temperature, 107, 127, 305, *see also* warmth
"temper disease", 146
terpene, 304, 340
tests on humans; barium test, 206; basal meatabolism test, 190, 197; blood tests, 175, 202; continuous performance test (CPT) 265, 266; digit-symbol substitution test (DSST), 265; "double-blind" experimentation, xxi, 218, 257, 263; hematological surveys, 363, 365; "intraindividual potency comparison", 376; physiological tests, 340; psychiatric examination, 363; psychiatric studies, xviii, 102, 292; psychological tests, 256, 259, 265, 267, 384; Rorschach test, 113; venous pressure test, 363
tetanic paroxysms, 26, 27, 28
tetanus, 1, 4, 23, 25, 26, 30, 123, 136, 139, 148, 161, 343, *see also* lock-jaw

tetrahydrocannabinol (THC), xxii, xiv, 167, 185, 188, 192, 206, 217, 256, 257, 258, 259, 263, 292, 349, 351, 352, 254, 356, 358, 360, 361, 363, 364, 365, 369, 370, 376, 378, 379, 381, 383, 392, 399, 402, 403, 404, 407, 410, 414, 415
tetrahydrocannabinol homolog, xxiii
tetrahydrocannabinol molecule, 370, 371
thalamic structures, 250
thalamotomy, 250
thalamo-cortical region, xx
therapeutic applications of marijauna, xv, xxiii, 83, 117, 122, 159, 292
therapeutic effects, 151, 384
therapeutic potentiaities, xiii, 93, 160, 251, 375
therapeutic properties, xiv, 317
thirst, xx, 84, 104, 196
throat, constriction of, 8
throat, dryness of, 35, 85, 103, 370, *see also*, dryness of lips, mouth and throat
tic douloureux, xvii, xxiv
time, altered sense of (due to marijuana), 43, 90, 91, 99, 100, 245, 315
tinct. strophanth., 142
Tinctura Chlorali et Potassii Bromidi Composita, 344
tincture of Cannabis Indica, 27, 138, 344
tincture of hemp, 10, 28, 30, 112
tinnitus aurium, 108, 147
tobacco, 7, 16, 24, 33, 40, 99, 242, 243, 365
tobacco cigarettes, 242, 261, 264
tolerance, minimal (from marijuana), xiii, xvii, 314, 365, 393
tolerance production, 115
tonic spasm, 83, 95, 148
torticollis, 148
toxic effects of marijuana, xviii, 146, 149, 197
toxicity, low, xiii, xvii, 151
tragacanth, powdered, 224
trans-tetrahydrocannabinol, 405, 414
Treasury Department, 345, 433, 435, 436, 437
tremor, muscle, 89, 97, 109, 184, 189, 192, 196, 364, *see also* oral tremor
tri-bromcannabinol, 317
trigeminal neuralgia, *see* neuralgia
trismus, 148

ultraviolet light, 379
Uniform State Narcotic Act, 428
University of Athens, 110
University of Capetown, 213
University of Illinois, 345, 348n., 402
University of Michigan, Dept. of Pharmacology, xxii
urea nitrogen, 200
urge to defecate, 184
urge to urinate, 211
urinalysis, 363
urinary excretion, 383
urine, 91, 203, 230, 237
urine output, 223, 252

urticaria, 152
U.S. Pharmacopoeia, 122, 291, 334, 358, 421, *see also* pharmacopoeia
uterine cancer, 154
uterine hemorrhage, 124, 343
uterine irritation, 154
uterine leucorrhoea, 124
uterus, 123, 124
Utrecht Psychiatric Clinic, 106

vagal centers, 298
vagi, 298
valerian (tincture), 129, 132
variability of strength of marijuana preparations, xiii, xvi, 24, 122, 148, 301
vascularity of the eyes, 7, *see* conjunctival suffusion
vasodilation, xx, 265
venipuncture, 228, 233, 240
venous pressure, 107
venous pressure tests, 363
vertigo, 89, 104, 111, 230, 337
vesical spasm, 154
veterinary medicine, 419
vision, blurring of, 184
visions, 73, 89, 106, 122

visions of angels, 185
visual hallucinations, 113, 228, *see also* hallucinations
visual images, 225, 227, 229, 248
visual perception, 228
volatile oil, *see* red oil
vomiting, 70, 71, 72, 84, 95, 104, 110, 128, 184, 190, 205, 210, 233, 296, 305, 306, 311, 316, 386

warmth, sensation of, 34, 35, 83, 85, 86, 184, 232
"weed", 427
Welfare Island Hospital, 192, 194, 196, 197, 345, 362, 365, 369
well-being, sense of, 185, *see also* euphoria
Western Lancet, 125
whooping-cough, 124
wine of hemp, 3, 10
wink reflex, 386
W.P.A., 193

zinc ethyl, 217
zinc phosphate, 153
zinc sulphate, 86

Tod H. Mikuriya, M.D.

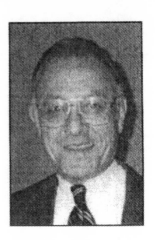

A graduate of Reed College, Portland, Oregon, and Temple University Medical School, Philadelphia, Dr. Mikuriya served a rotating internship at Southern Pacific General Hospital, San Francisco. He specialized in psychiatry at the Oregon State Hospital in Salem and completed his training at Mendocino State Hospital. His status is "eligible" by the American Board of Psychiatry and Neurology. He is certified in biofeedback by the American Association of Biofeedback Clinicians.

In private medical psychiatric consultative practice in Berkeley and the East Bay, he was an attending psychiatrist at Gladman Hospital from 1970 until 1991; Chair 1993–94 of the Department of Psychiatry, Eden Medical Center, Castro Valley, and attending psychiatrist at Laurel Grove, Vencor, Alameda County Medical Center, and San Leandro Hospitals until 2000. He was on the staff at Kindred Hospital San Leandro.

Mikuriya was Director of the Drug Abuse Treatment Center at the New Jersey Neuropsychiatric Institute, Skillman, NJ before appointment as director of non-classified marijuana research for the National Institute of Mental Health Center for Narcotics and Drug Abuse Studies.

A planner for Project Eden community drug abuse treatment program he set up the first methadone maintenance program in Alameda County.

Member of the California Medical Association, American Psychiatric Association (Life Member), American Society of Addiction Medicine, California Society of Addiction Medicine (certified Addiction Medicine Specialist and Medical Review Officer) and the Alameda-Contra Costa Medical Association, he served on the ACCMA Chemical Addictions Committee.

- Member, Biofeedback Society of California
- Member, Association for Advancement of Behavior Therapy
- Member, The International Society for the Study of Subtle Energies and Energy Medicine
- Member, Mensa
- Member, International Cannabinoid Research Society
- Member, International Association of Cannabis as Medicine
- He is Medical Coordinator for California Cannabis Centers. Author: Oakland Buyers' Cooperative protocols
- Member, Medical Marijuana Work Group, City of Oakland 8/96–
- Member, Medical Marijuana Task Force, California Society for Addiction Medicine and California Medical Association 4/20/97–
- Member, Advisory Board: Journal of Cannabis Therapeutics 2000-
- President, California Cannabis Research Medical Group 1999–

Dr. Mikuriya is the editor and publisher of *Marijuana: Medical Papers 1839-1972* and numerous papers on therapeutic cannabis and drug control policy. The most recent: "Medicinal Uses of Cannabis at a Buyers' Club: A Pilot Study," 12/94, Internet 2/96. He is the editor and publisher of Indian Hemp Drugs Report Centennial, Volume I: Policy, Social and Religious Customs (Last Gasp Press, San Francisco, 1994). Mikuriya is a coauthor of *Marijuana Medical Handbook: A Guide to Therapeutic Use* (Ed Rosenthal, Tod Mikuriya, M.D., and Dale Gieringer, Quick American Archives, Oakland, 1997.)